Jim
Pα

BIOPSY INTERPRETATION SERIES

BIOPSY INTERPRETATION

OF THE LIVER

2nd Edition

BIOPSY INTERPRETATION SERIES

Series Editor: Jonathan I. Epstein, MD

BIOPSY INTERPRETATION SERIES

BIOPSY INTERPRETATION OF THE LIVER

2nd Edition

Stephen A. Geller, MD
Chairman Emeritus and Professor of Pathology
Department of Pathology and Laboratory Medicine
Cedars–Sinai Medical Center
Professor of Pathology
David Geffen School of Medicine
University of California, Los Angeles
Los Angeles, California

Lydia M. Petrovic, MD
Professor of Pathology
University of Southern California
Los Angeles, California

Wolters Kluwer | Lippincott Williams & Wilkins
Health
Philadelphia · Baltimore · New York · London
Buenos Aires · Hong Kong · Sydney · Tokyo

Acquisitions Editor: Jonathan W. Pine, Jr.
Managing Editor: Sirkka Howes and Jennifer Verbiar
Production Editor: Kevin P. Johnson
Manufacturing Manager: Benjamin Rivera
Creative Director: Doug Smock
Compositor: Aptara Inc.
Printer: C & C offset China

530 Walnut Street
Philadelphia, PA 19106 USA
LWW.com

Printed in China

Library of Congress Cataloging-in-Publication Data

Geller, Stephen A., 1939-
  Biopsy interpretation of the liver / Stephen A. Geller, Lydia M. Petrovic. — 2nd ed.
    p. ; cm. — (Biopsy interpretation series)
  Includes bibliographical references and index.
  ISBN 978-0-7817-7468-0 (alk. paper)
  1. Liver—Biopsy. 2. Liver—Histopathology. I. Petrovic, Lydia M. II. Title. III. Series: Biopsy interpretation series.
  [DNLM: 1. Biopsy—methods. 2. Liver—pathology. 3. Liver Diseases—diagnosis. WI 700 G318b 2009]
  RC847.5.B56B55 2009
  616.3'6—dc22   2008056134

10 9 8 7 6 5 4 3 2

CCS0309

To Kate, David, Cathia, Lila, Jennifer Lee, William, and Alice.

   —Stephen A. Geller

To my parents, family, and friends.

   —Lydia M. Petrovic

CONTENTS

PREFACE

Since the time of the publication of the first edition of this book in 2004, Peter J. Scheuer, our teacher and friend, and one of the foremost hepatopathologists, has died, as have Dame Sheila Sherlock and Fenton Schaffner, two brilliant and renowned hepatologists. We dedicate this book to them.

Despite occasional suggestions to the contrary, hepatopathology remains vibrant, exciting and, most importantly, an integral part of the diagnosis and treatment of the patient with liver disease. Although the reasons for performing liver biopsies have slightly changed over the years, the need for their performance has not. Increasingly both the hepatopathologist and the general pathologist interested in the study of liver are called upon to comment about specific diagnoses and also about prognosis and treatment of both neoplastic and nonneoplastic liver diseases. The further development of immunohistochemistry, with many more antibodies available for biopsy evaluation, and the explosive growth of molecular pathology, allow the pathologist to provide considerably more information for patient care than ever before.

This book concentrates almost entirely on liver biopsy, with only fleeting attention to macroscopic features, resection samples, and electron microscopy, but does include considerable information about ancillary procedures useful in the study of liver biopsy. This is not a comprehensive treatise of liver pathology, but rather is intended to serve as a handbook useful at the microscope to study both common and uncommon hepatic disorders. The focus of the book continues to be practical and the authors hope that it proves useful to both the neophyte and the seasoned practitioner in their studies of liver diseases.

Stephen A. Geller, MD

Lydia M. Petrovic, MD

PREFACE TO THE FIRST EDITION

The contemporary playwright John Guare has, in Six Degrees of Separation, suggested that all people on earth can be linked by only six relationships. Were we to try, Guare indicated, we could in some way potentially identify six persons by whom we could connect to every other living human being. The connection might be relatively trivial or could be quite significant. So it is with pathology.

Pathology, as with all of Medicine, is a continuum of learning. Our teachers studied their craft with other teachers who themselves studied with their own teachers. In this way it is not difficult to identify invisible bonds with the great 19th century founders of pathology who pioneered in the study of diseases of the liver. With some effort, one could even delve further into the past.

We both have links with two of the world leaders of hepatopathology. Hans Popper (1903–1988) is widely acknowledged to be the founder of the modern discipline of hepatology and hepatopathology. Popper, and his longtime colleague and friend, Fenton Schaffner, wrote the first modern textbook of liver diseases, Liver: Structure and Function. This pioneering text combined clinical information, morphologic observations, and experimental studies. It remains a valuable source of information. One of the authors of this liver biopsy book (Stephen A. Geller) knew Hans Popper for 19 years—first as a resident, and then as colleague and friend.

Students from all over the world came to Hans Popper's laboratories at The Mount Sinai Hospital in New York during the third quarter of the 20th century to learn about liver diseases and liver pathology. Peter J. Scheuer was a lecturer at the Royal Free Hospital School of Medicine in London, when he determined to take a year's leave of absence to enhance his already considerable knowledge of liver pathology. He studied with Popper at Mount Sinai Hospital before returning to the Royal Free Hospital as hepatopathologist and, ultimately, Professor and Chairman of Histopathology; where the other author of this book (Lydia M. Petrovic) was a fellow in hepatic histopathology. Scheuer became, as Popper had been before him, the foremost hepatopathologist of the world; with his laboratory serving as a magnet for students coming from all countries. Since it was first published in the mid-1960's, Scheuer's text Liver Biopsy Interpretation, now in its 6th edition, has been an invaluable source of information for practicing pathologists confronted with the daunting task of evaluating liver biopsies.

Biopsy Interpretation of the Liver is intended to be a practical source of information to help in the understanding of diseases of the liver and, particularly, the histopathology of those diseases. It is meant to complement, rather than to replace, larger textbooks of hepatic diseases and hepatopathology, which should be studied for more detailed discussions of clinical phenomena, laboratory tests, pathogenesis, and therapy. This book is focused on the biopsy, and details of gross pathology are only mentioned when they augment the understanding of the biopsy features under discussion. Similarly, ultrastructural findings, immunopathology reactions, and molecular studies are not reviewed in detail; and other literature should be sought for the most complete and the most current information. Although some of the information in this book will change in the coming years, we hope it remains a useful and informative resource for those studying liver biopsies.

Stephen A. Geller, M.D.

Lydia M. Petrovic, M.D.

ACKNOWLEDGMENTS

We gratefully acknowledge the assistance and support of the publisher, Lippincott Williams & Wilkins. Jonathan Pine, Senior Executive Editor and Managing Editors Jean McHale and Jennifer Verbiar have been especially supportive, understanding, and patient. Jean McHale was particularly supportive in the early stages of the preparation of the second edition and was ably succeeded by Jennifer Verbiar, who greatly facilitated the completion of the book. Satvinder Kaur, Project Manager, Professional Publishing Group, Aptara, in Delhi, India, ably supervised the final stages of preparation.

We are also appreciative of our many colleagues, pathologists, hepatologists, and surgeons, who have provided valuable information, invaluable cases, and ongoing support. Residents and fellows often challenge concepts and dogma and our daily interactions with them have also imperceptibly, but significantly, added to the value of this book. We have also been supported by our respective families and friends. Writing and preparing any book for publication is a time-consuming, demanding activity that often requires that time be taken from life's other activities. This is no less true for a second edition than it is for a first, as we have updated text and references and added many new images. Finally, and certainly not least, many thousands of patients contributed to our love for and understanding of the study of liver diseases.

1

A BRIEF HISTORY OF LIVER BIOPSY

The study of the liver is at least as old as written history. The Assyro-Babylonian clay model of a liver in the British Museum is approximately 4,000 years old, and its carefully inscribed segments are remarkably similar to those obtained today with modern angiographic or postmortem injection studies (6). There is good evidence that this liver, and countless others like it, was used to predict the future. The art of predicting events from examination of the liver was known as hepatoscopy or haruspicy. In ancient times, the word *liver* was also used to imply strength in many languages all over the world, even in the Old Testament (3,5).

The practice of haruspicy spread to the Etruscans, the ancient Hebrews, and later to the Greeks and Romans. Similar rites have been used in modern times by people living in Borneo, Burma, and Uganda.

Gradually the liver took a lesser role in both the primitive medical practices and in the mythology of the common people as the heart and the brain, at various times, assumed importance. In galenic anatomy, the heart was thought to derive its nourishment from the brain, which was regarded as the progenitor for all other organs, and the liver was both underemphasized and incorrectly described. A thousand years after Galen (129–200), Vesalius (1514–1564), Fabricius (1537–1619), and William Harvey (1578–1657), among others, made significant contributions to the study of the anatomy of the liver and, in particular, about its vital vascular connections. It was not until the 17th and 18th centuries, however, that an accurate understanding of hepatic structure was obtained.

Glisson (1597–1677) was not the first to discover the capsule of the liver, but he did come remarkably close to deciphering the complexities of hepatic vasculature, and the relationship of the vessels to the biliary tree, by producing casts of the portal and hepatic veins, and then dissecting away the parenchyma. Malpighi (1628–1694) established the firm foundation for our studies of the structure of the liver with the use of a primitive microscope. He recognized the liver lobule, although he was not able to identify individual hepatocytes. Malpighi also identified the liver as the source of bile. He suggested, after carrying out a series of injection studies, that a sinusoidal network connected portal and hepatic venous systems.

In the 19th century, many scientists contributed to our knowledge of the liver. Paul Ehrlich, in 1884, and Lucatello, in 1885, both performed "puncture" of the liver through laparoscopes for various reasons (1). Histopathology studies were still in their infancy at this time, and tissues were mostly being obtained for chemical, rather than morphologic, studies. Needle puncture of the liver was performed repeatedly during the latter part of the 19th century and the first third of the 20th century, primarily for drainage of hepatic abscesses and hydatid cysts (4).

In 1938, the Vim-Silverman needle was introduced (7). At this time, histopathology was a dominant specialty in medicine, and major advances in the study of the pathology and the pathophysiology of the liver were possible. In 1958 the technique of liver biopsy was further refined with the introduction of the Menghini needle (4), which allowed for the recovery of a core of liver tissue with relatively little artifact induced by the procedure itself. The Menghini needle helped to dramatically expand the use of biopsy, both because it was safer and easier to use than the Vim-Silverman and because it provided tissue of sufficient quality to support sophisticated light microscopic, histochemical, ultrastructural, and immunohistochemical studies. Newer core needle biopsy devices, such as the Tru-cut biopsy and biopsy guns, have refined the technique.

In the 1920s, Martin and Ellis, at Memorial Sloane-Kettering Cancer Center in New York City, developed the technique of aspiration cytology (2). Over the years, aspiration cytology was only rarely applied to the study of liver diseases because the core biopsy was the focus of most diagnostic studies. In recent years, aspiration cytology has been increasingly used for the study of mass lesions.

For most disorders of the liver, percutaneous liver biopsy can yield a satisfactory specimen. Generally, the pathologist would like to have a specimen at least 2 cm long. Laparoscopic biopsy is useful for specific lesions that cannot easily be obtained with percutaneous sampling. Recently it has become practical to obtain specimens via jugular vein entry using a venous catheter through the right atrium and inferior vena cava into the hepatic vein. Transjugular biopsy is particularly useful when the patient has a bleeding diathesis or is markedly ascitic. This wedge biopsy technique, which depends on a biopsy forceps to obtain a sample, generally yields only liver fragments rather than a core, even with an experienced operator. Refinements of this technique have been described that do obtain cores, however. In some cases, particularly when architectural rather than cytologic features are important for evaluation, the usual fragmented transjugular biopsy may not be adequate, and core biopsy is necessary.

REFERENCES

1. Chen TS, Chen PS. Understanding the Liver. Westport, CT: Greenwood Press, 1991.
2. Martin HE, Ellis EB. Biopsy by needle puncture and aspiration. Ann Surg 1930;92: 169–181.

3. Mellinkoff SM. Some meanings of the liver. Gastroenterology 1979;76:636–638.
4. Menghini G. One-second needle biopsy of the liver. Gastroenterology 1958;35:190–199.
5. Popper H. Vienna and the liver. In: Hepatology: A Festschrift for Hans Popper. New York: Raven Press, 1985:1–14.
6. Popper H, Schaffner F. Liver: Structure and Function. New York: Blakiston, 1957:1–3.
7. Silverman I. A new biopsy needle. Am J Surg 1938;40:671–672.

2

INDICATIONS FOR LIVER BIOPSY

In the 1960s and 1970s, liver biopsy was the *sine qua non* for establishing the diagnoses of cirrhosis, extrahepatic biliary obstruction, and acute viral hepatitis. Those diagnoses are today generally easily established by characteristic clinical behavior; relatively specific laboratory tests, including serologic markers for hepatitis; and imaging studies, including various techniques for study of the biliary tree. As the indications for liver biopsy have changed, the practicing pathologist has become less familiar with many common disorders. The consulting pathologist to whom liver biopsies are referred may be the first to recognize histologically classic acute viral hepatitis, extrahepatic biliary obstruction, and even cirrhosis. In the last quarter century, liver transplantation has become a widely accepted and used procedure leading to increasing use of liver biopsies for various indications (1,3,6,7,13), with more and more posttransplant biopsies performed at local hospitals rather than transplant centers.

Liver biopsy is still performed for these conditions when the clinical behavior or the diagnostic procedures and test results are not typical. As an example, cirrhosis not yet expressing itself in terms of portal hypertension or impaired hepatic synthetic function can still be a clinically elusive condition and diagnosis may be established with liver biopsy performed either for a suspected liver disorder other than cirrhosis or for some entirely unrelated condition. In addition, liver biopsy serves in identifying etiologic factors, determining the stage of progression of a disease process, and evaluating the effects of therapy.

This chapter briefly reviews some of the indications for liver biopsy, with emphasis on clinical considerations. Indications for liver biopsy are as follows:

1. Abnormal liver tests not explained by other methods
   a. Granulomatous hepatitis. Granulomatous hepatitis is typically diagnosed only with liver biopsy (8). Granulomas may form because of infections, such as tuberculosis, and also as a consequence of a multisystem disorder, most often sarcoidosis. Many medications, including allopurinol, isoniazid, and phenylbutazone, cause hepatic granulomas. Schistosomiasis is, worldwide, the most commonly

encountered parasitic cause of granuloma. Foreign materials may reach the liver either directly during surgery or biopsy, via the bloodstream as in the case of the intravenous drug abuser, but also with inadvertent entry of foreign material after intravenous therapy, and also via the portal system from the intestines. Granulomas seen after liver transplantation can be problematic (9). Often, the cause of hepatic granulomas is not easily established. Biopsy still has an important role in providing a morphologic basis for a previously unexplained elevation of serum alkaline phosphatase and/or aminotransferases by reducing the necessity for further studies.

b. Unexplained chronic liver disease. Some patients may have chronic hepatitis but without the clinical history or serologic findings usually associated with the chronic hepatitides. Liver biopsy confirms the presence of the disorder and allows evaluation of its stage. Is there active necrosis? What is the extent of fibrosis?

c. Liver injury due to therapeutic drugs. Therapeutic drugs may cause a host of liver reactions other than granulomas (21,33), and patients may present with various signs and symptoms that mimic other liver disorders. As an example, the cardiac drug amiodarone may cause fever, elevation of aminotransferases, and malaise; in addition, clinical and histologic features identical to those of alcoholic hepatitis may be present (12).

2. Fevers of unknown origin. This application of liver biopsy has diminished in frequency because (a) some hepatotropic infections have become less common; (b) several new microbiologic and immunologic diagnostic methods have been developed; and (c) there is widespread use of increasingly sophisticated imaging procedures that allow for fine-needle aspiration (FNA) rather than core needle biopsy. Nevertheless, liver biopsy is often the way in which the diagnosis of a variety of diseases can be established. These include:

a. Mycobacterial disorders

i. *Mycobacterium hominis*. The number of cases of *M. hominis* tuberculosis has increased slightly in recent years, after having declined dramatically in the last half century.

ii. *Mycobacterium avium-intracellulare*. Liver biopsy is often helpful in patients with acquired immune deficiency syndrome (AIDS) who may have unexplained malaise, with or without temperature elevation (2,4,11,15,24).

b. Cytomegalovirus (CMV). CMV hepatitis is a significant risk for patients with AIDS, patients immunosuppressed after organ transplantation, and patients with immune deficiencies from other causes (29).

c. Histoplasmosis. Histoplasmosis can involve the liver as part of a disseminated infection, especially in immunodepressed patients, but may also occur as limited disease presenting with fever, elevation of serum alkaline phosphatase, with lesser elevation of transaminases. The bilirubin level is minimally elevated or normal. Generally, except in immunodepressed patients, well-formed granulomas and organisms can be demonstrated with the Gomori methenamine silver method (16).

d. Candidiasis. Although *Candida* lesions of the liver can be seen in immunodepressed individuals, we usually encounter it in patients with iatrogenic leukopenia, typically the leukemic patient undergoing treatment. Not uncommonly, the patient has had unexplained fever for some time, and imaging techniques demonstrate multiple small hepatic and splenic lesions. Characteristic *Candida* organisms are found in necrotic foci, which may have relatively scant inflammatory response.

e. Toxoplasmosis. *Toxoplasma gondii* hepatitis is rarely seen except in newborns or in persons with AIDS or another immune disorder, although subclinical cases may occur in young adults in a manner similar to that of infectious mononucleosis. Typically, there is a mild hepatitis with extensive infiltration of the sinusoids by lymphocytes (26). Sometimes marked necrosis and granulomas are visible. The organisms are rarely demonstrable in hematoxylin-eosin–stained sections.

f. Sarcoidosis. Generally, patients present with pulmonary disease. Sometimes patients may have fever alone, however, or in association with arthralgia. Liver biopsy almost always demonstrates the characteristic noncaseating epithelioid granulomas, with or without inflammatory cell infiltration of the surrounding parenchyma (8,26).

g. Brucellosis. The diagnosis of brucellosis is considered in inverse proportion to its incidence. The liver shows nonspecific reactive changes, including mild to moderate portal inflammation and Kupffer cell hypertrophy (5,26). Necrosis of hepatocytes is uncommon and focal. In the acute phase, there may be small granulomas (5).

h. Coccidioidomycosis. Coccidioidomycosis is a fungus common to the southwestern United States, generally presenting as pulmonary disease. Rarely, an unexplained febrile illness may prompt a liver biopsy. Focal necrosis without diffuse hepatitis may be seen (26).

i. Q fever. Q fever is caused by the rickettsial agent *Coxiella burnetii*. In addition to unexplained fever, patients complain of headaches and have symptoms consistent with hepatitis. A distinctive but not pathognomonic "fibrin ring granuloma" is seen, with a central droplet of fat surrounded by a delicate ring of brightly eosinophilic fibrin, which is itself surrounded by an inflammatory cell aggregate consisting mostly of lymphocytes but also having some polymorphonuclear leukocytes (23). A true hepatitis with hepatocellular necrosis and both lobular and portal accumulations of chronic inflammatory cells can be seen. Similar granulomas have been reported with CMV, leishmaniasis, Epstein–Barr virus, and even hepatitis A, as well as in association with allopurinol therapy and in Hodgkin lymphoma (17,22,31).

    j. Infectious mononucleosis. Rarely, hepatitis may be the presenting phenomenon. Dense accumulations of atypical lymphocytes, analogous to the Downey cells of blood smears, can be present in portal tracts and sinusoids (18,26). The infiltration may mimic acute leukemia and, rarely, may form aggregates suggestive of lymphoma. Hepatocyte necrosis is distinctly uncommon, but there may be mild cholestasis.

    k. Hodgkin lymphoma. Liver biopsy is only rarely performed as a part of a staging evaluation. Involvement of the liver by Hodgkin lymphoma may resemble nonspecific portal inflammation. Noncaseating granulomas can be seen in portal tracts and involving the lobule. The classic features of Hodgkin lymphoma, especially Reed–Sternberg cells, are almost never seen.

    l. Non-Hodgkin lymphoma. An abdominal lymphoma may present with fever and without peripheral nodal or thoracic disease, and liver biopsy may rarely be the first way in which the diagnosis is obtained. Alternatively, the patient with established lymphoma may have an unexplained fever, and tumor masses may not be seen with imaging techniques but may be found with liver biopsy or FNA. There has been increasing awareness of the association of hepatitis C with both intrahepatic and extrahepatic non-Hodgkin lymphoma (28).

    m. Metastatic carcinoma. Metastatic carcinoma, usually confirmed with imaging or other techniques, can rarely present as fever of unknown origin without an obvious mass. In these instances, liver biopsy sometimes establishes the diagnosis.

3. Systemic inflammatory or metabolic disorders. The liver biopsy in a vasculitis may be normal or difficult to interpret unless the typical vascular lesion is serendipitously sampled. Although the term "lupoid hepatitis" was previously used for patients with autoimmune hepatitis, liver involvement is distinctly unusual in patients with true systemic lupus erythematosus (10). In contrast, liver biopsy can be especially helpful in the study of metabolic disorders, providing sufficient tissue with which appropriate biochemical and ultrastructural studies can be performed. Even in adults, liver biopsy may be the most efficacious way to diagnose certain systemic disorders, such as Gaucher disease and amyloidosis.

4. Evaluation and staging of chronic liver diseases

    a. Cholestatic liver diseases

        i. Chronic obstructive biliary tract disease. Liver biopsy can determine the degree of damage. In particular, biopsy can show when irrevocable damage has occurred, at which time transplantation may be a consideration.

ii. Primary biliary cirrhosis. Liver biopsy is still *sine qua non* for both the diagnosis and staging of primary biliary cirrhosis. Liver biopsy helps in evaluating the efficacy of new drugs and is an integral part of clinical trials.

iii. Primary sclerosing cholangitis. Primary sclerosing cholangitis is principally diagnosed with imaging studies. The changes associated with primary sclerosing cholangitis are exceedingly variable and, despite radiologically determined disease, may not be seen in a given biopsy. Indeed, the characteristic periductal "onion skin" pattern of fibrosis or the ductopenic scar may not be seen even with multiple biopsies.

iv. Chronic cholestasis. Chronic cholestasis in the absence of biliary tract disease can occur with certain drugs, chronic hepatitis, alcoholic liver disease, Hodgkin lymphoma, metastasis, and idiopathic recurrent cholestasis (30).

b. Alcoholic liver disease. Liver biopsy is no longer the principal way to study alcoholic liver disease, although sometimes it is useful in establishing the diagnosis. In alcoholics considered for liver transplantation or in posttransplantation patients with unexplained liver test results, biopsy can provide evidence of continuing alcohol use.

c. Chronic hepatitis. The liver biopsy remains the key to the evaluation of chronic hepatitis (14,19,25,29). In the patient with clinical or biochemical evidence of liver disease for more than 6 months' duration, biopsy can determine the nature of the inflammatory process, provide prognostic guidelines, and often establish etiology. The efficacy of drugs used to manage forms of chronic hepatitis can be determined. In terms of recognition of fibrosis and transition to cirrhosis (staging), biopsy remains the best approach. Although the liver biopsy is not an absolute guide to prognosis in every case, it often provides the following:

i. An indication of the severity of the lesion at a given time, including the amount of inflammation and the degree and distribution of necrosis.

ii. Some information about cause, or at least exclusion of some etiologic factors.

iii. Information about irreversible architectural alterations, such as fibrosis to septum formation to cirrhosis.

iv. Recognition of incidental lesions.

d. Cirrhosis. Cirrhosis is a pathophysiologic alteration of the liver with both vascular septa, connecting portal and central venous systems, and regenerative nodules. This combination, septa plus nodules, is the basis of the signs and symptoms we recognize as cirrhosis (portal hypertension, decreasing catabolic function, and decreasing synthetic function).

Liver biopsy is useful for four principal reasons: (a) to confirm the clinical impression of cirrhosis where the diagnosis is not unequivocal (20,26); (b) to ascertain the cause of the injury; (c) to attempt to determine prognosis; and (d) to identify patients in whom clinical manifestations of cirrhosis are simulated, but in whom there may be some other condition, such as nodular hyperplasia or schistosomiasis. In addition, (e) the biopsy can document hepatocellular dysplasia and/or carcinoma.

The histopathologic diagnosis of cirrhosis is not always straightforward (20,26). The appreciation of nodule formation and, consequently, the diagnosis of cirrhosis by liver biopsy can be quite difficult, particularly if the sample obtained is suboptimal. Overdiagnosis can also occur, especially when cirrhosis is diagnosed (a) on the basis of fibrosis alone, (b) in the face of intact acinar architecture and without regenerative nodule formation, (c) when recent bridging necrosis is thought to be fibrosis, or (d) when capsular fibrosis appears to be intraparenchymal because of the way in which the tissue is oriented in histologic sections. This latter problem is particularly prevalent during examination of wedge biopsies of the liver, without obtaining deep parenchyma relatively far from the capsule.

The clinician should consider several useful features and concepts when establishing the diagnosis of cirrhosis:
  i. The liver tends to be hard or gritty when the needle enters.
 ii. Fragmentation is common in cirrhosis. Depending on the operator's technique, however, it may also occur with relatively normal liver and should not be regarded as diagnostic.
iii. Capsular fibrosis can simulate a septum. Evidence of regeneration should be sought if the putative septum is histologically close to the capsule.
 iv. Reticulin stain is particularly useful. Two-cell–thick liver plates of the regenerative nodule are well shown with reticulin. In fragmented specimens, isolated nodules often are circumscribed by reticulin fibers.
  v. Elastic stains, including Victoria blue and orcein, can be useful in distinguishing elastic-rich septa of cirrhosis from elastic-poor capsular tissue.
 e. Candidates for liver transplantation. Evaluation of the liver biopsy is not required before liver transplantation. Most chronic liver disease patients will be selected for transplantation because of clinical evidence of increasing liver function deterioration. In acute liver failure, liver biopsy may be contraindicated.

The donor liver may be evaluated to determine if conditions exist that may affect graft survival, such as excess steatosis.
5. Evaluation of liver injury caused by therapeutic drugs. It is not possible in this brief review to discuss in detail the responses of the liver to

therapeutic agents (33). The changes seen, either individually or in combination, include (a) steatosis and other cellular degenerative changes, (b) cholestasis, (c) lobular hepatitis, (d) chronic active hepatitis, (e) granulomatous hepatitis, (f) fulminant (massive) hepatitis, (g) destructive cholangitis, (h) sinusoidal dilatation, (i) veno-occlusive disease, (j) Budd–Chiari syndrome, (k) cirrhosis, (l) hepatocellular proliferation and hepatocellular neoplasia, and (m) nonhepatocellular neoplasia, such as that associated with angiosarcoma.

6. Diagnosis of space-occupying lesions. This is a traditional application for the liver biopsy and remains useful today. The FNA technique can often provide the diagnosis and spare the patient the slightly more traumatic biopsy. Core biopsy provides sufficient tissue for immunohistochemical studies conducted to determine the site of origin of an unknown primary.

   The core needle biopsy can also show changes of the uninvolved liver that reflect the presence of a mass lesion. Specimens from the vicinity of a mass typically show portal edema, proliferation of bile ductules, and infiltration by neutrophils, with focal and irregular sinusoidal dilatation. Changes are similar to those seen in extrahepatic biliary obstruction but are generally not accompanied by the characteristic clinical findings of biliary obstruction.

7. Unexplained hepatomegaly and/or mild hepatic dysfunction. The two most common findings when liver biopsy is performed for hepatomegaly, with or without mild liver dysfunction, are nonspecific steatosis and congestion. Usually these findings are not clinically helpful.

   a. Hepatocellular and/or pleomorphic hypertrophy may be seen as a nonspecific response to various medications. There is an increase in the amount of cytoplasm in the zone 3 (centrolobular) hepatocytes. The liver cells may resemble the "ground-glass" cells of hepatitis B carriers, but these "induction cells" do not react with Victoria blue, orcein, or monoclonal antibody to hepatitis B surface antigen.

   b. Congestion as an unexpected finding is most often caused by mild congestive heart failure. In some cases, however, congestion may be an early indication of venous outflow obstruction, as in early Budd–Chiari syndrome. The correct diagnosis may not be evident until the condition progresses and, even in retrospect, may not be apparent prior to the development of the characteristic zone 3 atrophy.

REFERENCES

1. Alshak, NS, Jiminez AM, Gedebou ML, et al. Epstein–Barr virus infections in liver transplantation patients: correlation of histopathology and semi-quantitative EBV-DNA by polymerase chain reaction (PCR). Mod Pathol 1993;24:1306–1312.

2. Beale TJ, Wetton CW, Crofton ME. A sonographic-pathologic correlation of liver biopsies in patients with the acquired immune deficiency syndrome (AIDS). Clin Radiol 1995;50:761–764.

3. Cakaloglu Y, Devlin J, O'Grady J, et al. Importance of concomitant viral infection during late acute liver allograft rejection. Transplantation 1995;59:40–45.

4. Cavicchi M, Pialoux G, Carnot F, et al. Value of liver biopsy for the rapid diagnosis of infection in human immunodeficiency virus-infected patients who have unexplained fever and elevated serum levels of alkaline phosphatase or gamma-glutamyl transferase. Clin Infect Dis 1995;20:606–610.

5. Cervantes F, Bruguera M, Carbonell J, et al. Liver disease in brucellosis: a clinical and pathological study of 40 cases. Postgrad Med J 1982;58:346–350.

6. Demetris AJ, Lasky S, Van Thiel DH, et al. Pathology of hepatic transplantation: a review of 62 adult allograft recipients immunosuppressed with cyclosporine-steroid regimen. Am J Pathol 1985;118:151–161.

7. Demetris AJ, Jaffe R, Sheahan DJ, et al. Recurrent hepatitis B in liver allograft recipients. Differentiation between viral hepatitis B and rejection. Am J Pathol 1986;125:161–172.

8. Ferrell LD. Hepatic granulomas: a morphologic approach to diagnosis. Surg Pathol 1990;3:87–106.

9. Ferrell LD, Lee R, Brixco C, et al. Hepatic granulomas following liver transplantation. Clinicopathologic features in 42 patients. Transplantation 1995;60:926–933.

10. Geller SA. Autoimmune hepatitis. Pathol State of the Art Rev 1994;3:57–76.

11. Geller SA, Said JW, Joshi VJ. Acquired immunodeficiency syndrome (AIDS). In: Damjanov I, Linder J, eds. Anderson's Pathology. 10th Ed. St. Louis: Mosby, 1996: 645–646.

12. Guigui B, Perrot S, Berry JP, et al. Amiodarone-induced hepatic phospholipidosis. Hepatology 1988;8:1067–1068.

13. Hanto DW, Snover DC, Noreen HJ, et al. Hyperacute rejection of a human orthotopic liver allograft in a presensitized recipient. Clin Transplant 1987;1:304–310.

14. International Working Party. Terminology of chronic hepatitis. Am J Gastroenterol 1995; 90:181–189.

15. Lebovics E, Thung SN, Schaffner F, et al. The liver in the acquired immunodeficiency syndrome: a clinical and histologic study. Hepatology 1985;5:293–298.

16. Lee RG. Non-alcoholic steatohepatitis: a study of 49 patients. Hum Pathol 1989;20:594–598.

17. Marazuela M, Moreno A, Yebra M, et al. Hepatic fibrin-ring granulomas. Hum Pathol 1991;22:607–613.

18. Popper H, Schaffner F. Liver: Structure and Function. New York: Blakiston, 1957:1–3.

19. Popper H, Schaffner F. The vocabulary of chronic hepatitis. N Engl J Med 1971;284: 1154–1156.

20. Popper H. Pathologic aspects of cirrhosis: a review. Am J Pathol 1977;87:228–264.

21. Popper H, Geller SA. Pathogenetic considerations in the histologic diagnosis of drug-induced liver injury. Progr Surg Pathol 1981;2:233–246.

22. Propst A, Propst T, Dietze O, et al. Development of granulomatous hepatitis during treatment with interferon-alpha 2b. Dig Dis Sci 1995;40:2117–2118.

23. Qizilbash AH. The pathology of Q fever as seen on liver biopsy. Arch Pathol Lab Med 1983;107:364–367.

24. Schaffner F. The liver in HIV infection. Progr Liv Dis 1990;9:505–522.

25. Scheuer PJ. Classification of chronic viral hepatitis: a need for reassessment. J Hepatol 1991;13:372–374.

26. Scheuer PJ, Lefkowitch JH. Liver biopsy interpretation. 5th Ed. London: WB Saunders, 1994.

27. Schlichting P, Fauerholdt L, Chistensen E, et al. Clinical relevance of restrictive morphologic criteria for the diagnosis of cirrhosis in liver biopsies. Liver 1981;1:56–61.
28. Schöllkopf C, Smedby KE, Hjalgrim H, et al. Hepatitis C infection and risk of malignant lymphoma. Int J Cancer 2008;122:1885–1890.
29. Sherlock S. Classifying chronic hepatitis. Lancet 1989;2:1168–1170.
30. Snover DC, Hutton S, Balfour HH, et al. Cytomegalovirus infection of the liver in transplant recipients. J Clin Gastroenterol 1987;9:659–665.
31. Snover DC. Biopsy diagnosis of liver disease. Baltimore: Williams & Wilkins, 1992.
32. Yamamoto T, Ishii M, Nagural H, et al. Transient hepatic fibrin-ring granulomas in a patient with acute hepatitis A. Liver 1995;15:276–279.
33. Zimmerman HJ. Hepatotoxicity. New York: Appleton-Century-Crofts, 1978.

3

TECHNICAL CONSIDERATIONS

Liver biopsy samples needed for study can be obtained percutaneously as a core with a biopsy needle, as a wedge or core either during open laparotomy or with the laparoscope, or with a biopsy forceps inserted through the jugular vein. Alternatively, fine-needle aspiration can be used. Each method has limitations; therefore, to avoid an unnecessary procedure or forestall the preparation of a sample that cannot provide the needed answer, the purpose of the biopsy should be determined before the method is chosen (1).

Percutaneous needle biopsy technique has proven to be the most useful method for obtaining liver tissue representative of diffuse liver disease and has been the standard for almost 50 years. Core needle biopsy does not provide the sought-after answer in all cases. Although the special utility of liver biopsy is based on the fact that the liver tends to react uniformly to a great variety of injuries and stimuli, it must be remembered that sampling error can occur in various hepatic disorders. For example, the changes of primary sclerosing cholangitis are not uniformly seen throughout the liver. Primary sclerosing cholangitis can usually be diagnosed with imaging studies, whereas a series of biopsies may fail to demonstrate typical changes. Similarly, characteristic inclusions of cytomegalovirus, in either the posttransplantation patient or the acquired immune deficiency syndrome patient, may not be seen in every section of liver prepared. Several serial sections may be required or a more sensitive technique, such as DNA in situ hybridization, may be required. Of course, tumor nodules, either deep or superficial, can be missed by the relatively blind percutaneous technique, even when performed with the aid of computed tomography.

SIZE MATTERS

An adequate specimen is necessary for the evaluation of diffuse liver disease. Hepatitis C patient biopsies are the most common. Grading and staging, whether using English language diagnosis or scoring system or both, is the standard of practice, used to determine the need for therapy as well as to evaluate prognosis. Ideally, the liver core sample should be obtained with a 16- or 14-gauge needle. The core should be at least 2.0 cm in total length and should include at least 10 complete portal tracts (e-Fig. 3.1).

Even with diffuse disease, percutaneous biopsy not meeting these criteria can prove insufficient. There is considerable difference in the samples obtained with biopsy needles because the needles themselves differ in many aspects. Biopsy needles vary in terms of the length of the sample obtained, the diameter of the sample obtained, and the degree of compression artifact. For example, smaller biopsy needles may not obtain sufficient numbers of portal tracts to appropriately evaluate the immune biliary disorders. In cirrhosis, a small needle may not obtain any septal structures and may yield only fragments of parenchyma, contributing to difficulty in establishing the correct diagnosis.

In our experience wedge biopsy, in the absence of a grossly recognizable lesion, and prompted by what the surgeon perceives to be an abnormal-appearing liver, is often disappointing. Wedge biopsy is the technique of choice for a focal lesion presenting at or immediately below the capsule. If a primary, generalized liver disorder is suspected, a needle biopsy should be performed, even in the intraoperative setting. In wedge biopsy samples, (a) the capsule may be thickened and relatively little diagnostically useful parenchyma obtained; (2) (b) capsule fibrosis extending into the liver may mimic cirrhosis (documentation of features clearly indicative of regeneration of hepatocytes is required); (c) there may be clusters of chronic inflammatory cells immediately below the capsule that can be misinterpreted as evidence of chronic hepatitis; and (d) acute inflammatory cells may be prominent throughout the lobule as a nonspecific sequel to laparotomy. Bile duct hamartomas (von Meyenburg complex) are relatively common and often multiple. They may attract the attention of the surgeon who will biopsy them suspecting metastasis. The lesions can then be misinterpreted by the unwary pathologist as metastatic carcinoma.

The principal indication for laparoscopic biopsy is to diagnose a focal lesion not easily obtained, because of location or size, with standard percutaneous liver biopsy or with computed tomography–guided aspiration. In the absence of a distinct nodule or mass, core needle biopsy should be obtained rather than wedge biopsy.

Transjugular biopsy is generally used for patients with generalized liver disease who have marked ascites or for those with severe thrombocytopenia or another coagulation disorder. The specimen obtained with transjugular biopsy forceps is often markedly fragmented and portal tracts may be absent, but the technique for obtaining core biopsies is available and the samples can be excellent (3–5). It is an excellent technique for the confirmation of a predominantly hepatocytic disorder.

Aspiration biopsy samples obviously do not demonstrate architectural changes, which are key in the recognition of many disorders. They have also proven to be of limited use in the diagnosis of diffuse inflammatory disorders of the liver and are most often obtained for the evaluation of a space-occupying lesion.

CARE AND HANDLING OF THE LIVER BIOPSY SPECIMEN

Although prompt fixation of the liver biopsy is vital to ensure optimal quality of the histologic section, forethought about the goals of the biopsy, including consultation by the clinician with the pathologist, can help to guarantee that all studies needed for diagnosis can be performed without the necessity of a second biopsy performed solely for the purpose of obtaining appropriately prepared tissue.

Formalin, the most common fixative used, is exceedingly stable, penetrates and adequately fixes tissues well, and is the most economical of fixatives. Furthermore, formalin allows for the subsequent application of many histochemical, immunohistochemical, and molecular procedures. The characteristics of tissues fixed in formalin are well known throughout the world, and the cytologic alterations subsequent to fixation are familiar in most settings.

In general, the pathologist decides on the fixative with which he or she is most comfortable; most hepatopathologists prefer fixation with 4% neutral buffered formalin. The core needle biopsy requires at least 2 to 3 hours for adequate fixation, although microwave processing can be used to reduce fixation time. The wedge biopsy can require as long as 12 hours for fixation, unless it is immediately sectioned into 1- to 2-mm-thick portions, in which case satisfactory fixation can be obtained in shorter periods.

The hepatologist or surgeon should be encouraged to ask certain questions prior to immersion of the tissue in fixative: Do I suspect a lymphoma? If so, I may want to obtain a fixative favored for the study of hematologic disorders. Will it also be useful to freeze tissues for immunohistochemical study of lymphocyte markers? Do I suspect Wilson disease? I may want to prepare tissue for electron microscopy. Do I suspect a bacterial disease? I may want to submit a small portion of tissue for microbiologic studies. Do I want to confirm the presence of hepatitis C, Epstein–Barr virus, or other viruses? I may want to save fresh tissue, or use formalin-fixed tissue, for polymerase chain reaction. Do I suspect a metabolic disorder? Which metabolic disorder? I may want to use more than one type of fixative. I may want to fresh-freeze some tissue for specialized histochemical studies as well as fix tissue for electron microscopy. Do I suspect a neoplasm? I may want a "touch print" for cytopathology studies. What kind of neoplasm? Do I need specialized histochemistry? Do I need electron microscopy?

Do I need to talk to the pathologist before I perform the biopsy? The correct answer to this question is often "yes."

Special Handling of Liver Biopsies and Aspirates

Too often the pathologist is asked to provide a definitive diagnosis on tissue that has been inappropriately obtained and prepared.

First, don't let the specimen dry or actively contribute to its drying! Biopsy samples should not be placed on dry gauze, paper towel, or cloth towel, all of which will dehydrate the individual hepatocytes (Fig. 3.1,

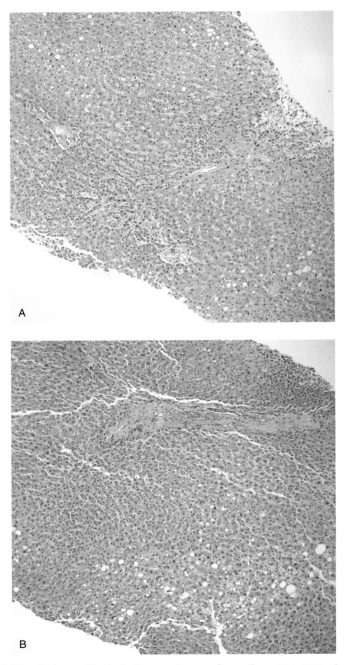

FIGURE 3.1 Drying artifact. Both samples are from the same case. **A** was promptly immersed in formalin. **B** was placed on a dry non-Telfa gauze for approximately 1 minute. Note the artifactually increased eosinophilia in **B**, as well as what appears to be increased nuclear cytoplasmic ratio (hematoxylin-eosin, original ×100).

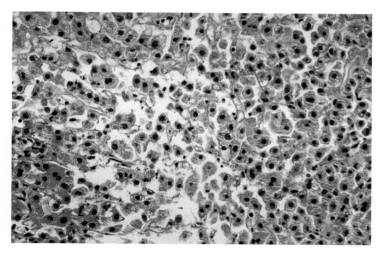

FIGURE 3.2 Image showing dissolution of liver architecture because of immersion of the specimen in saline for more than 15 minutes (hematoxylin-eosin, original ×200.)

e-Figs. 3.2–3.5). The sample should be kept on saline-moisturized Telfa gauze. However, biopsy samples should never be immersed in saline; this leads to artifactual hepatocyte swelling and disruption of architecture (Fig. 3.2, e-Figs. 3.6, 3.7). Samples for microbiologic studies should be obtained without drying the specimen; dry culture swabs also dehydrate cells and affect morphology. A portion of the biopsy core should be submitted separately for this purpose. Exposure to room temperature for more than a few minutes causes specimen drying. If fixation cannot be done immediately, the tissue should be kept cool either by placing it in a closed container in a refrigerator, not a freezer, or by placing a jar containing the tissue in a larger container with ice-cold water or ice cubes, not dry ice. A variant of drying artifact is sometimes seen in wedge biopsy because of cautery effect in which the sinusoids become irregularly dilated (Fig. 3.3).

Second, prompt fixation is vital! If special biochemical studies, such as those for metabolic disorders, are needed, a portion of the biopsy should be immediately placed in the −70°C freezer or in an isopentane holding container. Tissue can also be placed in an appropriate support medium, such as Zeus medium, and then frozen.

Third, various artifactual changes can be seen in the tissue section, most of which are easily recognized (e-Figs. 3.8–3.11).

Fourth, fine-needle aspiration specimens must also be handled promptly. Delay causes artifactual changes because of drying and can prevent accurate evaluation. The most useful portion often is in the needle hub, which should be flushed after preparation of the smear. A clot in the needle hub, where it joins the syringe, can be recovered by

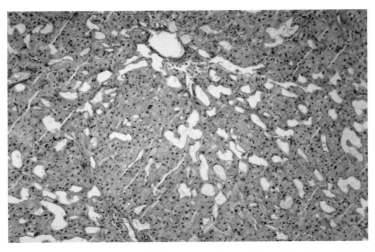

FIGURE 3.3 Cautery artifact. Sinusoidal spaces are irregularly and haphazardly dilated, and hepatocytes have irregular forms with loss of cytoplasm and relatively nuclear enlargement (hematoxylin-eosin, original ×100).

mechanically scraping it free with either a new needle or an orange-wood stick so as to prepare a "cell button" for paraffin embedding and sectioning (1).

REFERENCES

1. Geller SA, Pitman MD, Nichols WS. Cellular and molecular diagnostic techniques. In: Burt AD, Portmann BC, Ferrell LD, et al., eds. MacSween's Pathology of the Liver. 5th Ed. London: Churchill Livingstone, 2007:119–146.
2. Petrelli M, Scheuer PJ. Variation in subcapsular liver structure and its significance in the interpretation of wedge biopsies. J Clin Pathol 1967;20:743–748.
3. De Hoyos A, Loredo ML, Martinez-Rios MA, et al. Transjugular biopsy in 52 patients with an automated Tru-cut-type needle. Dig Dis Sci 1999;44:177–180.
4. Mammen T, Keshava SN, Eapen CE, et al. Transjugular liver biopsy: a retrospective analysis of 601 cases. J Vasc Interv Radiol 2008;19:351–358.
5. Soyer P, Fargeaudou Y, Boudiaf M, et al. Transjugular liver biopsy using ultrasonographic guidance for jugular vein puncture and an automated device for hepatic tissue sampling: a retrospective analysis of 200 consecutive cases. Abdom Imaging 2008;33:627–632.

4

ANATOMIC CONSIDERATIONS

The liver is the largest solid organ of the body, generally weighing between 1,200 and 1,500 g in the adult, accounting for approximately 2% to 5% of the total body weight (6). In the healthy neonate, the liver generally accounts for about 5% of body weight. The liver is regarded as mostly consisting of a dominant right and a lesser left lobe, separated by the falciform ligament, with smaller caudate and quadrate lobes. More significant in terms of modern surgical approaches, however, is the segmental anatomy based on vascular supply and biliary drainage (3,6,7,16–20).

Vascular supply variation occurs particularly with the caudate lobe. It may contribute to some variations in imaging appearance of the liver and, if both the abnormally supplied region and the remainder of the liver are sampled, can contribute to diagnostic confusion. The pathology and pathophysiology of most liver diseases can be well understood only if their microscopic structural basis is appreciated. The liver has a highly complex histologic structure with various elements (Table 4.1). It is a unique elaboration of the vascular system centered between the afferent and efferent vessels. Comprehension of the way in which the portal system eventually drains into the hepatic vein, and the unique structure of the liver plate, which allows for the most direct contact between the hepatocyte and the blood and its contents, is a key to understanding.

Blood enters the liver principally via the portal vein, which branches to become incorporated in the distinctive structural entities of the portal tract. Blood traverses the parenchyma via the sinusoids, where all of the hepatic functions take place, to reach the terminal hepatic venule ("central vein"), and then to hepatic veins, the inferior vena cava, and, ultimately, the heart. The portal veins are the largest vessels in the portal tracts and empty into periportal sinusoids through venules. The hepatic artery is a relatively minor contributor to hepatic blood flow; indeed, it is almost never considered as a potential contributing factor in most hepatic diseases.

THE PORTAL TRACT

The portal tract (Fig. 4.1, e-Figs. 4.1, 4.2) is a well-defined connective tissue structure composed primarily of type I collagen, which interfaces with

TABLE 4.1   **Microanatomy of the Liver**
Portal tract
Portal vein and venules
Hepatic artery and arterioles
Bile ducts
Bile ductules
Lymphatics
Lymphocytes and mast cells
Macrophages
Fibroblasts
Nerves
Parenchyma
Hepatocytes
Canaliculi
Canals of Hering
Sinusoids
Sinusoidal lining cells
Endothelial cells
Kupffer cells
Pit cells
Space of Disse
Stellate cells (lipocytes, cells of Ito)
Reticulin fibrils
Nerves
Terminal hepatic venule (central vein)

the limiting plate of hepatocytes. Each portal tract contains at least one small arterial branch, a portal vein branch, and a bile duct. The portal tract system can be thought of as a great oak tree with incalculable numbers of branch points, the first of which occurs at the hilum of the liver. Because of this pattern of progressive branching, the portal tracts exhibit a great range of sizes. Furthermore, when the pyramid-shaped portal tracts are randomly cut they may, in the two-dimensional histologic section, display variation of both shape and components. The largest portal tracts are round or triangular, the medium-sized portal tracts are mostly triangular, the smallest portal tracts tend to be triangular or branching, and the smallest terminal divisions are round or oval (18,20). In any given histologic section, a portal tract may appear triangular or quadrangular, or may even resemble a fibrous septum, and a disease process potentially affecting portal structures cannot be excluded if adequate sampling has not been obtained.

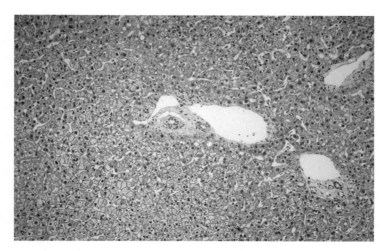

FIGURE 4.1 Photomicrograph of a normal portal tract showing portal vein, hepatic artery, and bile duct, along with the surrounding hepatic parenchyma directly abutting on the portal tract as a limiting plate of continuous hepatocytes. Note that there is only a sprinkling of lymphocytes (hematoxylin-eosin, original magnification ×200).

In the larger portal tracts, lymphatic channels and autonomic nerve fibers can be visualized. The lymphatic channels drain into the space of Disse, and their flow is opposite to that of blood but parallel to the bile system (18,20). Varying numbers of lymphocytes and rare mast cells are seen in the unaffected liver, but plasma cells and polymorphonuclear leukocytes are generally not seen. The finding of portal lymphocytes, even in significant numbers, should not be interpreted as evidence of chronic hepatitis in the absence of interface hepatitis ("piecemeal necrosis"). Mild portal inflammation without interface hepatitis can be seen with systemic illnesses, in association with drugs and toxins, adjacent to space-occupying lesions, and in individuals without historical, clinical, or biochemical evidence of liver disease ("normal") (Fig. 4.2).

Bile ducts in the smaller portal tracts, those generally seen in liver biopsies, are known as interlobular bile ducts, whereas those in large portal areas are called septal, or trabecular, ducts (Fig. 4.3). Interlobular bile ducts are lined by cuboidal or low columnar epithelium with an underlying basement membrane consisting of periodic acid–Schiff (PAS)–positive material that is resistant to diastase digestion. In the healthy liver, the duct epithelial cells are well demarcated with uniform round nuclei that are evenly spaced. The epithelial cells do not overlap, and there are no lymphocytes within the limits of the basement membrane. The epithelium of the septal duct also rests on a basement membrane but is tall columnar with a distinctly basal nuclear location and with an internal diameter of more than 100 mm (1,18,20).

In the normal portal tract, the bile duct tends to be adjacent to a hepatic artery branch of approximately the same size, so that the number

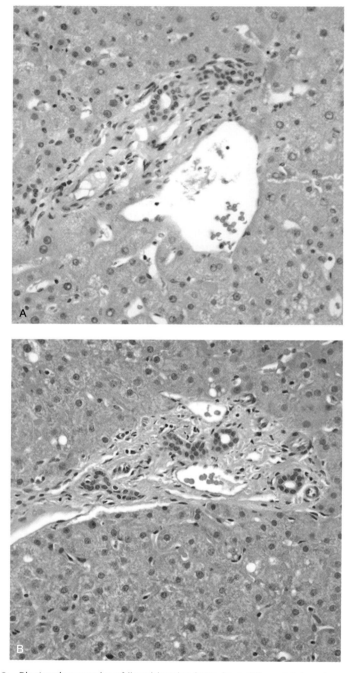

FIGURE 4.2   Photomicrographs of liver biopsies from four different living donors showing the great variability in the numbers of lymphocytes present in portal tracts in individuals who have no historical, clinical, or biochemical evidence for liver disease (**A,B,D**, hematoxylin-eosin, **C** Periodic acid-Schiff after diastase digestion, original magnification ×200) Note the presence of PAS-positive material in Kuppfer cells and portal macrophages in **C** and minimal "interphase hepatitis" in **D**.

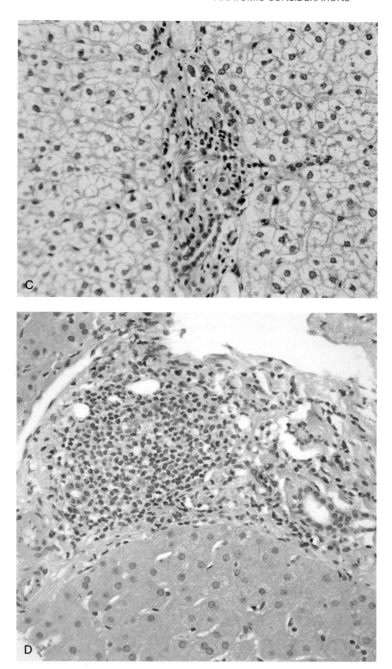

FIGURE 4.2   **(Continued)**

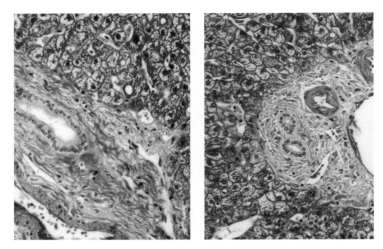

FIGURE 4.3   Photomicrographs showing interlobular bile ducts and septal bile ducts, taken at the same magnification for comparison purposes (Masson trichrome, original magnification ×200).

of bile ducts and the number of artery branches is usually equal or almost equal in a given section when at least four portal tracts are present for evaluation. Bile ducts can be immunohistochemically demonstrated with antibodies to high molecular weight cytokeratin polypeptides (Fig. 4.4).

The bile ductules, which are seen only when they proliferate (ductular reaction), are located at the periphery of the portal tracts and have a lumen size of less than 20 mm. They have a cuboidal epithelium and a

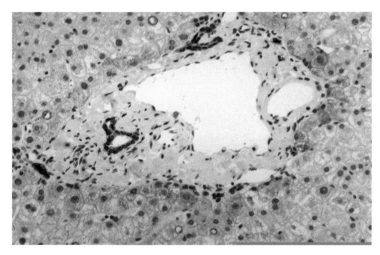

FIGURE 4.4   Bile ducts immunohistochemically demonstrated with antibodies to high molecular weight cytokeratin polypeptides (antikeratin AE 1/3, original magnification ×200).

basement membrane and may be accompanied by a tributary of the portal vein but not by a hepatic artery branch. After injury, the bile duct epithelium may also elaborate hormone polypeptides, which can be demonstrated immunohistochemically (18).

With age, the collagen fibers of the portal tract become increasingly dense, with newly formed type III collagen appearing as delicate light blue fibers, contrasting with the already present thick dark blue fibers of type I collagen. The hepatic artery may sometimes show changes of atherosclerosis in parallel with the aorta. The number of inflammatory cells also increases with age. The left lobe will tend to show more portal fibrosis than the right.

PARENCHYMA

The parenchyma consists primarily of hepatocytes that are arranged as one-liver-cell-thick anastomosing spongelike walls or plates (Fig. 4.5, e-Fig. 4.3), separated from each other by the sinusoids through which blood flows from the portal tracts to terminal hepatic venules. The normal function of the liver is to a great degree owing to the almost direct contact of the hepatocyte with the blood, allowing the efficient and direct removal from circulation of various substances, including normal metabolic products (endobiotics) as well as environmentally acquired substances (xenobiotics), and also allowing for the similarly unimpeded secretion of vital liver cell products, such as albumin and coagulation factors.

The one-cell-thick liver plate pattern prevails throughout the liver and helps to explain the efficiency of the hepatocyte, since it allows for each hepatocyte to be exposed on two sides to sinusoidal blood. Unlike vascular structures almost everywhere else in the body, the sinusoids do

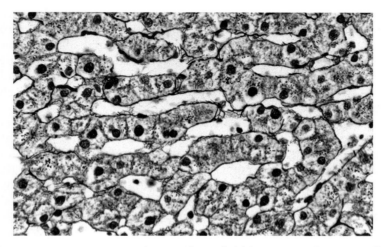

FIGURE 4.5   Hepatocytes arranged as one-liver-cell-thick, anastomosing, spongelike walls or plates, which are separated from each other by the sinusoids through which blood flows from the portal tracts to terminal hepatic venules (reticulin, original magnification ×100).

not have a basement membrane and the cell surface controls influx and efflux of substances almost entirely (18). In the usual histologic section, two- and even three-cell-thick areas are periodically seen; these represent the areas of anastomosis of liver plates. In healthy children, to the age of 5 or 6 years, the liver cell plates tend to be two-cells-thick.

Another variation is seen bordering the portal tracts where there is a continuous line of liver cells from which the liver cell plates extend; this is the limiting plate (18,20) (Fig. 4.1). The interface between the collagen of the portal tract and the hepatocytes of the limiting plate is, characteristically, an uninterrupted straight line. Despite its apparent homogeneity, however, the limiting plate is functionally heterogeneous. The hepatocytes near the apices of the portal triangle, where the blood supply leaves the portal tract, are truly periportal in terms of both location and function (see "Histologic Organization of the Liver" below), whereas those hepatocytes at the center of the limiting plate are relatively far from the blood supply and respond to injury as do the hepatocytes surrounding the terminal hepatic venule. It is for this reason that conditions that contribute to necrosis of hepatocytes surrounding the terminal hepatic venule (central vein), so-called centrolobular or Rappaport zone 3 necrosis, also cause necrosis of hepatocytes at the central portion of the limiting plate.

The sinusoids are separated from the hepatocytes by sinusoidal endothelial cells, Kupffer cells, Pit cells, and the space of Disse, which includes the perisinusoidal stellate cells (lipocytes, or Ito cells), reticulin fibers, and nerves (2–6,15,18,20). The sinusoids are generally empty in the usual liver biopsy, or they may contain a few red cells and rare white cells. In neonates, of course, hematopoietic foci are scattered throughout. Circulating megakaryocytes, not associated with myeloid metaplasia, can sometimes be seen, particularly in patients undergoing physiologic stress (e-Fig. 4.4).

The sinusoidal endothelial cell has a sievelike structure, with fenestra of approximately 1,000-Å diameter. These fenestra actively control the interchange between the blood and the perisinusoidal space by the contraction of cytoskeletal elements (8). The cytoskeletal activity is influenced by both endobiotics and xenobiotics. Although sinusoidal endothelial cells are not identical to other vascular endothelial cells (13), they share a wide range of biologic activities (18).

Kupffer cells (6,12,18,20) are slightly stellate. In the healthy liver they may not be easily differentiated from endothelial cells, although the nucleus of the Kupffer cell tends to be slightly more irregular and plumper. Since they function as macrophages fixed to the sinusoidal wall, Kupffer cells contain many kinds of materials, including foreign material as well as the products of injured or dead cells; consequently, they can usually be visualized by staining the section with PAS after diastase (dPAS) digestion to remove the hepatocyte glycogen, which may impede, but not prevent, Kupffer cell identification (Fig. 4.6). Kupffer cells can also be shown to contain nonspecific esterase, muramidase, peroxidase, and low concentrations of α1-antitrypsin.

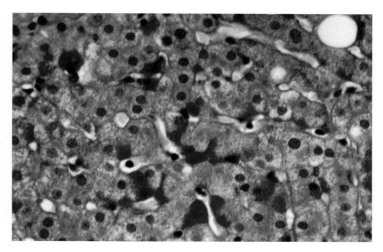

FIGURE 4.6   Kupffer cells stained with periodic acid–Schiff reagent, seen here after diastase digestion to remove glycogen from hepatocytes and highlight the Kupffer cells (diastase periodic acid–Schiff, original magnification ×200).

Pit cells are located on the endothelial lining (4). They correspond to large lymphocytes with natural killer activity and are considered to have a vital role in defense against viral infections as well as metastasis. They can be visualized only after immunohistochemical studies to demonstrate their CD56 and CD57 markers, as well as with the electron microscope.

The space of Disse is the area between the sinusoidal lining and the liver plate (6,7,18,20). It is generally not appreciated in liver biopsy samples unless there is an impediment to venous outflow, such as congestive heart failure. It is most likely because of heart failure at the time of death that the space of Disse is often seen in liver sections obtained at autopsy. The space of Disse contains the sinusoidal stellate cells (perisinusoidal lipocytes, Ito cells), reticulin fibers, and nerves. It is important to realize that although there is no basement membrane in the normal liver, various matrix components are present (11), including collagen types I, III, IV, and VI, fibronectin, laminin, tenascin, various proteoglycans, and trace amounts of collagen V. The reticulin fibers that are easily demonstrated with various common silver impregnation staining methods (Fig. 4.4, e-Fig. 4.3) have been shown to consist mostly of collagen type III, with attached fibronectin and glycoprotein (18,20). While the lack of a basement membrane contributes to the relatively free access of various molecules from the sinusoidal blood into the liver cell, and vice versa, these other structural elements may contribute to the modulation of the rate of passage of these substances. After liver cell injury, a basement membrane may form ("capillarization" of sinusoids); this is a characteristic of cirrhosis and helps to explain the diminished catabolic and anabolic liver cell activity inherent to that condition.

The sinusoidal stellate cell (perisinusoidal lipocyte, Ito cell, hepatic lipocyte, fat-storing cell) (5,18,20) is perisinusoidal, with cytoplasmic extensions that envelop the sinusoidal endothelial cells, similar to pericytes in other locations (2,5). This cell contains small droplets of fat in the cytoplasm, not usually visible with hematoxylin-eosin. The droplets are rich in vitamin A. Consequently, these cells can be recognized when studied with ultraviolet illumination, since vitamin A has a specific autofluorescence at 330 nm (5,8). The perisinusoidal cells are thought to have a role in regulating sinusoidal blood flow, but are also considered as the major cellular contributor to the maintenance of the normal liver matrix and also to the development of hepatic fibrosis (15). It is thought that hepatocytes, when damaged, may release proteins that, along with cytokines from inflammatory cells, macrophages, and platelets, contribute to activation, proliferation, and transformation of sinusoidal stellate cells, with the result that these cells synthesize and secrete various collagens and matrix substances at an accelerated rate. Quiescent stellate cells are not visualized on routine stains. However, activated stellate cells are highlighted with antibody to smooth muscle actin. In the normal liver, sinusoidal stellate cells can also elaborate enzymes needed to degrade matrix components; these enzymes may also be active in abnormal states to help modulate the degree of fibrosis.

The individual hepatocyte is a polygonal epithelial cell, approximately 25 mm in diameter, with abundant eosinophilic cytoplasm, a single round centrally placed nucleus with finely dispersed chromatin, and at least one nucleolus, with a well-defined plasma membrane. In the healthy young adult, only occasional hepatocytes are binucleate. The number of binucleate hepatocytes increases with age and also in response to various stimuli and injuries (9,14,21) (Fig. 4.7, e-Figs. 4.5–4.7). Nuclear variability,

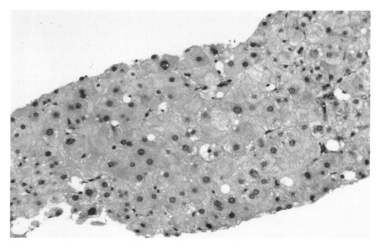

FIGURE 4.7   Liver biopsy from a 92-year-old woman showing increased numbers of binucleate hepatocytes (hematoxylin eosin, original magnification ×200).

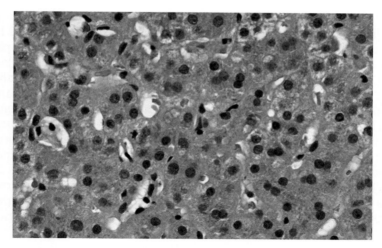

FIGURE 4.8   Liver biopsy from a 32-year-old woman who had been using oral contraceptive pills for 7 years and had a slight, otherwise unexplained, increase in serum transaminase values. There is variability in size and shape of hepatocytes, with many enlarged nuclei and increased numbers of binucleate hepatocytes. After she stopped taking the contraceptive pills, her transaminase values returned to reference range. Liver biopsy was not repeated (hematoxylin-eosin, original magnification ×200).

seen as larger, more irregular, and hyperchromatic nuclei, also occurs with age and after injury. This nonspecific finding, sometimes called "hepatocyte unrest," can also be a subtle sign of drug effect (21) (Fig. 4.8).

There are distinctive hepatocyte polar domains that differ morphologically and functionally (10,20). The sinusoidal domain of the plasma membrane has irregular microvilli, which greatly increase the surface area of the cell and enable it to better participate in exchange of substances with the blood that enters the space of Disse, within which the microvilli project. This portion of the plasma membrane is the site of receptors for glycoprotein, asialoglycoprotein, various peptides, hormones, growth factors, and immunoglobulin A, as well as multiple carrier-mediated transport processes. The sodium pump is at this region of the cells. This is also the site for endocytosis and for transmembrane proteins that recognize specific matrix components, such as laminin, collagen, and integrin (11).

The intercellular domain is specialized for intercellular adhesion but also for intercellular communication. Junctional complexes ensure the attachment and include desmosomes, tight junctions, and intermediate junctions. Intercellular communication occurs via gap junctions (8).

The bile canaliculus is a specialized portion of the intercellular domain, comprising approximately 15% of the hepatocyte plasma membrane, and is the beginning of the bile drainage system of the liver. The bile canaliculus is the portion of the hepatocyte that corresponds to the apex of an exocrine secretory cell. It is an intercellular space between two adjacent hepatocytes, isolated from the rest of the intercellular space by tight junctions. The bile canaliculus is approximately 1 mm in diameter and is not easily recognized with the light microscope unless distended as a part of parenchymal cholestasis. The bile canaliculi form a chicken wire–like network (18,20) in the center of the liver cell plate and connect to small portal bile ductules via the canals, or ducts, of Hering. Bile canaliculi can also be recognized with polyclonal antibody to carcinoembryonic antigen.

The canal of Hering connects the bile canaliculus to the bile ductule. The canal of Hering is lined partly by biliary epithelial cell and partly by hepatocyte and is thought to be the site of origin for the proliferating bile ductules that are seen after liver injury.

The canalicular domain of the hepatocyte has recently been shown to have at least three adenosine triphosphate–dependent export carriers: a leukotriene, a bile salt carrier (gp 110), and a multidrug export carrier (gp 170) (7).

Each hepatocyte is filled with an array of organelles, including smooth and rough endoplasmic reticulum, more than 1,000 mitochondria, approximately 300 lysosomes, an equal number of peroxisomes, approximately 50 Golgi complexes, and an organized cytoskeleton (7). Sometimes the cytoplasm has poorly defined eosinophilic and basophilic areas that most commonly are light microscopic indications of smooth and rough endoplasmic reticulum. Rough endoplasmic reticulum is more easily appreciated in hematoxylin-eosin–stained sections as indistinct basophilic granules or fibers, which become more prominent in association with some xenobiotics, including many drugs, even at therapeutic levels. In liver cell regeneration, as in the cirrhotic liver, mitochondria-rich cells can be recognized as slightly enlarged, intensely eosinophilic, slightly granular hepatocytes. In the normal liver cell, mitochondria cannot be seen.

The normal hepatocyte also contains abundant glycogen, which is not seen with hematoxylin-eosin but is easily demonstrated with the PAS reaction. Glycogen can also be seen as vacuoles that herniate into the nucleus and appear, in routine sections, to be optically clear intranuclear inclusions with a thicker-than-usual nuclear membrane (Fig. 4.9, e-Figs. 4.8, 4.9). These "glycogen nuclei" or "glycogenated nuclei" are present in small numbers in individuals free of recognizable disease and are located in periportal (zone 1) hepatocytes but are present in greater numbers in persons with Wilson disease, diabetes mellitus, prolonged congestive heart failure, and some other disorders; they can also be seen in increased numbers in adolescents and elderly people. With the electron microscope they are seen to consist of smooth endoplasmic reticulum distended with rosettes of glycogen.

The cytoplasm of the perivenular (zone 3) hepatocytes contains uniform fine, refractile, gold–brown granules of lipofuscin. This "wear-and-tear" pigment becomes more prominent with age and progressively is seen in midzonal (zone 2) and periportal (zone 1) hepatocytes. The granules tend to be oriented along the canalicular domain of the hepatocyte

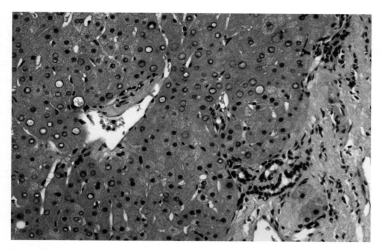

FIGURE 4.9 Glycogen ("glycogenated") nuclei in the liver biopsy of a 75-year-old man (hematoxylin eosin, original magnification ×400).

(Fig. 4.10). Lipofuscin can be stained with the Ziehl–Neelson method, usually used to demonstrate acid-fast bacilli.

Other normal cell constituents, such as albumin and many enzymes, can be demonstrated with special histochemical or immunohistochemical methods (12,18,20).

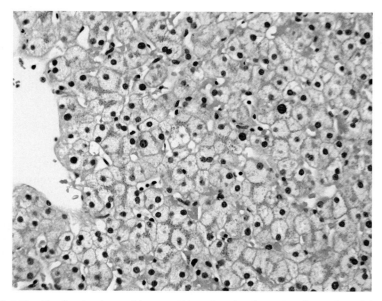

FIGURE 4.10 Lipofuscin pigment in zone 3 hepatocytes (hematoxylin-eosin, original magnification ×200).

The hepatocyte has an orderly cytoskeleton, which includes microtubules, microfilaments, and intermediate filaments, and which can also be visualized using immunohistochemical methods (8). Microtubules are formed from tubulin and involved in the secretion of proteins into the plasma. They are present throughout the cytoplasm but are most prominent in the region of the Golgi apparatus and along the sinusoidal plasma membrane. Microfilaments consist of myosin and actin and are particularly concentrated around the bile canaliculus, where they are involved with bile secretion and with the functioning of sinusoidal surface microvilli. Intermediate filaments are cytokeratins that extend from the plasma membrane to the perinuclear zone. Hepatocytes normally have cytokeratins 8 and 18 but, after injury, may acquire subtypes 7 and 19 (12,18). Intermediate filaments form an irregular meshlike network, which extends from the plasma membrane to the perinuclear zone, where they are in greatest concentration. They are thought to be the principal microfilament responsible for the spatial organization of the hepatocyte.

TERMINAL HEPATIC VENULE

The terminal hepatic venules (central veins) collect all of the blood that traverses the sinusoids. The terminal hepatic venules are the smallest efferent veins and are an integral part of the hepatic parenchyma. There is no direct connection between the terminal hepatic venules and the vessels contained within the portal tracts, requiring, in the normal liver, that blood traverse the parenchyma to leave the liver. The terminal hepatic venule has a thin wall lined by endothelial cells and is not surrounded by collagen in the normal state, although interrupted islands of collagen can be seen in the subintima of the larger venules, in an otherwise normal liver, as they approach the hepatic vein (Fig. 4.11, e-Fig. 4.10). The terminal hepatic venules empty into three main hepatic veins. The intrahepatic portion of the hepatic veins, which are without valves as are the terminal hepatic venules, then empty directly into the inferior vena cava.

HISTOLOGIC ORGANIZATION OF THE LIVER

The precise definition of the smallest structural and functional unit of the liver remains controversial. The Kiernan and Mall models, developed in the 19th and early 20th century, were based on the distribution pattern of the hepatic blood vessels with the terminal hepatic venule regarded as the center of the lobule (central vein) and is the pattern seen in subhuman mammals, such as the pig (Fig. 4.12, e-Figs. 4.11, 4.12). Today the Rappaport concept of the hepatic acinus is widely regarded as the functional unit of the liver. In this model, the acinus is a complex entity whose center is the portal tract and whose sinusoids are drained by neighboring terminal hepatic venules (16,20). This model remains the most useful for understanding the pathology of the liver but may not be entirely accurate in terms of the biology of the liver (10).

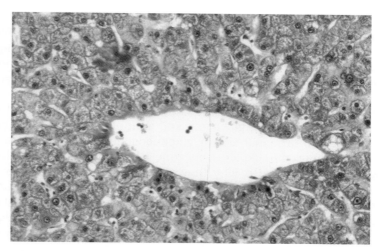

FIGURE 4.11 Terminal hepatic venule (central vein) showing interrupted islands of collagen in the subintima (van Giesen, original magnification ×200).

In the Rappaport scheme, the hepatocytes of each acinus have been designated as belonging to one of three zones in terms of their relationship to the portal tract and particularly in relationship to the blood flow emanating from the apices of the portal triangle. The zones reflect functional variations of the hepatocytes because they are farther from the portal tract (9), but they are not readily identified in routine histologic material. Those in the one third nearest to the apex of the portal tract are zone 1 (formerly

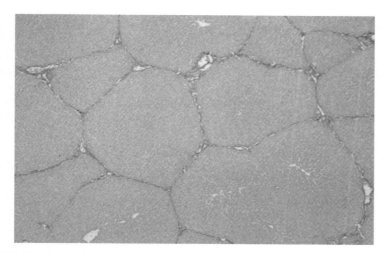

FIGURE 4.12 Photomicrograph of pig liver showing the classic hepatic lobule, with the terminal hepatic venule (central vein) at the center (periodic acid–Schiff, original magnification ×100).

called "periportal"), and those in the one third farthest away, and closest to the terminal hepatic venule, are zone 3 (formerly called "pericentral" or "centrolobular"), with the intervening, and less easily identified, one third called zone 2 (formerly called "midzonal"). In this way, also the hepatocytes at the angle formed by the junction of the limiting plates are zone 1, whereas those in the middle of the limiting plate are zone 3.

Zone 1 hepatocytes are exposed to the blood when it has the highest content of oxygen, insulin, glucagon, and amino acids, and these zone 1 liver cells are the principal site of gluconeogenesis and glycolysis. This activity has been used to explain why zone 1 hepatocytes have the highest metabolic activity and also why they are the first sites of regeneration. Protein synthesis occurs mostly in zone 1, and transaminases, glutamyl transpeptidase, alcohol dehydrogenase, and other enzymes are most easily demonstrated in this zone (12). In contrast, glutamine synthetase, required for the conversion of ammonia and glutamic acid to glutamine, is predominantly found in perivenular zone 3.

The functional activity of the hepatocytes has also been shown in experimental settings to be determined by the microenvironment of the hepatocytes. For example, when blood flow is altered by retrograde perfusion of the liver, the perivenular zone 3 becomes the site of maximal activity for some of the previously zone 1 functions, such as gluconeogenesis and glycolysis. Similarly, when isolated hepatocytes are transplanted to the spleen, they lose some of their enzyme productivity; this loss is reversible when they are returned to the milieu of the liver.

Anatomic Structures Contributing to the Misdiagnosis of Cirrhosis

With age, the left lobe of the liver may become increasing fibrotic and atrophic (e-Figs. 4.13, 4.14) and can be misinterpreted as representing cirrhosis. The liver capsule itself is often overrepresented in left lobe biopsies and is also sometimes obtained with right lobe biopsies. Capsule fibrous tissue can extend into the parenchyma and can even seem to be encircling portions of the lobule, mimicking a regenerative nodule and septa formation (e-Figs. 4.15–4.21). This is particularly a problem with wedge biopsies, which should be discouraged except for focal disease, such as tumors. Transjugular biopsies often include a portion of the hepatic vein wall (e-Figs. 4.22, 4.23).

REFERENCES

1. Baptista D, Bianchi L, de Groote J, et al. Histopathology of the intrahepatic biliary tree. Liver 1983;3:161–175.
2. Bioulac-Sage P, Lafon ME, Saric J, et al. Nerves and perisinusoidal cells in human liver. J Hepatol 1990;10:105–112.
3. Bismuth H, Houssin D, Castaing D. Major and minor segmentectomies "réglées" in liver surgery. World J Surg 1982;6:10–24.

4. Bouwens L, Wisse E. Pit cells in the liver. Liver 1992;12:3–9.

5. Bronfenmajer S, Schaffner F, Popper H. Fat-storing cells (lipocytes) in human liver. Arch Pathol 1966;82:447–453.

6. Dawson JL, Tan KC. Anatomy of the liver. In: Millward-Sadler GH, Wright R, Arthur MJP, eds. Wright's Liver and Biliary Diseases: Pathophysiology, Diagnosis, and Management, vol. 1, 3rd Ed. London: WB Saunders, 1992:3–11.

7. Desmet VJ. Organization principles. In: Arias IM, Boyer JL, Fausto N, et al., eds. The Liver: Biology and Pathobiology. 3rd Ed. New York: Raven Press, 1994:3–14.

8. Feldmann G. The cytoskeleton of the hepatocyte: structure and functions. J Hepatol 1989;8:380–386.

9. Gumucio JJ. Hepatocyte heterogeneity: the coming of age from the description of a biological curiosity to a partial understanding of its physiological meaning and regulation. Hepatology 1989;9:154–160.

10. Lamers WH, Hilberts A, Furt E, et al. Hepatic enzymic zonation: a reevaluation of the concept of the liver acinus. Hepatology 1989;10:72–76.

11. Martinez-Hernandez A, Amenta PS. The hepatic extracellular matrix. I. Components and distribution in normal liver. Virchows Arch A Pathol Anat Histopathol 1993;423:1–11.

12. Millward-Sadler GH, Jezequel A-M. Normal histology and ultrastructure. In: Millward-Sadler GH, Wright R, Arthur MJP, eds. Wright's Liver and Biliary Diseases: Pathophysiology, Diagnosis, and Management, vol. 1, 3rd Ed. London: WB Saunders, 1992:12–42.

13. Petrovic LM, Burroughs A, Scheuer PJ. Hepatic sinusoidal endothelium: Ulex lectin binding. Histopathology 1989;14:233–243.

14. Popper H. Aging and the liver. In: Popper H, Schaffner F, eds. Progress in Liver Diseases, vol. 8. Orlando: Grune & Stratton, 1986:659–683.

15. Ramadori G. The stellate cell (Ito-cell, fat-storing cell, lipocyte, perisinusoidal cell) of the liver: new insights into pathophysiology of an intriguing cell. Virchows Arch B Cell Pathol 1991;61:147–158.

16. Rappaport AM, Borowy ZJ, Lougheed WM, et al. Subdivision of hexagonal liver lobules into a structural and functional unit. Role in hepatic physiology and pathology. Anat Rec 1954;119:11–34.

17. Rappaport AM. The microcirculatory acinar concept of normal and pathological hepatic structure. Beitrage Pathol 1976;157:215–243.

18. Roskams T, Desmet VJ, Verslype C. Development, structure and function of the liver, In Burt AD, Portmann BC, Ferrell LD, eds. MacSween's Pathology of the Liver. 5th Ed. London: Churchill Livingstone, 2007:1–73.

19. Soyer P. Segmental anatomy of the liver: utility of a nomenclature accepted worldwide. AJR Am J Roentgenol 1993;161:572–573.

20. Suriawinata AA, Thung SN. Liver. In: Mills SE, ed. Histology for Pathologists. 3rd Ed. Philadelphia: Lippincott Williams & Wilkins, 2007;685–703.

21. Watanabe T, Tanaka Y. Age-related alterations in the size of human hepatocytes: a study of mononuclear and binucleate cells. Virchows Arch B Cell Pathol 1982;39:9–20.

5

EXAMINATION OF THE LIVER BIOPSY

Despite great improvements in diagnostic imaging procedures and immuno-logic testing, liver biopsy remains invaluable in establishing diagnoses, in staging, in monitoring the progression of various liver diseases (including chronic hepatitis and primary biliary diseases), and in monitoring the effects of therapy. In liver transplantation patients, day-to-day assessment may be necessary to evaluate immunosuppressive therapy, to detect surgical compli-cations or to identify recurrent disease (3). Similarly, patients with chronic hepatitis due to hepatitis B or hepatitis C virus infection treated with antivi-ral agents should have pretreatment and posttreatment biopsies to docu-ment the initial degree of inflammatory activity and the stage of the disease, as well as to assess the changes that may come with treatment.

TECHNICAL CONSIDERATIONS

Histochemical Stains

Hematoxylin-eosin is the standard stain for the initial study of the liver biopsy. In our practice we routinely prepare two widely separated sec-tions, approximately 100 μm apart, to be stained with hematoxylin-eosin. In addition, a panel of special stains are applied to the interven-ing sections, including Masson trichrome, reticulin silver stain, periodic acid–Schiff (PAS) after digestion with diastase (dPAS), and Perls Prussian blue stain for iron. Reticulin can be useful in separating capsule tissue from cirrhotic septa, with septa rich in reticulin fibers and capsule lacking them, and Victoria blue for screening for hepatitis B surface antigen (HBsAg) and copper-associated protein. Certain modifications and differences in various departments do exist, however. For example, the orcein stain (Shikata) or aldehyde fuchsin (Gomori) may be used instead of Victoria blue. These stains also demonstrate elastic fibers and phagocytosed material; for specific indications, vari-ous immunohistochemical and molecular techniques may have to be applied.

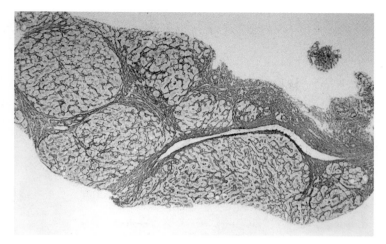

FIGURE 5.1 Extensive bridging fibrosis and developing cirrhosis is highlighted with the reticulin silver stain (original magnification ×100).

Trichrome Stains

For the evaluation of type I collagen, Masson trichrome stain or Mallory chromotrope aniline blue are commonly used. Normal liver shows only a small amount of collagen in portal tracts and a narrow rim of collagen around larger terminal hepatic venules. Trichrome stain is useful for determining the presence of increased amount of collagen, as well as for the determination of the extent of fibrosis. Pericellular fibrosis is also easily seen with trichrome stain. Mallory material and giant mitochondria are also highlighted with this stain (18,19).

Reticulin Silver Impregnation

Type III collagen is highlighted by reticulin silver preparation. Reticulin stain is particularly useful in delineating the liver cell plate structure and in studying the overall architectural pattern of the lobule (acinus). Regeneration with increased thickness of liver cell plates, as well as collapse of the underlying reticulin network in acute hepatic necrosis, is also highlighted with reticulin silver preparation (2,6,15,18) (Figs. 5.1, 5.2).

Periodic Acid–Schiff Reaction

The PAS reaction demonstrates mucopolysaccharides of various kinds, including glycogen. Diastase (PAS/D) removes glycogen from the tissue, allowing for the easier recognition of various mucopolysaccharide compounds. For example, digested material in Kupffer cells is highlighted by PAS; the finding of many PAS-positive Kupffer cells can be the only evidence of a

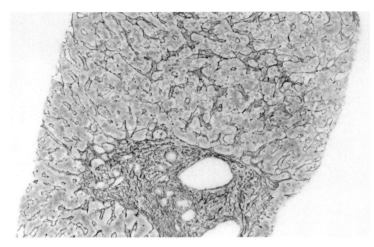

FIGURE 5.2 Thickening of the liver cell plates in liver regeneration (reticulin silver stain, original magnification ×200).

recent, but resolved, hepatitis in which the Kupffer cells contain the partially digested hepatocyte cell membrane remnants (Fig. 5.3). Similarly, portal macrophages will react with this method. In general, PAS without diastase is not useful in studying adult liver diseases.

PAS/D highlights the characteristic globules of α1-antitrypsin deficiency, characteristically found in zone 1 (periportal/periseptal) hepatocytes.

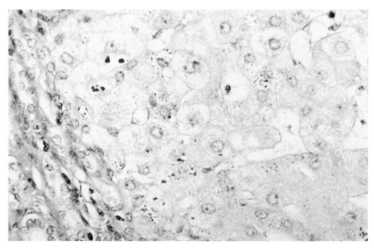

FIGURE 5.3 Intracellular globules in α1-antitrypsin deficiency. **A.** Periodic acid–Schiff (PAS) after digestion with diastase (dPAS, original magnification ×400). **B.** Immunohistochemical reaction for α1-antitrypsin (avidin-biotin-peroxidase immunoperoxidase, original magnification ×200).

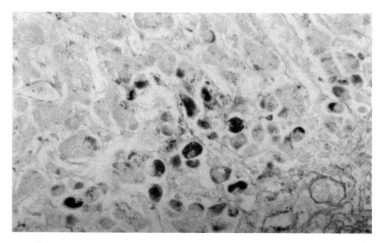

FIGURE 5.4   Hepatocytes containing intracytoplasmic hepatitis **B** surface antigen are stained blue with Victoria blue (original magnification ×200).

They have a striking fuchsia color (Fig. 5.3), and their presence can be confirmed with monoclonal antibody.

In pediatric pathology, PAS and PASD are helpful in excluding various metabolic diseases, such as glycogenosis IV. Abnormal amylopectin-like glycogen in glycogenosis IV is only partially digested with diastase, and the finding of intense reactivity with PAS and partial and irregular reactivity after diastase digestion is virtually diagnostic. PAS is also helpful in evaluating bile duct basement membrane, especially in destructive biliary diseases, such as primary biliary cirrhosis. In contrast, there is generally no destruction of the basement membrane in primary sclerosing cholangitis.

Victoria Blue

Victoria blue stain is used to screen for HBsAg (Fig. 5.4) and also demonstrates copper-associated protein and elastic fibers. Elastic fibers are present in a cirrhotic septa but not in scars. As another example, collapsed liver parenchyma does not have elastic fibers. The rare developmental disorder termed congenital hepatic fibrosis looks like cirrhosis in biopsy but also lacks elastic fibers. Victoria blue, orcein (Shikata), and Gomori aldehyde fuchsin are equivalent. With orcein, reaction products are brown-black rather than blue, and with aldehyde fuchsin they are fuchsia-purple.

Hemosiderin

Perls stain is used to detect stainable tissue hemosiderin. Semiquantitative analysis can be virtually diagnostic. When the amount of hemosiderin suggests genetic hemochromatosis, quantitative iron analysis and histologic iron index may be needed (see Chapter 15).

Copper

Rhodanine and rubeanic acid are special stains commonly applied in those cases where the accumulation of copper and copper-associated protein is suspected, including Wilson disease and chronic cholestasis. A modification of the rubeanic acid method allows for same-day staining (4). However, these stains are not especially sensitive, and copper assay of hepatic tissue is the standard for establishing the diagnosis of Wilson disease (see Chapter 16).

IMMUNOHISTOCHEMICAL STAINS AND MOLECULAR BIOLOGY

Identification of Viral Material in Tissue

HEPATITIS B. Immunoperoxidase methods using antibodies to both HBsAg and hepatitis B core antigen (HBcAg) are readily available. HBsAg may be present diffusely or focally in the cytoplasm and sometimes may also have membranous expression. HBcAg is expressed in the liver cell nuclei in most cases, but both intranuclear and granular intracytoplasmic expression may be simultaneously present, especially with high levels of viral replication (Fig. 5.5).

The most reliable and highly specific method to demonstrate hepatitis B virus DNA is the polymerase chain reaction (PCR). Patients with hepatitis B virus infection may also be infected with D or delta virus, in the form of superinfection or coinfection. The viral antigen can also be immunohistochemically detected in the tissue and has intranuclear expression very similar to that of HBcAg (18).

HEPATITIS C. There is no reliable immunohistochemical method to demonstrate hepatitis C virus in formalin-fixed paraffin-embedded tissue. A commercially available antibody that gives consistent results in paraffin-embedded tissue, rather than frozen section material, is not available (Fig. 5.6). Hepatitis C virus antigen can be demonstrated in cryostat-prepared sections, but the antibody for this is not widely available. In situ hybridization is useful for detection of replicating and nonreplicating viral proteins. PCR in tissue samples, reverse transcriptase PCR (RT-PCR), and RT-PCR in situ can all be used for the detection of hepatitis C virus RNA, but these techniques are used selectively (12,17).

CYTOKERATINS. Immunohistochemical reactions for low molecular weight (CAM 5.2) and high molecular weight (AE 1/3) keratins are useful in the evaluation of bile ducts and ductules in various conditions, including cholangiopathies and congenital or acquired bile duct paucity, as well as in demonstrating chronic (ductopenic) rejection (Fig. 5. 7). The expression of some cytokeratins, particularly CAM 5.2, may be helpful in evaluating liver tumors (8,9,20).

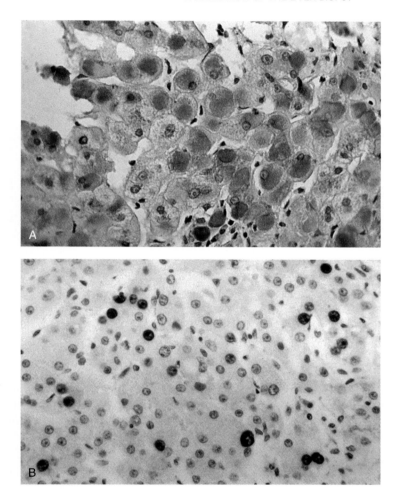

FIGURE 5.5 Immunohistochemical reactions for **A** hepatitis B surface antigen and **B** hepatitis B core antigen; respective intracytoplasmic and intranuclear expression is present (avidin-biotin- peroxidase immunoperoxidase, original magnification ×200).

One of the newer markers that is helpful in differentiating hepatocellular carcinoma and cholangiocarcinoma or metastatic adenocarcinoma is a hepatocyte monoclonal antibody (Hep, Hepar 1) (15).

Immunofluorescent Studies

Immunofluorescent studies requiring frozen material are only rarely needed for diagnostic purposes. When humoral allograft rejection is suspected, immunofluorescent analysis is needed to demonstrate tissue deposition of immunoglobulin G (IgG), IgA, IgM, C3, and C1q components of complement, as well as fibrinogen. Fibrinogen deposition is also present in

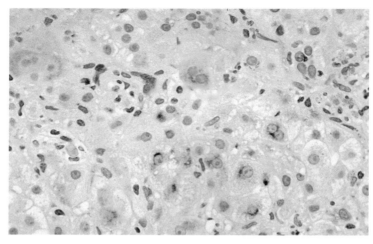

FIGURE 5.6   Immunohistochemical reaction for hepatitis C viral (envelope NS4) antigen. Intracytoplasmic expression is seen (avidin-biotin-peroxidase immunoperoxidase, original magnification ×400).

cases of eclampsia (Fig. 5.8), preeclampsia, and HELLP (hemolysis, elevated liver function, and low platelets) syndrome.

Molecular Pathology

Molecular techniques can demonstrate the causative agent in many viral infections. In situ hybridization is particularly sensitive for the demonstration of cytomegalovirus. The Epstein–Barr virus–associated EBER-1 gene can also

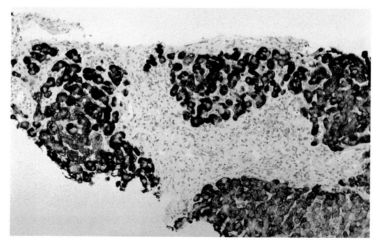

FIGURE 5.7   Almost complete absence of interlobular bile ducts in this example of ductopenic rejection. Immunoperoxidase method for mixed keratins (AE 1/3 original magnification ×200).

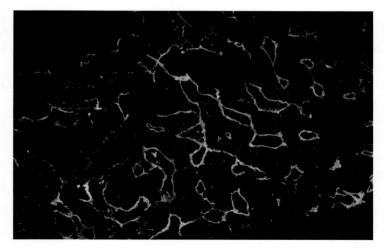

FIGURE 5.8 Perisinusoidal fibrinogen deposition in a case of eclampsia (immunofluorescent method, original magnification ×400). (See Color Figure 5.11 following page 46.)

be demonstrated in patients with posttransplantation lymphoproliferative disorder (16).

Electron Microscopy

Ultrastructural examination is rarely needed in the study of adult liver biopsies. Ultrastructural studies are particularly helpful for metabolic disorders (e.g., in glycogenosis IV (Fig. 5.9)).

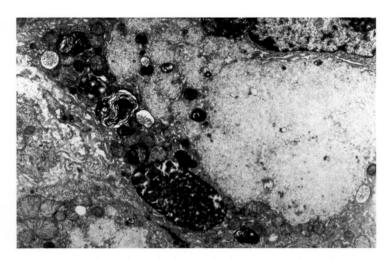

FIGURE 5.9 Non-membrane-bound abnormal glycogen (amylopectin) in a case of glycogenosis IV (electron microscopy, original magnification ×10,000).

TABLE 5.1	Histopathologic Considerations in Evaluation and Interpretation of the Liver Biopsy

1. Type of biopsy
   Needle (core): percutaneous, ultrasound or computed tomography–guided
   Transjugular
   Wedge
   Resection
2. Size of the biopsy
3. Adequacy of the sample (14–16 gauge, 2.5 cm, >10 portal tracts)
   Possible artifacts
4. Site of the biopsy (subcapsular, deep parenchyma, perihilar)
5. Overall architecture
   Retained
   Partially or completely distorted
6. Portal tracts
   Normal (normal structures present)
   Inflammation (type, extent, interface hepatitis)
   Edema
   Fibrosis (extent, pattern)
   Bile duct (type of injury, inflammation, loss, bile ductular proliferation)
   Vascular structures (inflammation, thrombosis)
7. Lobules (acinar changes)
   Degenerative and regenerative changes
   Inflammation (type, extent, zonal distribution)
   Necrosis (type, zonal distribution, extent)
   Sinusoids (inflammation, dilatation, deposits)
8. Central vein (terminal hepatic venule)
   Size
   Inflammation
   Fibrosis

New techniques, including computer-assisted morphometry, flow cytometry, static cytometry image analysis, and neural network analysis can be performed on either fixed or unfixed liver tissue. However, these methods are not widely available and are usually applied for research purposes (1,5,7,13).

TABLE 5.2	Key Clinical Information for Liver Biopsy Evaluation

1. Age, Sex
2. Immunocompetent or immunocompromised patient (status posttransplantation, AIDS)
3. Viral serologies (hepatitis A, B, C, D, E, G)
4. Relevant chemical values
5. Autoantibodies (AMA, ANA, SMA, LKM)
6. Platelet count (usually decreased in cirrhosis)
7. Duration of symptoms and relevant laboratory findings
8. Medications (recent or other longstanding)
9. Other treatment (total parenteral nutrition, hemodialysis, immunosuppressive agents, radiotherapy)
10. Imaging studies

AMA, antimitochondrial antibody; *ANA*, antinuclear antibody; *SMA*, smooth muscle antibody; *LKM*, liver-kidney microsomal (antibody).

GENERAL APPROACH TO THE LIVER BIOPSY

A systematic approach to the evaluation of the liver biopsy is vital to ensure that important diagnostic findings are not overlooked. The topographic and biologic relationships of morphologic changes generally provide correct and clinically meaningful diagnoses.

We initially evaluate the liver biopsy without clinical information and subsequently correlate morphologic findings with clinical data. Once the general diagnosis or at least the differential diagnosis has been reached, clinical information is vital. For example, diagnosis may require knowledge of viral serologies, autoantibodies, medications, and imaging studies. Features to be assessed on the liver biopsy are summarized in Table 5.1, and the clinical information that may be useful in liver biopsy interpretation is summarized in Table 5.2. We use a worksheet (Fig. 5.10 for nontumor cases.

Our approach is to, in effect, follow the blood flow. We begin with the portal tract and its component structures, then study the lobular including the limiting plate of hepatocytes, and complete our examination at the terminal hepatic venule (central vein).

Subcapsular liver biopsies, both needle and wedge, may be misleading and exhibit changes not present in the remainder of the parenchyma (9,13). This is particularly important in cases of chronic hepatitis, in which a subcapsular biopsy can be misinterpreted as showing cirrhosis (Fig. 5.11 The subcapsular region is also a common site for bile duct hamartomas

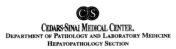

CEDARS-SINAI MEDICAL CENTER.
DEPARTMENT OF PATHOLOGY AND LABORATORY MEDICINE
HEPATOPATHOLOGY SECTION

LIVER BIOPSY WORK SHEET

S-0 _____ - _____

Study biopsy before reviewing history, and then again after

Liver tests:

ALT		Bilirubin T/D	
AST		Albumin	
AlkPh		ProTime / INR	
GGT		Platelets	

Other tests, if indicated (e.g. γ globulin, ferritin, 24-hr Cu, etc):

History:

Clinical Dx:

Microscopic findings:

Biopsy adequate _____ Biopsy suboptimal _____

Diagnosis:

Form No. 9182 (Rev. 6/13/07)

FIGURE 5.10 Worksheet used to record clinically relevant data and other information in the review of liver biopsies with inflammatory changes.

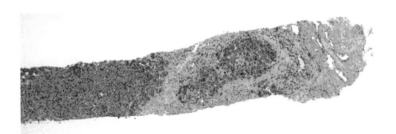

FIGURE 5.11 Subcapsular liver parenchyma showing fibrosis and mild chronic inflammation, imparting a pseudonodule appearance. The findings were present only in this region. The remainder of the liver parenchyma is unremarkable (trichrome, original magnification ×100).

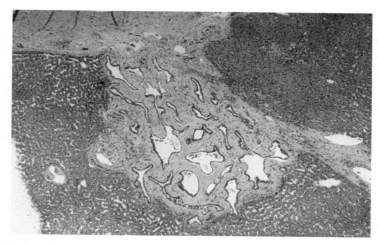

FIGURE 5.12 Subcapsular von Meyenburg complex. Irregular bile duct–like structures are in a fibrous background (hematoxylin-eosin, original magnification ×200).

(von Meyenburg complex), bile duct adenomas, and peribiliary gland hamartomas (Fig. 5.12). These benign lesions may be misinterpreted as metastatic adenocarcinoma, especially with frozen section examination (Fig. 5.13).

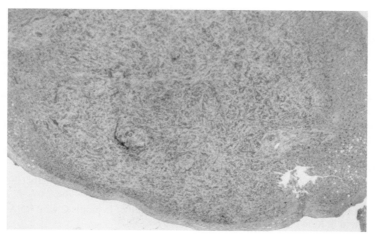

FIGURE 5.13 Intraoperative consultation (frozen section) histology section showing subcapsular peribiliary gland hamartoma (hematoxylin-eosin, original magnification ×200).

REFERENCES

1. An C, Petrovic LM, Reyter I, et al. The application of image analysis and neural network technology to the study of premalignant and malignant liver lesions. Hepatology 1997;26: 1224–1231.
2. Bianchi L. Liver biopsy interpretation in hepatitis. I. Presentation of critical morphological features used in diagnosis (glossary). Pathol Res Pract 1983;178:2–19.
3. Demetris AJ, Belle SH, Hart J, et al. Intraobserver and interobserver variation in the histopathological assessment of liver allograft rejection. Hepatology 1991;14:751–755.
4. Emanuele P, Goodman FD. A simple and rapid stain for copper in liver tissue. Ann Diagn Pathol 1998;2:125–126.
5. Erler BS, Hsu L, Truong HM, et al. Image analysis and diagnostic classification of hepatocellular carcinoma using neural networks and multivariate discriminant functions. Lab Invest 1994;71:446–451.
6. Gerber MA, Thung SN. Histology of the liver. Am J Surg Pathol 1987;11:709–722.
7. Hata K, Van Thiel DH, Herberman RB, et al. Phenotypic and functional characteristics of lymphocytes isolated from liver biopsy specimens from patients with active liver disease. Hepatology 1992;15:816–823.
8. Lau SK, Prakash S, Geller SA, Alsabeh R. Comparative immunohistochemical profile of hepatocellular carcinoma, cholangiocarcinoma and metastatic adenocarcinoma. Hum Pathol 2002;33:1175–1181.
9. Maharaj B, Maharaj RJ, Leary WP, et al. Sampling variability and its influence on the diagnostic yield of percutaneous needle biopsy of the liver. Lancet 1986;1:523–525.
10. McAffee JH, Keeffe EB, Lee RG, et al. Transjugular liver biopsy. Hepatology 1992;15: 726–732.
11. Nuovo GJ, Lidonnici K, McConnell P, et al. Intracellular localization of polymerase chain reaction (PCR)–amplified hepatitis C cDNA. Am J Surg Pathol 1993;17:683–690.
12. Orsatti G, Thiese ND, Thung SN, et al. DNA image cytometric analysis of macroregenerative nodules (adenomatous hyperplasia) of the liver: evidence in support of their preneoplastic nature. Hepatology 1993;17:621–627.
13. Petrelli M, Scheuer PJ. Variation in subcapsular liver structure and its significance in the interpretation of wedge biopsies. J Clin Pathol 1967;20:743–748.
14. Petrovic LM. Benign hepatocellular tumors and tumor-like lesions. In: Ferrell LD, ed. Diagnostic Problems in Liver Pathology. London: Hanley and Belfus, 1994.
15. Randhawa PS, Jaffe R, Demetris AJ, et al. Expression of Epstein–Barr virus–encoded small RNA (by the EBER-1 gene) in liver specimens from transplant recipients with post-transplantation lymphoproliferative disease. N Engl J Med 1992;327:1710–1714.
16. Savage K, Dhillon AP, Brown D, et al. HCV by PCR of liver in autoimmune hepatitis. Hepatology 1992;16:590.
17. Scheuer PJ. General considerations. In: Scheuer PJ, Lefkowitch JH, eds. Liver Biopsy Interpretation. 5th Ed. London: WB Saunders, 1994:1–10.
18. Snover DC. Technical aspects of the evaluation of liver biopsies. In: Snover, ed. Biopsy Diagnosis of Liver Disease. Baltimore: Williams & Wilkins, 1992:2–23.
19. Van Eyken P, Sciot R, Paterson A, et al. Cytokeratin expression in hepatocellular carcinoma: an immunohistochemical study. Hum Pathol 1988;19:562–568.
20. Yamada G, Nishimoto H, Endou H, et al. Localization of hepatitis C viral RNA and capsid protein in human liver. Dig Dis Sci 1993;38:882–887.

6

EMBRYOLOGY AND DEVELOPMENTAL CONSIDERATIONS

Embryologic issues arise relatively rarely in the interpretation of the liver biopsy. However, problems relating to prenatally acquired conditions, unrelated to disorders of embryogenesis, are not uncommon.

Anomalies of the liver manifest principally in terms of liver shape and position, as well as vascular variations (12,20). Although ectopia of the entire liver is exceedingly rare, liver tissue may be found in various places throughout the abdomen and even in the lung (25). The biliary tree is the principal site of abnormality in association with documented chromosomal disorders (12).

DEVELOPMENT OF THE LIVER AND INTRAHEPATIC BILIARY STRUCTURES

Parenchymal Development

Development of the human liver and biliary tract begins as a hepatic anlage at the 18th day of gestation, when the embryo is 2.5 mm in length (9), becoming more prominent in the third to fourth week as the hepatic diverticulum from the ventral distal foregut (12,26,29). The cephalic portion (pars hepatica) differentiates to become the liver, and the caudal portion (pars cystica) matures into the gallbladder and cystic duct.

The septum transversum mesenchymal cells form the connective tissue elements of the hepatic stroma, as well as the capsule (e-Figs. 6.1, 6.2). Near the end of the fourth week, the hepatic diverticulum acquires a T shape, creating the early right and left liver lobes (9). The mesodermal cells also form endothelial-lined spaces.

Initially, the liver plates are three to five cells thick. These decrease to two-cell-thick plates at the time of birth. After the fifth year of life, the normal plates are one cell thick. At 3 months, bile formation begins. The canaliculus appears in the 10-mm embryo as a differentiated zone of the intercellular surface of the liver and has its typical appearance by 7 to

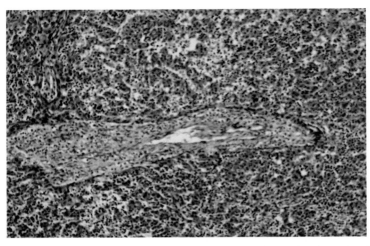

FIGURE 6.1 Image of developing liver showing ductal plate formation (hematoxylin-eosin, original magnification ×200).

8 weeks. Selected mitochondrial, microsomal, and lysosomal enzymes are demonstrable in liver cells by the eighth week.

Primitive hepatocytes express cytokeratins 8, 18, and 19 (40,41). It has been suggested that these cells, precursors to the mature hepatocytes, give rise to the intrahepatic biliary system (11,33,34). Intrahepatic bile ducts develop progressively from the hilum, beginning at the eighth week. Portal vein extensions push into the primitive parenchyma, and the septum transversum mesenchyme induces the transformation of embryonic hepatocytes into ductal cells (12,15,23,35,36). The epithelial cells first transform into single- and then double-cell layered tubular structures, the so-called ductal plate (Fig. 6.1, e-Figs. 6.3–6.6) (8,10,35,36). At 5 to 6 weeks gestational age, a lumen forms between the two layers of the ductal plate, with the formation of true duct structures. These grow into the mesenchyme and further transform to become bile ducts. Cytokeratins, as well as the adhesion glycoprotein laminin, are thought to play a key role in this process (35–37,41). Progenitor cells have the potential for expressing multiple cytokeratins (37). The periportal mesenchymal sheath diminishes, and the newly formed ducts are incorporated into the portal tracts. Eventually, an arterial plexus envelops the ducts. True interlobular ducts are rare at 13 weeks but develop throughout gestation and even during the neonatal period (29). Ductal plate structures may persist, even at 40 weeks' gestation, and in some portal tracts there may not be an individual mature bile duct accompanying the most peripheral portal vein branches (9,10,41). Instead, the portal veins may be surrounded by a layer of cytokeratin-rich cells in ductal plate arrangement.

Vascular Development

During the fifth week, the paired vitelline veins penetrate the primitive hepatic cords to form primitive sinusoids. The hepatic veins form from modifications of the vitelline veins. The portal vein results from multiple anastomoses between the caudal left and right vitelline veins. Some of the channels eventually atrophy, contributing to the tortuosity of the portal vein.

The ductus venosus forms as an enlargement of the sinusoids. The ductus is a potential conduit to the hepatic vein and inferior vena cava; since its diameter is less than 15% that of the umbilical vein, however, most of the blood flow is diverted through the liver parenchyma (14). A sinus intermedius connects the lobes, but the most highly oxygenated umbilical blood preferentially perfuses the left lobe.

Hepatic artery and portal vein development proceed from the hepatic hilum to the periphery. Portal vein extensions, with their accompanying cuff of mesenchyme within which bile ducts form, permeate the parenchyma. Arterial twigs become abundant by the last trimester (29).

Intrahepatic Hematopoiesis

Hematopoietic cells first appear in the fifth week, reaching a peak during the third month. The peak of hematopoietic activity is during the third month, diminishing progressively during the last trimester. In the normal infant, there is virtually no hematopoiesis by age 7 days (12).

Lymphocytes appear in the liver by 6 or 7 weeks' gestation and, after the 20th week, account for more than 20% of mononuclear cells (17).

Iron, demonstrable as hemosiderin, is seen in the fetal liver in both ductal plate cells and the developing limiting plate; the amount varies considerably throughout gestation, increasing as hematopoiesis progressively decreases and reaching peak concentrations at the end of gestation (9,28). Copper and zinc are also stored in these cells (13).

ABNORMALITIES OF THE BILE DUCT SYSTEM

Ductal Plate Malformation

Ductal plate malformations are defects of the portal tract and its component structures, especially the bile duct system, arising during the formation and modification of the ductal plate. Failure of remodeling results in persistence of the embryologic ductal plate, the "ductal plate malformation." This may appear in a biopsy as a ring of bile duct–like structures arrayed circumferentially at the periphery of the portal tract, generally with a central portal vein or groups of veins (Fig. 6.2, e-Fig. 6.7). The ring may be complete or incomplete (10). Typically, excess of mesenchymal tissue and ectasia of ducts is seen.

Conditions thought to be associated with ductal plate malformation are congenital hepatic fibrosis (Fig. 6.3, e-Figs. 6.8–6.13), bile duct hamartomas

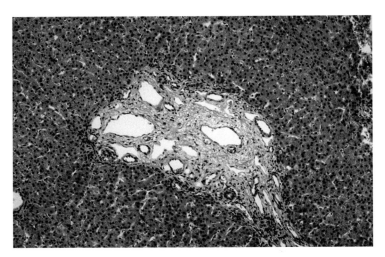

FIGURE 6.2   Image of a liver biopsy from an adult with ductal plate malformation, showing peripherally arranged bile ducts and splayed portal vein segments ("pollard-tree" pattern). (hematoxylin-eosin, original magnification ×200)

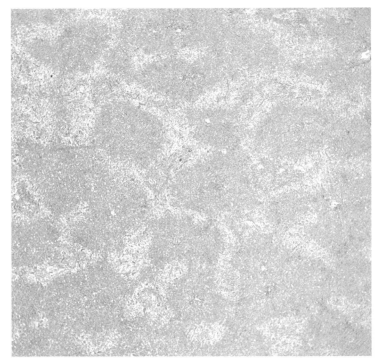

FIGURE 6.3   Image of congenital hepatic fibrosis, diffuse form, from a child with portal hypertension, showing portal tracts with increased numbers of abnormally developed bile ducts, with fibrosis within portal tracts and also linking portal tracts (hematoxylin-eosin, original magnification ×40).

(von Meyenburg complexes) (e-Figs. 6.14–6.17), Caroli disease (e-Fig. 6.18), and Caroli syndrome, infantile polycystic disease, Meckel-Gruber syndrome, renal-hepatic-pancreatic dysplasia (Ivemark syndrome), and Beckwith-Wiedemann syndrome (7,10,12). Ductal plate and renal tubular differentiation share genetic determinants, and single-gene defects can give rise to such varied entities as congenital hepatic fibrosis, Caroli disease and syndrome, and autosomal recessive and autosomal dominant polycystic kidney disease (7).

Recognition of these entities is important because their presence in liver biopsy specimens can be misinterpreted as metastatic, well-differentiated, desmoplastic adenocarcinoma.

Congenital Hepatic Fibrosis

Congenital hepatic fibrosis was originally described in association with autosomal recessive polycystic kidney disease but can occur as an isolated entity (Fig. 6.3, e-Figs. 6.8–6.13). Patients usually have hepatosplenomegaly and portal hypertension, but there are four patterns of expression: (a) portal hypertension, (b) cholangitis without portal hypertension, (c) cholangitis and portal hypertension, and (d) latent cholangitis, generally discovered incidentally either during an unrelated surgical procedure or at autopsy. Symptoms of cholangitis are due to associated Caroli disease.

Microscopically, the picture can be variable (7,10). In the focal form, abnormally formed bile ducts are in irregularly shaped portal tracts with prominent fibrous tissue. The bile ducts can be multiple and appear branching or stellate. In the diffuse form the portal tracts are linked by fibrosis (Fig. 6.4). In both forms, ductal plate malformation is seen at the portal tract periphery. Inflammation is generally mild. Portal veins may appear hypoplastic, but arterioles are prominent. Degeneration of the biliary duct epithelium and mild cholestasis can also be seen. Congenital hepatic fibrosis can be limited to one lobe (19). The intervening hepatic parenchyma and the terminal hepatic venule are unremarkable.

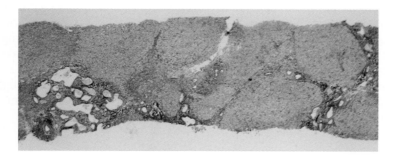

FIGURE 6.4 Image of congenital hepatic fibrosis, incomplete form, from an adult, also with a bile duct hamartoma (von Meyenburg complex) (trichrome, original magnification ×100).

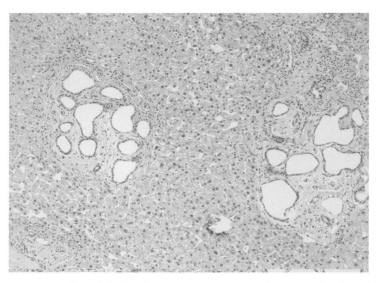

FIGURE 6.5 Image of two bile duct hamartomas (von Meyenburg complex) found inciden-tally in a liver biopsy obtained from a patient with chronic hepatitis. There are irregularly dilated bile ducts surrounded by dense fibrous tissue (hematoxylin-eosin, original magnifi-cation ×200).

The biopsy features suggesting the diagnosis are as follows: (a) fibrotic portal tracts containing few or no inflammatory cells; (b) increased numbers of prominent, often focally ectatic, bile ducts; (c) multiple small portal vein trib-utaries; (d) prominent arterioles; and (e) conspicuous, often irregularly ectatic, ductulelike structures encircling the portal tract. Other ductal plate malforma-tion changes, such as bile duct hamartoma (Fig. 6.5) can also be seen.

Bile Duct Hamartoma (von Meyenburg Complex)

The small, benign lesions of bile duct hamartoma, often visible grossly as tiny white liver nodules, are composed of groups of dilated bile ducts embedded in connective tissue (Figs. 6.4, 6.5, e-Figs. 6.14–6.17). The ducts may contain polypoid epithelial projections. Bile duct hamartomas are most often seen in the otherwise unremarkable liver but may be associated with congenital hepatic fibrosis and Caroli disease. They may be single or multiple, and sometimes are immediately adjacent to a normal portal tract. The pattern of ductal plate malformation is seen only rarely. The ectatic ducts may contain bile or even small calculi (30). Recent evidence suggests that bile duct hamartomas communicate with the bile duct system (11). Cholangiocarcinoma may rarely arise (5).

Caroli Disease and Caroli Syndrome

The Caroli lesion is characterized by congenital dilatation, fusiform or sac-cular, of the larger intrahepatic bile ducts, generally at multiple sites. The ducts maintain continuity with the biliary tree. Caroli disease is not associated with other histologic abnormalities. In Caroli syndrome, the changes of congenital hepatic fibrosis are also seen. Caroli syndrome is significantly more common than Caroli disease.

Caroli disease is thought to be caused by ductal plate malformation affecting the large bile ducts (e-Fig. 6.18), whereas Caroli syndrome occurs when the entire bile duct system is affected. Patients with Caroli disease most often have repeated attacks of cholangitis, often complicated by the development of calculi and by abscess formation and sepsis. Cholangiocarcinoma may ensue (38). The liver biopsy may be normal or may show the changes of an ascending cholangitis.

In Caroli syndrome with congenital hepatic fibrosis, the cholangitic episodes are often accompanied by portal hypertension. The liver biopsy may appear normal, may show cholangitic changes, or may show the typical changes of congenital hepatic fibrosis.

Caroli disease and Caroli syndrome may be associated with autosomal recessive polycystic kidney disease and choledochal cysts.

Biliary Atresia

The biliary atresias have generally been considered to be related development disorders since they may occur together. It may be that isolated extrahepatic biliary atresia is an acquired disease, perhaps caused by intrauterine infection (27).

In contrast, isolated intrahepatic biliary atresia is most likely truly developmental, caused by a primary defect in the bile secretory mechanism at the level of hepatocyte with secondary loss of bile ducts (8,39). Indeed, in Zellweger (cerebrohepatorenal) syndrome, a peroxisomal disorder results in abnormal bile acid metabolism and may also be associated with the histologic picture of intrahepatic biliary atresia (8).

EXTRAHEPATIC BILIARY ATRESIA. Extrahepatic biliary atresia (EHBA) occurs in approximately 1 in 10,000 births and is more common in females than in males (9). Clinical manifestations include jaundice persisting beyond the physiologic period, acholic stools, and hepatomegaly. EHBA may occur with other disorders, such as galactosemia, α1-antitrypsin deficiency, and small bowel atresia, and with several malformations. The polysplenia syndrome occurs in 11% of patients with EHBA. Differentiation from other forms of neonatal cholestasis may be difficult (2,3). Imaging studies or direct examination of biliary structures establishes the diagnosis.

In type I EHBA, the common bile duct is affected while the cystic duct and hepatic ducts remain patent. In type IIa, the common hepatic duct is obliterated, but the cystic duct and common bile duct are unaltered. In type IIb, the cystic duct, common hepatic duct, and common bile duct are all affected, but the gallbladder is unremarkable and, typically, the hepatic ducts at the hilum are cystically dilated. In type III (uncorrectable) extrahepatic biliary atresia, there is absence or atresia of the common, hepatic and cystic ducts, and the hilar ducts are not cystically dilated, making anastomosis to the small intestine impossible. Liver biopsy can be helpful.

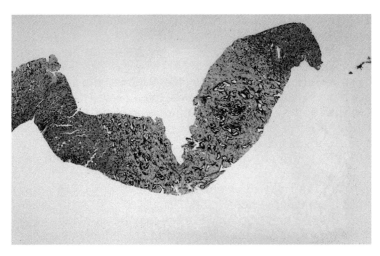

FIGURE 6.6   Image of early stage of extrahepatic biliary atresia, showing spherical enlargement of the portal tract, caused by edema and dilatation of lymphatic channels, with ductular proliferation at the periphery of the portal tract (hematoxylin-eosin, original magnification ×200).

During the stage of ductular reaction, the portal tract shows typical changes of extrahepatic biliary obstruction, with edema and dilatation of lymphatic channels contributing to the characteristic rounding of the portal tracts (Fig. 6.6), and with ductular proliferation at the periphery of the portal tract. Inflammation involving polymorphonuclear leukocytes as well as lymphocytes follows. A stage of portal bile duct destruction follows, with epithelial cell vacuolization, necrosis, atrophy, and changes of repair, along with interruption of basement membrane and permeation by inflammatory cells. This characteristic stage generally occurs after 6 weeks, but its time of onset is highly variable.

Prior to the stage of ductular reaction, the biopsy shows hepatocytic and canalicular bile stasis, with little or no inflammation and only rare necrotic hepatocytes. Extramedullary hematopoiesis may persist. A few hydropic hepatocytes may be seen, and there may be scattered multinucleated giant cells.

During the stage of ductular reaction, the parenchymal changes may be dominant, with extensive hepatocyte necrosis and florid giant cell transformation of hepatocytes, suggesting the diagnosis of neonatal giant cell hepatitis (Fig. 6.7).

Portal and periportal fibrosis develops, with fibrous septa irregularly dissecting through the liver. Portal inflammatory changes diminish at this stage, but bile plugs become more prominent and there are more extensive changes secondary to the accumulation of bile, with feathery degeneration (cholestasis) of hepatocytes, frank necrosis, and small bile lakes. Dilated ductules contain bile concretions. Periductal fibrosis may be concentric, resembling that seen in primary sclerosing cholangitis. In the third month, fibrosis links portal tract to portal tract, and portal hypertension may

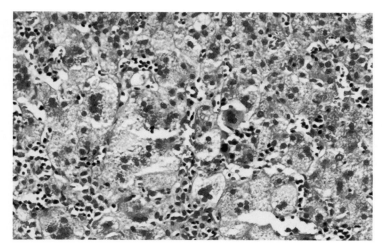

FIGURE 6.7   Image of stage of ductular reaction of extrahepatic biliary atresia, with marked cholestasis and florid giant cell formation suggesting the diagnosis of giant cell hepatitis (hematoxylin-eosin, original magnification ×200).

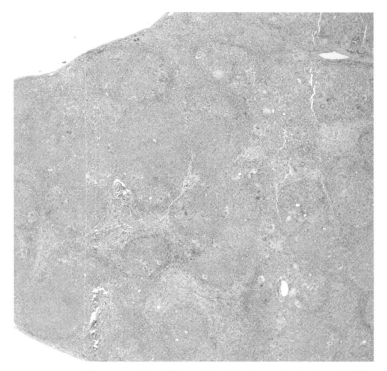

FIGURE 6.8   Image of the (secondary biliary) cirrhotic stage of extrahepatic biliary atresia, showing fibrous septa connecting portal areas, with changes of chronic cholestasis, including cholate stasis of zone 1 hepatocytes imparting the appearance of marked cell swelling (hematoxylin-eosin, original magnification ×40).

TABLE 6.1	Histopathology of Extrahepatic Biliary Atresia

Prediagnostic stage
    Hepatocytic and canalicular cholestasis
    Rare hydropic hepatocytes
Early stage (stage of ductular reaction)
    Progressively severe cholestasis
        Extensive hepatocyte necrosis
        Extensive giant cell transformation
    Portal edema
    Portal lymphatic ectasia
    Ductular proliferation
    Portal inflammation
        Acute and chronic inflammatory cells
        Bile duct destruction
Precirrhotic stage
    Progressive portal and periportal fibrosis
        May have concentric periductal fibrosis
    Diminishing portal inflammation
    Increasingly severe cholestasis
        Bile plugs increasingly prominent
        Hepatocytic cholate stasis (feathery degeneration)
        Hepatocyte necrosis
        Small bile lakes
Secondary biliary cirrhosis

ensue, although there are not yet regenerative changes of hepatocytes with formation of nodules and the full clinical picture of cirrhosis may not be seen. After 12 weeks, the fibrosis is accompanied by regeneration and typical secondary biliary cirrhosis is seen (Fig. 6.8). Bile ducts may be partially or completely obliterated. In as many as 25% of cases, the liver biopsy shows the pattern of ductal plate malformation (31).

The stages of evolution of fully developed secondary biliary cirrhosis as a sequel to extrahepatic biliary atresia are summarized in Table 6.1.

INTRAHEPATIC BILIARY ATRESIA (PAUCITY OF INTERLOBULAR BILE DUCTS). Paucity of interlobular bile ducts may be associated with extrahepatic anomalies ("syndromatic") or may be isolated ("nonsyndromatic").

Syndromatic paucity (e-Figs. 6.17–6.29) was first described by Alagille as a disorder morphologically distinct from other causes of cholestasis in infancy and childhood (1). Alagille syndrome, or arteriohepatic dysplasia, is the most common form of familial intrahepatic cholestasis. Cholestasis is severe in infancy and childhood but improves, and potentially even resolves, with age. Cirrhosis is uncommon. Extrahepatic anomalies can be seen, including pulmonary artery stenosis or hypoplasia, thickening of the junction of Descemet membrane with the endothelium of the anterior chamber of the eye (posterior embryotoxon), and abnormalities of vertebral bodies. Skeletal abnormalities can be seen. There may be a characteristic facies (1,3,4). A chromosomal anomaly, del(20p), has been demonstrated in some patients (6). There may be growth retardation and/or mental retardation, as well as impaired sexual development (3).

Nonsyndromatic paucity of interlobular bile ducts (e-Fig. 6.3) is less common than the syndromatic variant and is a heterogeneous group of disorders. There may be associated congenital rubella, α1-antitrypsin deficiency, Turner syndrome, Down syndrome, trisomy 17-18, congenital syphilis, and familial trihydroxycoprostanic acid excess. Cirrhosis develops in as many as 50% of patients. A variant in adults is termed idiopathic adulthood ductopenia (16).

Histologic diagnosis requires biopsy sufficiently large to contain at least five complete portal tracts (3,24). Immunohistochemical methods to stain high molecular weight keratins facilitate visualization of interlobular bile ducts (40) (Fig. 6.9). In normal newborns, the ratio of interlobular ducts to the number of portal tracts is between 0.9 and 1.8, although a ratio less than 0.9 may be seen in premature newborns when the liver biopsy is performed before the 38th week of gestation (22). The diagnosis of paucity is established when the ratio is less than 0.5 (3). Portal tracts generally appear somewhat hypoplastic, and the total number may be reduced (18). Cholestasis is

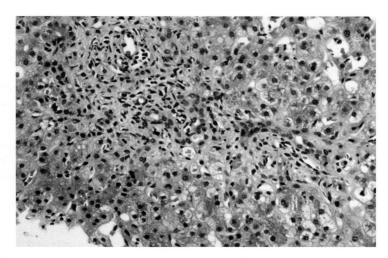

FIGURE 6.9 Image of a liver biopsy from a patient with paucity of interlobular bile ducts, showing adjacent portal tracts lacking bile ducts, with peripheral ductal reaction (proliferation). (hematoxylin-eosin, original magnification ×200).

hepatocellular rather than canalicular. Portal and perisinusoidal fibrosis may be apparent (21). Changes generally occur after infancy. Inflammatory destruction of bile ducts is observed more often in the nonsyndromatic variant. Extrahepatic bile ducts are patent but may be hypoplastic. Endoscopic retrograde cholangiography can demonstrate focal dilatation of segments of the biliary tree, resembling primary sclerosing cholangitis.

COMBINED EXTRAHEPATIC AND INTRAHEPATIC BILE DUCT ATRESIA. Cases demonstrating features of both extrahepatic biliary atresia and paucity of interlobular bile ducts have been described (32,41), rarely associated with ductal plate malformation (31). In most infants with extrahepatic biliary atresia, however, the intrahepatic changes may be secondary because of the obstruction of bile outflow.

REFERENCES

1. Alagille D, Odièvre M, Gautier M, et al. Hepatic ductular hypoplasia associated with characteristic facies, vertebral malformations, retarded physical, mental and sexual development and cardiac murmur. J Pediatr 1975;86:63–71.
2. Alagille D. Cholestasis in the first three months of life. In: Popper H, Schaffner F, eds. Progress in Liver Diseases, vol. 6. New York: Grune & Stratton, 1979:471–485.
3. Alagille D, Odievre M. Liver and Biliary Tract Disease in Children. New York: John Wiley and Sons, 1979:68–93.
4. Alagille D, Estrada A, Hadchouel M, et al. Syndromatic paucity of interlobular bile ducts (Alagille syndrome or arteriohepatic dysplasia): review of 80 cases. J Pediatr 1987;110:195–200.
5. Burns C, Kuhns JG, Wieman TJ. Cholangiocarcinoma in association with multiple biliary microhamartomas. Arch Pathol Lab Med 1990;114:1287–1289.
6. Byrne JLB, Harrod MJE, Friedman JM, et al. Del (20p) with manifestation of arteriohepatic dysplasia. Am J Med Genet 1986;24:673–678.
7. D'Agata IDA, Jonas MM, Perez-Atayde AR, et al. Combined cystic disease of the liver and kidney. Semin Liver Dis 1994;14:215–228.
8. Desmet VJ. Cholangiopathies: past, present, and future. Semin Liver Dis 1987;7:67–76.
9. Desmet VJ. Embryology of the liver and intrahepatic biliary tract, and an overview of malformations of the bile duct. In: McIntyre N, Benhamou J-P, Bircher J, et al., eds. Oxford Textbook of Clinical Hepatology, vol. 1. New York: Oxford University Press,1991:498–519.
10. Desmet VJ. Congenital diseases of intrahepatic bile ducts: variations on the theme "ductal plate malformation." Hepatology 1992;16:1069–1083.
11. Desmet VJ. What is congenital hepatic fibrosis? Histopathology 1992;20:465–477.
12. Dimmick JE. Hepatobiliary system. In: Dimmick JE, Kalousek DK, eds. Developmental Pathology of the Embryo and Fetus. Philadelphia: JB Lippincott Co, 1992:545–578.
13. Dubois AM. The embryonic liver. In: Rouiller C, ed. The Liver. New York: Academic Press, 1963:1–39.
14. Emery JL. The distribution of hematopoietic foci in the infantile human liver. J Anat 1956;90:293–311.
15. Enzan H, Ohkita T, Fujita H, et al. Light and electron microscopic studies on the development of the periportal bile ducts of the embryo. Acta Pathol Jpn 1974;24:427–447.
16. Faa G, Van Eycken P, Demelia L, et al. Idiopathic adulthood ductopenia presenting with chronic recurrent cholestasis. J Hepatol 1991;12:44–20.
17. Gale RP. Immune development in human fetal liver. In: Gale RP, Touraine J-L, Lucarelli G, eds. Fetal Liver Transplantation. New York: Alan R. Liss, 1985:73–88.

18. Hadchouel M, Hugon RN, Gautier M. Reduced ratio of portal tracts to paucity of intrahepatic bile ducts. Arch Pathol Lab Med 1978;102:402–403.

19. Hausner RJ, Alexander RW. Localized congenital hepatic fibrosis presenting as an abdominal mass. Hum Pathol 1978;9:473–476.

20. Hutchins GM, Moore DW. Growth and asymmetry of the human liver during the embryonic period. Pediatr Pathol 1988;8:17–24.

21. Kahn E, Daum F, Markowitz J, et al. Nonsyndromatic paucity of interlobular bile ducts: light and electron microscopic evaluation of sequential liver biopsies in early childhood. Hepatology 1986;6:890–901.

22. Kahn E, Markowitz J, Aiges H, et al. Human ontogeny of the bile duct to portal space ratio. Hepatology 1989;10:21–23.

23. Koga A. Morphogenesis of intrahepatic bile ducts of the human fetus. Light and electron microscopic study. Z Anat Entwicklungsgesch 1971;135:156–184.

24. Labrecque DR, Mitros FA, Nathan RJ, et al. Four generations of arteriohepatic dysplasia. Hepatology 1982;2:467–474.

25. Mendoza A, Voland J, Wolf P, et al. Supradiaphragmatic liver in the lung. Arch Pathol Lab Med 1986;110:1085–1086.

26. Moore KL. The developing human. 4th Ed. Philadelphia: WB Saunders, 1988.

27. Morecki R, Glaser JH, Johnson AB, et al. Detection of reovirus type 3 in the porta hepatis of an infant with extrahepatic biliary atresia: ultrastructural and immunocytochemical study. Hepatology 1984;4:1137–1142.

28. Oyer CE, Rogers BB, Singer DB. A histologic survey of iron positive cells in fetal and neonatal livers utilizing morphometry and a semiquantitative grading method. Pediatr Pathol 1989;9:798.

29. Peters RL. Early development of the liver: a review. In: Fisher MM, Roy CC, eds. Pediatric Liver Disease. New York: Plenum Publishing, 1983:1–15.

30. Popper H, Schaffner F. Liver: Structure and Function. New York: McGraw-Hill, 1957:587.

31. Raweily EA, Gibson AAM, Burt AD. Abnormalities of intrahepatic bile ducts in extrahepatic biliary atresia. Histopathology 1990;17:521–527.

32. Riely C. Familial intrahepatic cholestatic syndromes. Semin Liver Dis 1987;7:119–133.

33. Ruebner BH, Blankenberg TA, Burrows DA, et al. Development and transformation of the ductal plate in the developing human liver. Pediatr Pathol 1990;10:55–68.

34. Sell S. Is there a liver stem cell? Cancer Res 1990;50:3811–3815.

35. Shah KD, Gerber MA. Development of intrahepatic bile ducts in humans: immunohistochemical study using monoclonal antibodies to cytokeratin. Arch Pathol Lab Med 1989;113:1135–1138.

36. Shah KD, Gerber MA. Development of intrahepatic bile ducts in humans. Arch Pathol Lab Med 1990;114:598–600.

37. Stosiek P, Kasper M, Karsten U. Expression of cytokeratin 19 during human liver organogenesis. Liver 1990;10:59–63.

38. Takei M, Yoda H, Kamijo N, et al. A case of Caroli's disease with hepatolithiasis, choledocholithiasis, and cholangiocarcinoma. Gastroenterol Jpn 1991;26:224–229.

39. Valencia-Mayoral P, Weber J, Cutz E, et al. Possible defect in the bile secretory apparatus in arteriohepatic dysplasia (Alagille's syndrome); a review with observations on the ultrastructure of the liver. Hepatology 1984;4:691–698.

40. Van Eyken P, Sciot R, Van Damme B, et al. Keratin immunohistochemistry in normal human liver. Cytokeratin pattern of hepatocytes, bile ducts and acinar gradient. Virchows Arch A Pathol Anat Histopathol 1987;412:63–72.

41. Van Eyken P, Sciot R, Callera F, et al. The development of the intrahepatic bile ducts in man: a keratin immunohistochemical study. Hepatology 1988;8:1586–1595.

7

NONSPECIFIC REACTIONS
OF THE LIVER

Liver biopsy can demonstrate various alterations that are not specifically diagnostic (Table 7.1). Recognition and understanding of these phenomena is important so they are not misinterpreted as primary liver disease with subsequent unnecessary and potentially harmful therapies.

INCIDENTAL LIVER BIOPSY FINDINGS DURING SURGICAL PROCEDURES

Not uncommonly, a liver biopsy may be obtained as part of a cholecystectomy, either open or laparoscopic (6) or, more recently, during a gastroplasty operation for morbid obesity. Most often biopsies show only features suggestive of a mild, chronic, nonspecific inflammation (hepatitis), including minimal or mild mononuclear inflammatory cell infiltrate in the portal tracts, sometimes even with mild portal fibrosis (Fig. 7.1). Occasionally, rare foci of parenchymal necrosis and a few scattered large fat droplets in liver cells are seen (10). In the morbidly obese, steatosis can be marked (e-Fig. 7.1), with changes of nonalcoholic fatty disease (NAFLD) or nonalcoholic steatohepatitis (NASH) (see Chapter 21). Biopsy obtained during surgical procedures can also show changes of primary liver disease that may not have been clinically recognized prior to surgery.

"Surgical Hepatitis"

Biopsy obtained at the end of an abdominal surgical procedure, either as a core needle biopsy or, more often, as a wedge biopsy, can have clusters of polymorphonuclear leukocytes irregularly distributed in sinusoids (Fig. 7.2, e-Fig. 7.2) (1). These clusters, so-called surgical hepatitis, can be seen in any area but are most often seen in zone 3, near the terminal hepatic venule (central vein), or immediately beneath the liver capsule. It is thought that surgical hepatitis is caused by foci of anoxia within the liver or possibly by mechanical injury, perhaps from surgical retractors. Occasional true liver cell necrosis with rare acidophilic body formation can also be seen, but there is no true hepatitis.

TABLE 7.1	**Nonspecific Histopathologic Changes Sometimes Seen in Liver Biopsy**

1. Mild and focal inflammatory infiltrate in the portal tracts, mild portal fibrosis
2. Focal (rare) liver cell necrosis or occasional acidophilic bodies
3. "Surgical hepatitis"
4. Prominent Kupffer cells
5. Kupffer cell pseudogranuloma
6. Extramedullary hematopoiesis
7. Circulating megakaryocytes
8. Microgranulomas or occasional noncaseating epithelioid granulomas
9. Focal, mild macrovesicular steatosis
10. Sinusoidal dilatation (focal and without zonal distribution)
11. Mild bile duct epithelial change
12. Lipofuscin pigment
13. Hemosiderin in Kupffer and sinusoidal endothelial cells

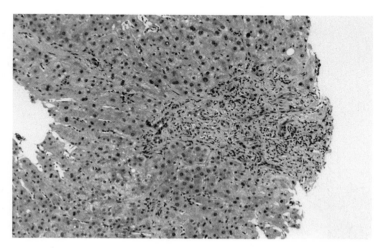

FIGURE 7.1   Photomicrograph of a liver biopsy obtained at the time of laparoscopic chole-cystectomy. Mild nonspecific portal chronic inflammation and mild fibrosis are present. Occasional large fat droplets are present in the parenchyma (hematoxylin-eosin, original magnification ×100).

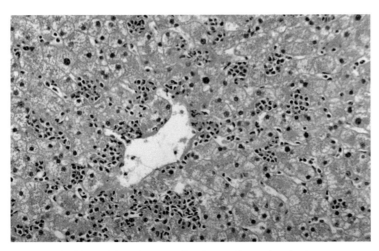

FIGURE 7.2 "Surgical hepatitis." Clusters of polymorphonuclear leukocytes are present in zone 3 of the acinus (hematoxylin-eosin, original magnification ×200).

Nonspecific Reactive Change (Nonspecific Reactive Hepatitis)

Hepatic inflammation may be prominent with various extrahepatic, systemic, and febrile conditions (7). A mild portal tract inflammatory cell infiltrate, usually lymphocytes, without interface hepatitis ("piecemeal necrosis") is seen (Fig. 7.3, e-Fig. 7.3) (10). Necrotic hepatocytes (acidophilic bodies) can

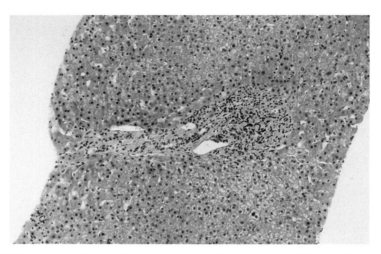

FIGURE 7.3 Nonspecific reactive change of the liver, showing mild portal tract chronic inflammatory cell infiltration, with a few lymphocytes in sinusoids (hematoxylin-eosin, original magnification ×100).

uncommonly be seen, and Kupffer cells are prominent. The term "reactive change" is preferable to "reactive hepatitis" so the erroneous diagnosis "chronic hepatitis" is not applied. Distinguishing between this nonspecific, reactive change and residual, resolving acute viral hepatitis or mild, smoldering chronic hepatitis is clearly important, and clinical correlation is imperative. Some cases of nonspecific reactive change follow prior hepatitis, either viral or drug, or another etiologic factor.

Febrile Illnesses

In protracted febrile illnesses, including fever of unknown origin, increased numbers of polymorphonuclear leukocytes circulate through the liver, prominently in sinusoids and, to a lesser degree, portal tracts. Zone 3 (centrilobular) sinusoidal dilatation is sometimes seen in the absence of other significant histopathologic findings.

Kupffer Cell Reactivity

Kupffer cells are often indistinguishable from sinusoidal endothelial cells (see Chapter 4). Kupffer cells react to various stimuli, both intrahepatic and systemic, and are seen as prominent sinusoidal lining cells (Fig. 7.4, e-Figs. 7.4, 7.5). This feature alone is entirely nonspecific and must be evaluated in the context of more specific findings. For example, Kupffer cells may be prominent in primary hepatic diseases (e.g., primary biliary cirrhosis). Kupffer cells often show ceroidlike material representing degraded cell membrane material, which can be highlighted with periodic acid–Schiff (PAS) after diastase digestion (PAS/D) as well as with Victoria blue, which likely reflects binding of Victoria blue to disulfide bonds of intracellular degradation products. Indeed, PAS/D to demonstrate phagocytosed

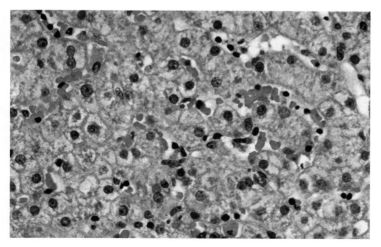

FIGURE 7.4 Prominent Kupffer cells in an otherwise normal liver (hematoxylin-eosin, original magnification ×400).

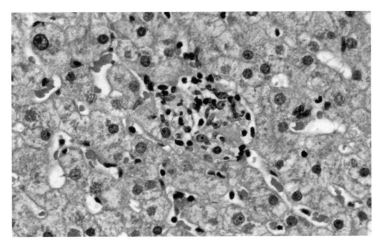

FIGURE 7.5   Kupffer cell pseudogranuloma (microgranuloma) (hematoxylin-eosin, original magnification ×400).

material in enlarged Kupffer cells can help to document a recent hepatitis when there is no longer significant lobular or parenchymal inflammation.

Kupffer Cell Pseudogranuloma

Sometimes Kupffer cells are distributed in small clusters and may have the appearance of microgranulomas, particularly concentrated around terminal hepatic venules (zone 3) (Fig. 7.5). They also often contain lipofuscin and ceroid pigments.

Extramedullary Hematopoiesis

Extramedullary hematopoiesis (EMH) as a nonspecific reactive phenomenon occurs more often in children but can be seen at any age. EMH can be seen in various primary liver tumors, including benign tumors such as adenoma and hepatocellular carcinoma and hepatoblastoma. EMH is entirely nonspecific and its significance unclear in the absence of an underlying hematologic disorder. EMH can follow transplantation, particularly combined liver–kidney transplantation, without any correlating hematologic factors (e.g., preoperative or postoperative hemoglobin values), rejection, or type of immunosuppression (Fig. 7.6) (2,9).

Circulating Megakaryocytes

The identification of isolated megakaryocytes in hepatic sinusoids is not necessarily EMH and does not indicate their origin in the liver. Rather, it may reflect the release, under conditions of stress, of megakaryocytes from the bone marrow into the peripheral blood and, consequently, throughout the circulatory system. Isolated circulating megakaryocytes in sinusoids are

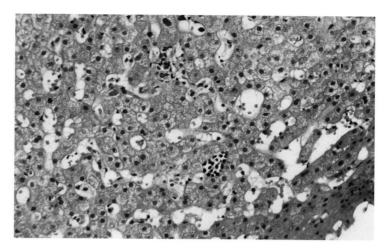

FIGURE 7.6 Extramedullary hematopoiesis in a patient following liver transplantation (hematoxylin-eosin, original magnification ×200).

not infrequently seen in the early posttransplantation period (Fig. 7.7, e-Fig. 7.6) (8).

Granulomas

Noncaseating and nonnecrotizing epithelioid granulomas and microgranulomas are sometimes seen without evidence of other infectious or noninfectious granulomatous diseases (see Chapter 12) (3,8,11).

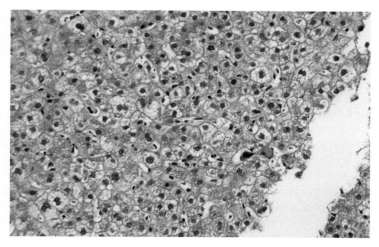

FIGURE 7.7 Sinusoidal megakaryocytes in a patient following liver transplantation (hematoxylin-eosin, original magnification ×400).

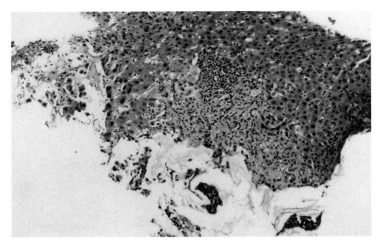

FIGURE 7.8 Vicinity of mass lesion. Focal sinusoidal dilatation and portal tract infiltration, including polymorphonuclear leukocytes, with mild portal tract edema (hematoxylin-eosin, original magnification ×200).

Steatosis

Mild, often focal, macrovesicular steatosis is seen in some liver biopsies without obesity, diabetes mellitus, alcohol or drug toxicity, or other known specific association (10).

Vicinity of Mass Lesion

Changes that occur adjacent to liver masses, both neoplastic and nonneoplastic, include focal sinusoidal dilatation and variable degrees of bile ductular reaction (proliferation) with cholestasis accompanied by variable numbers of polymorphonuclear leukocytes (Fig. 7.8, e-Figs. 7.7, 7.8). Portal tracts can sometimes be edematous. These changes mimic large bile duct obstruction (5).

Bile Duct Epithelial Injury

Although the finding of bile duct epithelial injury is an important diagnostic feature of several hepatic disorders, including cholangiopathies (e.g., primary biliary cirrhosis, primary sclerosing cholangitis), acute allograft rejection, and graft versus host disease, bile duct injury, including frank necrosis, also occurs without a specific, identifiable etiologic factor. Mild and focal biliary epithelial irregularity, overlapping nuclei, and cytoplasmic vacuolization are seen. It is important, however, that these do not progress and do not cause bile duct destruction and loss. Mild bile duct epithelial injury is common in hepatitis C virus infection (see Chapters 8 and 9), and chronic hepatitis should always be considered. Bile duct injury

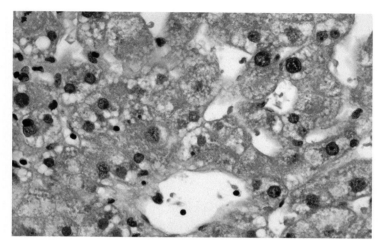

FIGURE 7.9   Lipofuscin pigment in zone 3 and zone 2 hepatocytes (hematoxylin-eosin, original magnification ×400).

also follows exposure to some drugs and toxins. Variable degrees of bile duct damage are common, both in simian monkeys with experimentally induced immune deficiency disease and in humans with acquired immune deficiency syndrome (4,6). The mechanism of injury remains obscure, although at least some degree of immunologically mediated response has been implicated.

Pigments

LIPOCHROME. Various pigments are seen in liver biopsy, the most common of which is lipochrome (lipofuscin). This "wear and tear" pigment is first in zone 3 hepatocytes adjacent to the terminal hepatic venule but with increasing age progresses from zone 3 to involve all hepatocytes (Fig. 7.9, e-Figs. 7.9, 7.10). It can also be seen in Kupffer cells. Individuals with chronic illnesses demonstrate lipofuscin pigment in excess of that expected for their age.

Hemosiderin

Hemosiderin is sometimes seen in Kupffer cells and sinusoidal endothelial cells with no clear explanation for its presence and in the absence of disorders usually associated with liver iron deposition (Fig. 7.10) (see Chapter 15). Patients who imbibe alcoholic beverages to excess have sinusoidal endothelial cells with hemosiderin. Hepatocytes may or may not show iron deposition in these cases. Bile duct epithelial cells can also show mild iron deposition, and the diagnosis of hemochromatosis should be considered even though the amount of hemosiderin is much less than in genetic hemochromatosis.

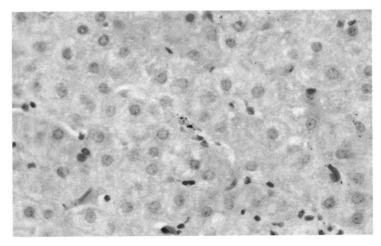

FIGURE 7.10   Hemosiderin granules are in sinusoidal cells (Perls stain, original magnification ×400).

REFERENCES

1. Christoffersen P, Poulsen H, Skei E. Focal liver cell necrosis accompanied by infiltration of granulocytes arising during operation. Acta Hepatosplenol 1970;17:240–245.

2. Collins RH, Anastasi J, Terstappen LWMM, et al. Donor-derived long-term multilineage hematopoiesis in a liver-transplant recipient. N Engl J Med 1983;328:762–765.

3. Drebber U, Kasper HU, Ratering J, et al. Hepatic granulomas: histological and molecular pathological approach to differential diagnosis – a study of 442 cases. Liver Int 2008 Feb 26 [Epub ahead of print].

4. Gerber MA, Chen ML, Hu FS, et al. Liver disease in rhesus monkeys infected with simian immunodeficiency virus. Am J Pathol 1991;139:1081–1088.

5. Gerber MA, Thung SN, Bodenheimer HC Jr, et al. Characteristic histological triad in liver adjacent to metastatic neoplasm. Liver 1986;6:85–88.

6. Michel S, Lipsky R, Morgenstern L. "Routine" liver biopsy in upper abdominal surgery. Arch Surg 1977;112:959–961.

7. Popper H, Schaffner F. Liver: Structure and Function. New York: McGraw-Hill, 1957.

8. Sartin JS, Walker RC. Granulomatous hepatitis: a retrospective review of 88 cases at the Mayo Clinic. Mayo Clin Proc 1991;66:914–918.

9. Schlitt JH, Schafers S, Deiwick A, et al. Extramedullary erythropoiesis in human liver grafts. Hepatology 1995;21:689–697.

10. Tran TT, Changsri C, Shackleton CR, et al. Living donor liver transplantation: histological abnormalities found on liver biopsies of apparently healthy potential donors. J Gastroenterol Hepatol 2006; 21:381–383.

11. Zoutman DE, Ralph ED, Frei JV. Granulomatous hepatitis and fever of unknown origin. An 11-year experience of 23 cases with three years' follow-up. J Clin Gastroenterol 1991; 13:69–75.

8

ACUTE VIRAL HEPATITIS

Acute viral hepatitis (AVH) is the term commonly applied for the hepatitides caused by hepatotropic viruses: A (HAV), B (HBV), C (HCV), D (delta), E (HEV), and F (HFV) (Table 8.1) (6,7,8,69). The etiologic factors in some cases of community-acquired and posttransfusion hepatitis remains unclear. Hepatitis G virus (HGV), a flavivirus, may be the basis of at least some of those cases (4,7,35,38). Nonhepatotropic viruses can also cause clinical and histologic manifestations of acute hepatitis, particularly in the immunocompromised patient, including cytomegalovirus (CMV), Epstein–Barr virus (EBV), adenovirus (in children), and herpes simplex virus (HSV) (Table 8.2) (12,22,27,31,41,45,47,57,66). Both the clinical and the histologic pictures of viral hepatitis can be produced by various drugs and toxic agents (81). The list of those products is long and ever-expanding (discussed in more detail in Chapter 11). As one example of the nonspecificity of the histologic picture, drug toxicity can appear to be AVH with subsequent evolution to autoimmune hepatitis (2).

Patients usually present with icterus, although anicteric forms are common. Historically, liver biopsy findings were crucial in determining further management of a jaundiced patient. Advanced imaging methods and sophisticated laboratory tests, including serologic and molecular tests for almost all of the viruses that can cause hepatitis, generally allow for the establishment of the correct diagnosis in liver biopsy.

ACUTE HEPATITIS WITH FOCAL NECROSIS

The parenchymal histopathologic changes seen in AVH are distinctive but not entirely specific. Portal tracts show varying degrees of chronic inflammatory cell infiltrate, but the dominant features are in the lobule/acinus. At low magnification, the biopsy is distinctive (Fig. 8.1). Typically the liver has a disordered or "dirty" appearance (Fig. 8.1, e-Figs. 8.1–8.6). In fully developed acute hepatitis, the changes are predominantly in zone 3 of the acinus (centrilobular, perivenular) and, to a lesser extent, in zone 1 (periportal).

Zone 3 hepatocytes show ballooning degeneration apoptotic cell necrosis and acidophilic (Councilman-like) body formation (Fig. 8.2).

TABLE 8.1	The Hepatotropic Viruses		
Virus	Type	Spread	Chronic
Hepatitis A (HAV)	RNA virus (picornavirus)	Fecal-oral	No
Hepatitis B (HBV)	DNA virus (hepadnavirus)	Parenteral, perinatal, sexual	Yes
Hepatitis C (HCV)	RNA virus (Flavivirus)	Parenteral, sexual, sporadic	Yes
Hepatitis D (HDV)	RNA virus ("defective virus")	Superinfection, coinfection with HBV	Yes
Hepatitis E (HEV)	RNA virus (Calicivirus)	Fecal-oral, epidemic, sporadic	No
Hepatitis F (HFV)	RNA virus (togalike virus)	? Parenteral, sporadic	No
Hepatitis G (HGV)	RNA virus (Flavilike virus)	Parenteral, vertical, sporadic	?

Ballooned hepatocytes have distended, pale eosinophilic, and finely granular cytoplasm. Nuclei may appear hyperchromatic and pleomorphic. Acidophilic bodies result from cell death either from cell injury or apoptosis, genetically programmed cell death at least partly controlled by the bcl-2 oncogene. Acidophilic bodies can be numerous and are recognized as refractile, deeply eosinophilic bodies, sometimes still with remnants of

TABLE 8.2	Nonhepatotropic Viruses That Can Affect the Liver
Virus	Hepatic Manifestation
Herpes simplex	Hepatitis, necrotizing hepatitis
Herpes zoster	Necrotizing hepatitis
Cytomegalovirus	Hepatitis, neonatal giant cell hepatitis
Epstein–Barr	Hepatitis, granulomas, lymphoproliferative disorder
Adenovirus group	Necrotizing hepatitis
Enterovirus (B coxsackie)	Hepatitis, hemorrhagic necrosis
Measles (rubeola)	Hepatitis
Rubella	Neonatal hepatitis
Parvovirus	Hepatocyte ballooning

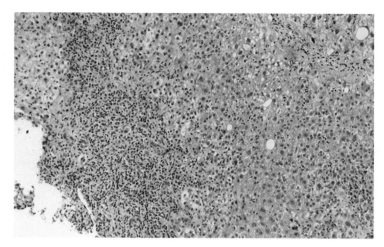

FIGURE 8.1 Low-magnification photomicrograph of acute viral hepatitis, with extensive lobular inflammation and liver cell necrosis with liver cell disarray (hematoxylin-eosin, original magnification ×100).

nuclear chromatin. Acidophilic bodies are often surrounded by mostly T lymphocytes, implicating a role for immunologically mediated cell injury and death (Fig. 8.3) (78). So-called naked acidophilic bodies may also be seen (Fig. 8.4). After cell death, there are transiently seen areas of dropout in which the liver plate structure is temporarily maintained despite the loss

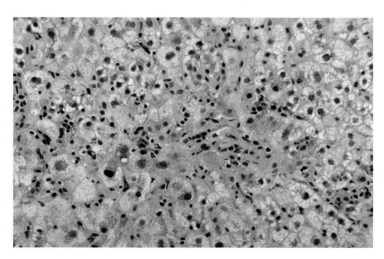

FIGURE 8.2 Acute viral hepatitis with moderately severe lobular inflammation and liver cell necrosis with numerous acidophilic (Councilman-like) bodies (hematoxylin-eosin, original magnification ×200).

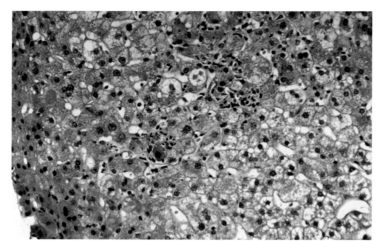

FIGURE 8.3   Acidophilic bodies surrounded by lymphocytes (hematoxylin-eosin, original magnification ×200).

of one or more hepatocytes, best demonstrated with reticulin stain. The debris from dead cells is phagocytosed by Kupffer cells, which, in acute viral hepatitis, are often enlarged and contain periodic acid–Schiff (PAS)–positive material, best seen after diastase digestion (PAS/D) to remove glycogen (e-Fig. 8.7). The destruction and loss of many liver cells leads to extensive liver plate disarray and subsequent confluent, bridging, or submassive and massive necrosis.

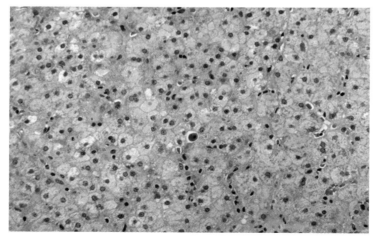

FIGURE 8.4   So-called naked acidophilic bodies, without surrounding lymphocytic infiltrate (hematoxylin-eosin, original magnification ×200).

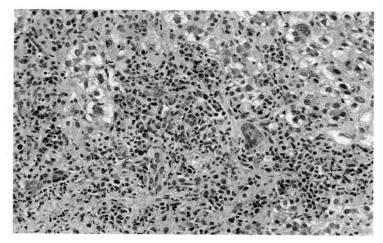

FIGURE 8.5   Acute viral hepatitis with necrosis that involves multiple acini (confluent necrosis) (hematoxylin-eosin, original magnification ×200).

"AVH with confluent necrosis" is the term used when focal necroses become numerous, coalesce, and cause cell loss in large areas of liver parenchyma (Fig. 8.5). Confluent necrosis can involve multiple acini and take the form of acute hepatitis with multiacinar (panacinar, submassive, massive) necrosis (Fig. 8.6, e-Figs. 8.8–8.10).

Bridging necrosis typically involves all three zones of the acinus, forming necroinflammatory bridges between portal and perivenular areas

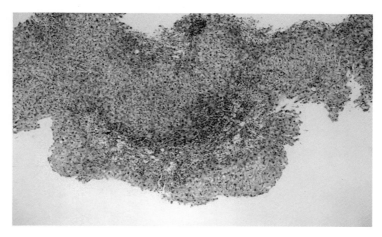

FIGURE 8.6   Acute viral hepatitis with bridging necrosis (hematoxylin-eosin, original magnification ×100).

(centroportal). However, bridging necrosis can also exist between portal tracts (portoportal). Although morphologically similar, the pathogenetic mechanisms of these two types of bridging necrosis seem to be different. Furthermore, because of the vascular shunting between the two vascular systems in centroportal bridging, this type of necrosis has more significant negative prognostic value in both acute and chronic hepatitis. AVH with bridging necrosis has a generally worse prognosis and is associated with high risk for progression to chronic hepatitis and ultimately cirrhosis. Patients with extensive bridging necrosis can die weeks to months after the onset of hepatitis with the clinical picture of subfulminant liver failure (e-Figs. 8.11–8.13). Complete recovery following acute hepatitis with bridging necrosis is not unusual, however.

When large numbers of adjacent liver cells undergo necrosis, the underlying reticulin network undergoes collapse (Fig. 8.7). Collapse, with hematoxylin-eosin, is indistinguishable from newly formed fibrous septa but is appreciated with reticulin stain as compressed fibers (64). True septa include elastic fibers, demonstrable with elastic fiber stains as well as with Victoria blue or orcein. There are no elastic fibers in recently developed collapse (64).

In addition to degenerative changes and acidophilic body formation, AVH has variable degrees of lobular (parenchymal) inflammation with mature T lymphocytes, with some histiocytes and occasional plasma cells (Fig. 8.8) (78, 79). The infiltrate in patients with acute hepatitis A may be particularly rich in plasma cells (1). Kupffer cells are also reactive and prominent in acute hepatitis, whether viral or drug induced.

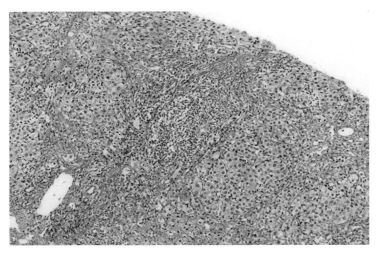

FIGURE 8.7 Acute viral hepatitis with bridging necrosis and collapse of the underlying reticulin network (reticulin silver, original magnification ×100).

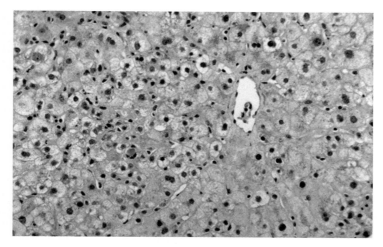

FIGURE 8.8   Acute viral hepatitis with lobular inflammation. The inflammatory cell infiltrate is predominantly lymphocytic with some histiocytes and occasional plasma cells (hematoxylin-eosin, original magnification ×200).

Multinuclear giant cells can be seen (Fig. 8.9). This occurs often in children (giant cell hepatitis), in whom it may be caused by various infectious and noninfectious factors, but may also be seen in AVH in adults, including hepatitis C (16,34). A clinically severe hepatitis with parenchymal giant cells can have paramyxoviruslike particles demonstrable with electron microscopy (59). Acute forms of autoimmune hepatitis may also show significant numbers of syncytial cells.

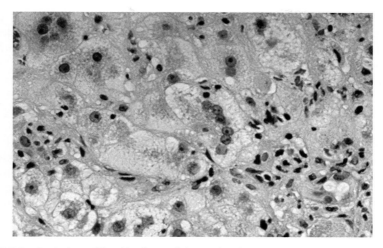

FIGURE 8.9   Acute hepatitis with giant cell formation (hematoxylin-eosin, original magnification ×400).

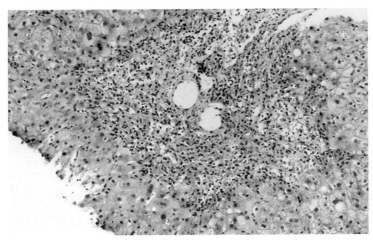

FIGURE 8.10 Acute hepatitis with relatively mixed inflammatory cell infiltrate, composed of mononuclear cells, but also including eosinophils and polymorphonuclear leukocytes (hematoxylin-eosin, original magnification ×200).

Portal tracts in AVH are generally mildly expanded, with an inflammatory infiltrate of lymphocytes, histiocytes, some plasma cells, and, rarely, few polymorphonuclear leukocytes and eosinophils (Fig. 8.10). If polymorphonuclear leukocytes and/or eosinophils predominate, etiologic factors for hepatitis other than viral should be considered, especially drugs or toxins. Interface hepatitis ("piecemeal necrosis") is characterized by the spilling of inflammatory cells from the portal tract into the limiting plate hepatocytes and is seen in various forms of acute viral hepatitis. Interface hepatitis has been thought to be associated with a greater potential for progressive disease and ultimate development of chronic hepatitis, but it is not as important in this regard as confluent necrosis.

The severity and progression of viral hepatitis is related more to cause than to the inflammatory pattern. Both AVH A and E can have severe liver inflammation, including interface hepatitis, but neither of these progresses to chronicity.

Mild cholestasis, generally confined to canaliculi, is seen in some forms of acute hepatitis (Fig. 8.11). Sometimes true cholestatic variants of hepatitis occur, however, and there may be clinically prolonged cholestasis.

Classically, three rather distinct stages of AVH are recognized: (a) early, (b) fully developed (weeks, rarely months), and (c) late, residual, or resolving hepatitis. In general, biopsy is now performed only in the late stage of acute viral hepatitis when there is concern that a relatively prolonged clinical course and/or persistence of biochemical abnormalities might be caused by another disorder.

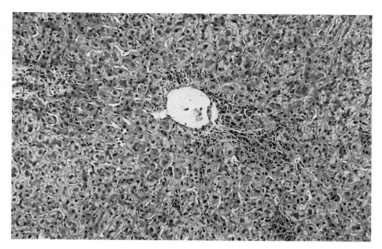

FIGURE 8.11   Acute hepatitis with cholestatic component. Cholestasis is predominantly in zone 3 of the acinus and is intracanalicular (hematoxylin-eosin, original magnification ×100).

Late, the usual parenchymal changes subside, with only rare focal necroses and/or clusters of PAS/D-positive macrophages indicating phagocytosis of cellular debris after necrosis (Fig. 8.12), most prominent in zone 3, where necrosis is most active. These macrophages contain pale brown, lipid-rich ceroid that can be stained with Perls method, resembling hemosiderin but generally paler. These mild, nonspecific changes can persist for months and may resolve without sequela.

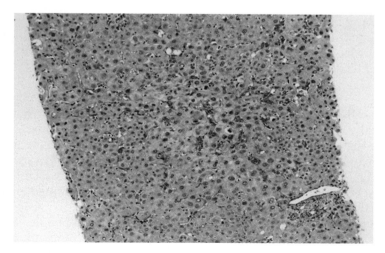

FIGURE 8.12   Resolving acute hepatitis with numerous macrophages containing a mixture of ceroid and hemosiderin pigment (periodic acid–Schiff reaction, after diastase digestion, original magnification ×200).

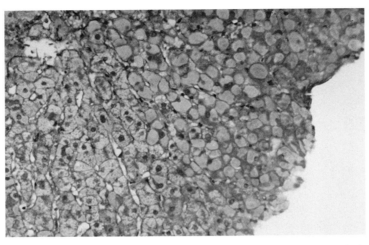

FIGURE 8.13   Hepatitis B surface antigen–containing hepatocytes ("ground-glass" cells) (hematoxylin-eosin, original magnification ×400).

Complete resolution is likely in most AVH cases. Fewer than 1% of hepatitis A, B, or C patients have a fulminant course and, without liver transplantation, may die.

AVH B, C, and D can all progress to chronicity, particularly HCV. HBV patients can also become carriers, who generally are without significant clinical manifestations but harbor the virus. The liver may appear to be quiescent, without inflammation but with abundant hepatitis B surface antigen HBsAg–containing hepatocytes, "ground-glass" cells, recognizable with hematoxylin-eosin, and highlighted with Victoria blue, orcein, or anti-HBsAg immunostain (Fig. 8.13).

Differential diagnosis of AHV includes the various hepatotropic and other viruses that can cause hepatitis, acute autoimmune hepatitis, and drug-induced hepatitis.

Type A Hepatitis

HAV is a linear, single-stranded RNA hepatotropic virus, transmitted by fecal-oral contamination. Immunoglobulin M (IgM)–type anti-HAV antibody in the serum reflects recent infection. Viral genomic material (HAV RNA) may be demonstrated in the tissue with in situ hybridization (71). Serum IgG-type anti-HAV antibodies indicate previous exposure. There are no carrier or chronic forms of HAV infection, although relapsing hepatitis has been described.

Hepatitis A is usually mild, especially in younger people. In older patients, however, the course may be more severe and fulminant and can lead to death. At one time, as many as 85% of all people in the United States demonstrated IgG antibodies against HAV. The number of seropositive individuals has dramatically declined. Travelers from Western countries

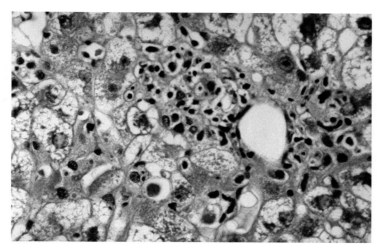

FIGURE 8.14 Acute viral hepatitis A, showing characteristic zone 3 (centrilobular) parenchymal necrosis (hematoxylin-eosin, original magnification ×400).

to endemic areas may have high susceptibility (Fig. 8.14) (1,3,30). Two distinct histologic patterns have been recognized, although overlapping features are commonly seen.

The periportal variant of hepatitis A has portal and periportal inflammation (interface hepatitis). The inflammatory infiltrate is often plasma cell–rich, and differentiation from autoimmune hepatitis is difficult without data. Generally, mild zone 3 (perivenular) cholestasis is seen.

In the cholestatic variant, zone 3 cholestasis predominates with little inflammation, often misinterpreted as drug or toxic cholestasis caused by drug or toxic injury (e-Figs. 8.14–8.19) (1,65,72).

Microvesicular steatosis and fibrin ring granulomas, generally associated with Q fever, have also been described in association with HAV infection (55). In fulminant cases, the pattern is that of submassive and massive necrosis.

Type B Hepatitis

With HBV, a hepadna virus, transmission is parenteral, sexual, and vertical from infected mothers to newborns. Vertical transmission is particularly high in endemic areas.

The infectious virion, the Dane particle, is a 42-nm structure, contains a 27-nm core with circular, incompletely double-stranded DNA surrounded by an envelope of viral surface material. The complete virion is assembled in the endoplasmic reticulum of liver cells. Other organs and tissues in the body, including lymphocytes, also contain viral DNA material.

Histologically, acute hepatitis B is not significantly different from the other forms of AVH (1). There may be acute hepatitis with focal, confluent,

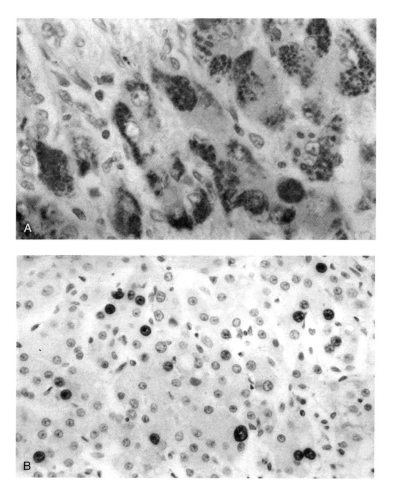

FIGURE 8.15   Chronic hepatitis B virus infection. **A.** Intracytoplasmic hepatitis B surface antigen (HBsAg) (immunoperoxidase with anti-HBsAg, original magnification ×200). **B.** Intranuclear distribution of hepatitis B core antigen (HBcAg) (immunoperoxidase with anti-HBcAg, original magnification ×200).

or submassive and massive necrosis. HBsAg-containing (ground-glass) cells are usually not seen in acute forms of hepatitis B. Both HBsAg and hepatitis B core antigen (HBcAg) can be detected in the tissue in chronic forms of hepatitis B by applying immunohistochemical methods (Fig. 8.15A,B). HBcAg is mostly intranuclear, except when the concentration of virus is very high, in which case cytoplasmic staining will also be apparent (44). HBsAg, in the cytoplasm, is also demonstrated with histochemical methods, using Victoria blue (Fig. 8.15C), orcein (Shikata), or aldehyde fuchsin (Gomori) methods.

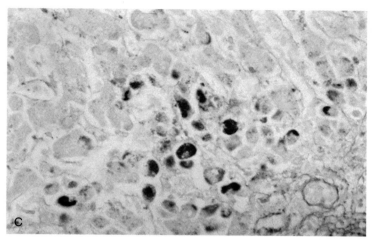

FIGURE 8.15 **(Continued)** **C.** Intracytoplasmic hepatitis B surface antigen (Victoria blue, original magnification ×400).

The chronic hepatitis B patient with acute exacerbation may have (a) superinfection with other viruses including delta, A, and C; (b) HBV reactivation; (c) superimposed drug-induced hepatitis; and (d), in patients being treated, interferon withdrawal or discontinuance.

The mechanism of cell injury is not entirely clear. The injury is immunologically mediated, including cytotoxic T cells, and natural killer (NK) cells. Although HBV does not have direct cytotoxic effect in the immunocompetent setting, recurrent hepatitis B after liver transplantation may reflect direct viral-induced cytotoxicity (19,84).

Type D (Delta) Hepatitis (HDV)

Infection with hepatitis D virus (HDV) occurs either as coinfection or as superinfection in a patient with existing HBV infection (9,11,62). In most cases the course is more severe and often fulminant. In some liver transplantation patients, HDV develops without HBV, suggesting that HDV can sometimes replicate in the absence of HBV, is not directly cytopathic, and does not necessarily require HBV to cause liver cell injury (14,36,51,60).

The viral antigen HDAg can be immunohistochemically demonstrated in the patients with superinfection or coinfection with HDV. Its expression is intranuclear, similar to that of HBcAg (33). The presence of viral RNA can be confirmed with in situ hybridization (40).

Severe acute delta virus hepatitis has been described in Venezuelan Indians (56). Significant portal inflammation is always seen, along with extensive microvesicular steatosis or spongiocytic change, in addition to focal lobular necrosis with acidophilic body formation (10,80). The liver cell nuclei containing HDAg are homogeneous and finely granular

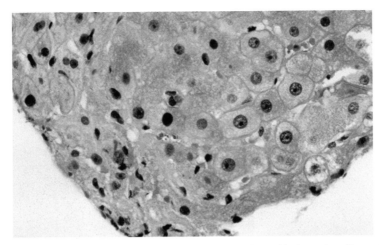

FIGURE 8.16   So-called sanded nuclei in hepatitis D virus hepatitis (hematoxylin-eosin, original magnification ×400).

("sanded") (Fig. 8.16), resembling the ground-glass cell of hepatitis B (43).

Type C Hepatitis

Acute forms of hepatitis C infection in the immunocompetent setting resemble other forms of virally induced acute hepatitis but are only rarely biopsied. The role of HCV in fulminant hepatitis is somewhat controversial (82,87). These patients have (a) portal tract enlargement and inflammation, often with lymphoid aggregates or true lymphoid follicles (Fig. 8.17);

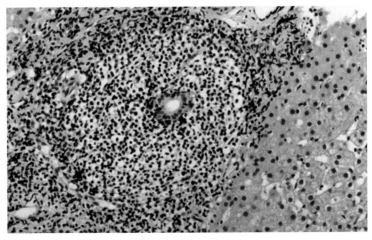

FIGURE 8.17   Hepatitis C virus infection with typical lymphoid aggregate formation in portal tracts (hematoxylin-eosin, original magnification ×200).

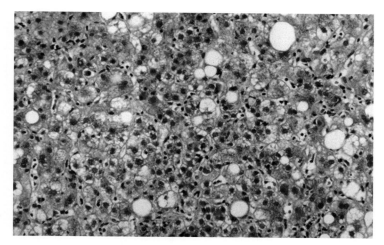

FIGURE 8.18   Lobular changes in hepatitis C virus infection with both lobular inflammation and focal liver cell necrosis, including acidophilic body formation (hematoxylin-eosin, original magnification ×200).

(b) generally mild lobular, sinusoidal inflammation, mostly lymphocytes, with only focal hepatocyte necrosis and spotty acidophilic body formation (Fig. 8.18); and (c) variable predominantly macrovesicular steatosis (Fig. 8.19) (8,18). There may also be (d) mild bile duct injury (Fig. 8.20), including vacuolation of the cytoplasm, overlapping nuclei, and nuclear pleomorphism, (e) prominent Kupffer cells, and (f) cholestasis. Despite this,

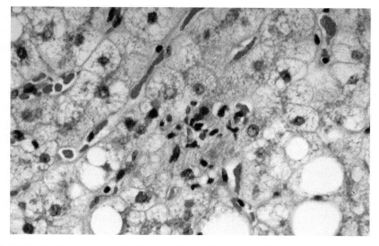

FIGURE 8.19   Macrovesicular steatosis in hepatitis C virus infection (hematoxylin-eosin, original magnification ×400).

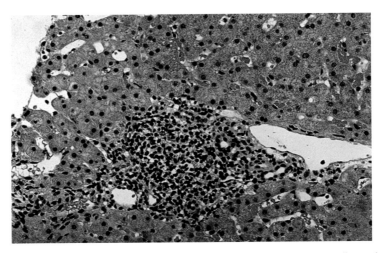

FIGURE 8.20 Mild portal inflammation with mild bile duct injury (hematoxylin-eosin, original magnification ×200).

HCV-associated antigens cannot be reliably demonstrated in tissue (23,30) and in situ hybridization methods do not show viral genome in bile duct epithelium or in liver cells. Reverse transcriptase polymerase chain reaction in situ has been used in a few selected cases to show viral genomic material in Kupffer cells, as well as in hepatocyte cytoplasm where the virus is localized to the area at the interface between the nucleus and cytosol (29,51,53). The most reliable method for detection of HCV in serum and in formalin-fixed, paraffin-embedded tissues, however, is the standard polymerase chain reaction (29,54,88).

In patients with recurrent HCV infection following liver transplantation, early histopathologic features of hepatitis may be very subtle. Recurrent forms of hepatitis in the posttransplantation setting are discussed in Chapter 25.

Type E Hepatitis

HEV infection is common in Asia, Africa, and Latin America, and only occasionally is seen in Western countries. Transmission is fecal-oral, similar to HAV (6,15,26,58,69,74,87). The RNA virus is nonenveloped single-stranded, 27 to 34 nm in diameter. Viral particles may be present in feces, bile ducts, and sinusoidal cells of patients with severe infection (8,70).

Histopathologic features of material obtained during several epidemics of HEV include portal and periportal inflammation and variable degrees of intracanalicular cholestasis, which can mimic large duct obstruction with liver cell rosette formation and extensive bile ductular proliferation (8,15).

Type F Hepatitis

Some patients with fulminant hepatitis have intranuclear 60- to 70-nm togalike virus particles seen ultrastructurally (3). After liver transplantation, some patients develop acute liver failure with similar viral particles in the graft in even greater abundance than in the native liver (18). The explanted livers showed extensive necrosis, collapse, cholestasis, and significant inflammatory infiltrate composed of lymphocytes and numerous plasma cells (18).

Hepatitis G Virus

HGV has been found in transfused patients who developed viral hepatitis, when no other agent was demonstrable. HGV, an RNA flavilike virus (4,7), is structurally closely related to HCV, with approximately 30% homology (29,35,38,67).

Most patients in whom HGV is demonstrable have an associated hepatitis. However, in some there is no elevation of transaminase values, and they could be healthy carriers or in a quiescent stage. The role of HGV infection in fulminant hepatitis and carcinogenesis is unclear (63,85) (e-Fig. 8.28). Some patients are also coinfected with HBV and HCV. In 6% to 10% of HGV patients other parenterally transmitted hepatotropic viruses can be identified, perhaps reflecting common risk factors such as intravenous drug use and multiple blood transfusions (37). Histopathologic features characteristic for HGV infection in humans have not been well delineated.

TT Virus Hepatitis

TT virus (TTV) is a recently discovered, nonenveloped, single-stranded DNA virus (48), discovered in the serum of patients with transfusion-transmitted hepatitis. TTV has been implicated in at least some cases of fulminant liver failure, cryptogenic chronic hepatitis, and cryptogenic cirrhosis. The highest carrier rate has been found in Japan, but the virus is found throughout the world. TTV is most frequently transmitted by blood transfusion, but other means of transmission exist. TTV DNA can be found in the bile and stool (50).

Herpes Simplex Virus

Hepatic HSV infection is almost exclusively seen in immunocompromised patients, including malnourished children, posttransplantation patients, and patients treated with corticosteroids and other forms of immunosuppressive medication (13,22,42,45). HSV hepatitis also occurs during pregnancy. In disseminated forms, transaminase and bilirubin values are markedly elevated, and there may be associated disseminated intravascular coagulopathy (DIC).

The liver has patchy coagulative necrosis, with no particular zonal distribution. Necrosis can be extensive with massive hepatic necrosis. Inflammation is usually not prominent (57,68).

Two types of viral intranuclear inclusions have been recognized in association with HSV infection, usually in hepatocytes at the periphery of the necrotic area: eosinophilic Cowdry type A and basophilic Cowdry type B. The intranuclear inclusions may be highlighted with Feulgen stain. A specific immunostain is available.

Cytomegalovirus

CMV hepatitis occurs mostly after renal and liver transplantation (53,73). Biopsy is often necessary to distinguish acute cellular rejection from CMV, since they can be clinically similar (53). Posttransplantation CMV hepatitis is discussed in Chapter 25.

In immunocompetent individuals, CMV produces an infectious mononucleosislike syndrome with mild hepatitis. Biopsy shows focal hepatocyte necrosis with sinusoidal lymphocytic infiltration. Mild bile duct injury is seen. Noncaseating epithelioid cell granulomas and ring granulomas of the type usually associated with Q fever occur (39). In contrast to posttransplant CMV, viral antigens are generally not demonstrable and viral inclusions are not seen.

CMV causes giant cell hepatitis in neonates with prominent cholestasis and inflammation, and easily demonstrable viral inclusions, mostly intranuclear, seen as amphophilic spherical masses surrounded by a clear halo. Intracytoplasmic inclusions, appearing as multiple, small, amphophilic, poorly defined inclusions, without halo, are also seen. There may be mild infiltration by polymorphonuclear leukocytes and lymphocytes around individual cells, but inflammation is generally not prominent (66). The intranuclear and intracytoplasmic inclusions represent aggregated virions, demonstrable immunohistochemically or with the electron microscope. Obliterative cholangitis with subsequent paucity of bile ducts has also been described (20).

Epstein–Barr Virus

EBV hepatitis occurs in immunocompetent and immunocompromised individuals, as well as after liver transplantation (e-Figs. 8.20–8.26). Posttransplantation EBV hepatitis is discussed in Chapter 25.

Biochemical hepatitis is relatively common in infectious mononucleosis, although clinical hepatitis is generally not seen. Jaundice is rare (41,80) (e-Fig. 8.27). Biopsy shows a diffuse sinusoidal lymphocytic infiltrate with varying degrees of portal inflammation. The lymphocytes are infected B cells, activated T lymphocytes, and NK cells. When inflammation is marked, apoptotic hepatocytes are seen focally (Fig. 8.21). When the infiltrate is prominent there can be many atypical lymphocytes, in parallel with the appearance of Downey cells in the

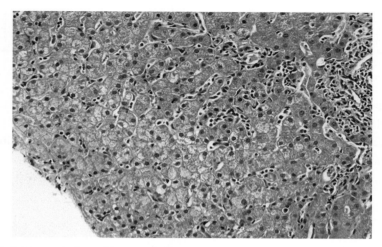

FIGURE 8.21 Acute hepatitis caused by Epstein–Barr virus. Numerous lymphocytes are arranged in a linear pattern in the sinusoids (hematoxylin-eosin, original magnification ×200).

peripheral blood, and the diagnosis of a malignant lymphoproliferative disorder can be erroneously made. Noncaseating epithelioid granulomas can be seen, and there may be varying degrees of macrovesicular steatosis (47).

Measles

Measles (rubeola) hepatitis is generally not a clinically important component in the patient infected with measles; particularly in adults, however, hepatitis can be prominent. Liver biopsy is virtually never obtained (3,10,21,43).

Rubella

Childhood rubella can be associated with a significant hepatitis, especially in neonates, in whom the histologic picture of giant cell hepatitis is seen. There may be massive necrosis, but generally involvement is milder with focal necrosis, cholestasis, and lymphocytic infiltration (86).

Varicella Zoster Virus

Hepatitis in association with varicella zoster is exceedingly rare (57,66).

Coxsackie Virus

Group B coxsackie virus usually causes a multisystem infection in neonates, leading to hemorrhagic necrosis of the liver. In adults, clinically demonstrable Coxsackie virus hepatitis is rare (23,24). There may be acinar zone 3 cholestasis, ballooning of hepatocytes, rare foci of hepatocyte necrosis, and mild infiltration of portal tracts and sinusoids by mononuclear cells and occasional polymorphonuclear leukocytes.

TABLE 8.3	Nonhepatotropic Viruses Causing Hemorrhagic Fevers and Involving the Liver	
Virus	Disease	
Flaviviridae	Yellow fever, dengue	
Arenaviridae	Lassa fever, Argentinean hemorrhagic fever	
Filoviridae	Ebola fever, Marburg fever	
Bunyaviridae	Rift Valley fever, hemorrhagic fever with renal syndrome	
Hantaan virus	Crimean-Congo hemorrhagic fever	

Other Viruses

Hepatitis has rarely been associated with adenovirus, echovirus, and parvovirus infections in both immunocompetent and immunocompromised children as well as in immunocompromised adults (5,12,27,31,32,50).

Exotic Hepatotropic Viruses

The exotic viruses are multisystem infections in which the liver serves as a primary target (Table 8.3). These infections tend to have similar clinical presentations and can be fatal. Biopsy findings include extensive coagulative necrosis and formation of acidophilic bodies. Although virtually never seen in Western society, they may rarely be encountered as more individuals travel to countries where these viruses are still active.

Lassa Fever

Lassa fever, caused by an RNA virus, manifests as a hemorrhagic fever in western and central Africa. It is transmitted by contact with rodent excrement (17). Patients present with fever, exudative pharyngitis, gastrointestinal symptoms, and coagulation disorders and develop hepatomegaly and right upper quadrant pain, with elevated transaminase, but normal bilirubin, values (39). Biopsy shows multiple foci of coagulative necrosis with numerous acidophilic bodies. Portal inflammatory infiltrates are relatively mild. Viral particles are seen with electron microscopy (17).

Yellow Fever

Yellow fever, a multisystem infection caused by an RNA arbovirus, is transmitted by the *Aedes aegypti* mosquito in parts of Africa, South America, and the Caribbean (76). Patients present with high fever, gastrointestinal hemorrhage, severe coagulopathy, and renal failure. Inflammatory cells are not prominent, although mononuclear cells may be seen as a mild portal infiltrate (Fig. 8.22, e-Figs. 8.29–8.32). The liver

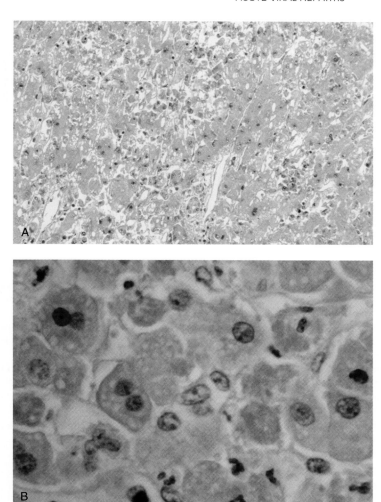

FIGURE 8.22   **A.** Yellow fever showing many zone 2 and 3 acidophilic (Councilman) bodies with scanty inflammatory response (hematoxylin-eosin, original magnification ×100). **B.** High magnification of acidophilic (Councilman) bodies (original magnification ×400).

characteristically shows innumerable acidophilic (Councilman) bodies, mostly in zone 2 with extension to zone 3 (Fig. 8.22B). Nucleoli are enlarged, and there may be true nuclear inclusions (Torres bodies). There is mild microvesicular steatosis and Kupffer cell hyperplasia. An antibody for yellow fever viral antigen has been developed but is not commercially available.

Ebola Virus

Ebola virus disease has occurred in epidemic proportions in sub-Saharan Africa, particularly in Zaire, Sudan, and Uganda, and is associated with high mortality. Ebola virus has also been recovered from monkeys brought from the Philippines to the United States. The clinical course and biopsy findings are similar to that of Lassa fever (28).

Marburg Virus

Marburg virus disease was first reported in people in contact with African green monkeys and has been described in Uganda, Kenya, and South Africa. There is a 25% mortality rate. The clinical course and biopsy findings are similar to that of Lassa fever (28,59).

REFERENCES

1. Abe H, Beninger PR, Ikejiri N, et al. Light microscopic findings of liver biopsy specimens from patients with hepatitis type A and comparison with type B. Gastroenterology 1982;82:938–947.
2. Abraham C, Hart J, Locke SM, et al. A case of indomethacin-induced acute hepatitis developing into chronic autoimmune hepatitis. Nat Clin Pract Gastroenterol Hepatol 2008;5(3):172–176. [Epub 2008 Jan 29.]
3. Ackerman Z, Flugelman MY, Wax Y, et al. Hepatitis during measles in young adults: possible role of antipyretic drugs. Hepatology 1989;10:203–206.
4. Aikawa T, Sugai Y, Okamoto H. Hepatitis G infection in drug abusers with chronic hepatitis C. N Engl J Med 1996;334:195–196.
5. Anand A, Gray ES, Brown T, et al. Human parvovirus infection in pregnancy and hydrops fetalis. N Engl J Med 1987;316:183–186.
6. Anon. The A to F of viral hepatitis. Lancet 1980;336:1158–1160.
7. Anon. Hepatitis G? Lancet 1991;337:1070.
8. Asher LVS, Innis BL, Shrestha MP, et al. Virus-like particles in the liver of a patient with fulminant hepatitis and antibody to hepatitis E virus. J Med Virol 1990;31: 229–233.
9. Bonino F, Brunetto MR, Negro F, et al. Hepatitis delta virus, a model of liver cell pathology. J Hepatol 1991;13:260–266.
10. Britfeld V, Hasida Y, Sherman FE, et al. Fatal measles infection in children with leukemia. Lab Invest 1973;28:279–291.
11. Caredda F, Rossi E, d'Armino Monforte A, et al. Hepatitis B virus–associated coinfection and superinfection with D agent: indistinguishable disease with different outcome. J Infect Dis 1985;151:925–928.
12. Carmichael GP, Zahradnik JM, Moyer GH, et al. Adenovirus hepatitis in an immunosuppressed adult patient. Am J Clin Pathol 1979;71:352–355.
13. Chase RA, Pottage JC Jr, Haber MH, et al. Herpes simplex viral hepatitis: two case reports and review of the literature. Rev Infect Dis 1987;9:329–333.
14. Cole SM, Gowans EJ, Macnaughton TB, et al. Direct evidence for cytotoxicity associated with expression of hepatitis delta virus antigen. Hepatology 1991;13:845–851.
15. De Cock KM, Bradley DW, Sanford NL, et al. Epidemic non-A, non-B hepatitis in patients from Pakistan. Ann Intern Med 1987;106:227–230.

16. Devaney K, Goodman ZD, Ishak KG. Postinfantile giant-cell transformation in hepatitis. Hepatology 1992;16:327–333.

17. Edington GM, White HA. The pathology of Lassa fever. Trans R Soc Trop Med Hyg 1972;66:381–389.

18. Fagan EA, Ellis DS, Tovey GM, et al. Toga virus–like particles in acute liver failure attributed to sporadic non-A, non-B hepatitis and recurrence after liver transplantation. J Med Virol 1992;38:71–77.

19. Feray C, Zignego AL, Samuel D, et al. Persistent hepatitis B virus infection of mononuclear blood cells without concomitant liver infection. The liver transplantation model. Transplantation 1990;49: 1155–1158.

20. Finegold MJ, Carpenter RJ. Obliterative cholangitis due to cytomegalovirus: a possible precursor of paucity of intrahepatic bile ducts. Hum Pathol 1982;13:662–665.

21. Gavish D, Kleinman Y, Morag A, et al. Hepatitis and jaundice associated with measles in young adults. An analysis of 65 cases. Arch Intern Med 1983;143:674–677.

22. Goodman ZD, Ishak KG, Sesterhenn IA. Herpes simplex hepatitis in apparently immunocompetent adults. Am J Clin Pathol 1986;85:694–699.

23. Gregor GR, Geller SA, Walker G, et al. Coxsackie hepatitis in an adult with ultrastructural demonstration of the virus. Mt Sinai J Med 1975;43:575–580.

24. Hosier DM, Newton WA. Serious coxsackie infection in infants and children: myocarditis, meningoencephalitis and hepatitis. Am J Dis Child 1958;96:251–267.

25. Hu KQ, Yu CH, Vierling JM. One-step RNA polymerase chain reaction for detection of hepatitis C virus RNA. Hepatology 1994;18:27–275.

26. Jameel S, Durgapal H, Habibullah CM, et al. Enteric non-A, non-B hepatitis: epidemics, animal transmission, and hepatitis E virus detection by the polymerase chain reaction. J Med Virol 1992;37:263–270.

27. Janner D, Petru AM, Belchis D, et al. Fatal adenovirus infection in a child with acquired immunodeficiency syndrome. Pediatr Infect Dis J 1990;9:434–436.

28. Johnson KM. Marburg and Ebola viruses. In: Mandell GL, Douglas RG, Bennett JE, eds. Principles and Practice of Infectious Diseases. 3rd ed. New York: Churchill Livingstone, 1990:1303–1305.

29. Kanda T, Yokosuka O, Ehata T, et al. Detection of GBV-C RNA in patients with nonA-E fulminant hepatitis by reverse transcription polymerase chain reaction. Hepatology 1997;25:1261–1265.

30. Khuroo MS, Teli MR, Skidmore S, et al. Incidence and severity of viral hepatitis in pregnancy. Am J Med 1981;70:252–255.

31. Krilov LR, Rubin LG, Frogel M, et al. Disseminated adenovirus infection with hepatic necrosis in patients with human immunodeficiency virus infection and other immunodeficiency states. Rev Infect Dis 1990;12:303–307.

32. Krous HF, Dietzman D, Ray CG. Fatal infections with echovirus types 6 and 11 in early infancy. Am J Dis Child 1973;126:842–846.

33. Lau JYN, Hansen LJ, Bain VG, et al. Expression of intrahepatic hepatitis D viral antigen in chronic hepatitis D virus infection. J Clin Pathol 1991;44:549–553.

34. Lau JYN, Koukoulis G, Mieli-Vergani G, et al. Syncytial giant-cell hepatitis—a specific disease entity? J Hepatol 1992;15:216–219.

35. Leary TP, Muerhoff AS, Simons JN, et al. Sequence and genomic organization of GBV-C: a novel member of the Flaviviridae associated with human non-A-E hepatitis. J Med Virol 1996;48:60–67.

36. Lefkowitch JH, Goldstein H, Yatto R, et al. Cytopathic liver injury in acute delta virus hepatitis. Gastroenterology 1987;92:1262–1266.

37. Lin HH, Kao JH, Chen PJ, et al. Mechanism of vertical transmission of hepatitis G. Lancet 1996;347:1116.

38. Linnen J, Wages J, Zhang-Keck Z-Y, et al. Molecular cloning and disease association of hepatitis G virus: a transfusion-transmissible agent. Science 1996;271:505–508.
39. Lobdell DH. 'Ring' granulomas in cytomegalovirus hepatitis. Arch Pathol Lab Med 1988;112:540–544.
40. Lopez-Talavera JC, Buti M, Casacuberta J, et al. Detection of hepatitis delta virus RNA in human liver tissue by non-radioactive in situ hybridization. J Hepatol 1993;17: 199–203.
41. Markin RS, Linder J, Zuerlein K, et al. Hepatitis in fatal infectious mononucleosis. Gastroenterology 1987;93:1210–1217.
42. Marrie TJ, McDonald ATJ, Conen PE, et al. Herpes simplex hepatitis: use of immunoperoxidase to demonstrate the viral antigen in hepatocytes. Gastroenterology 1982;82: 71–76.
43. McLellan RK, Gleiner JA. Acute hepatitis in an adult with rubeola. JAMA 1982;247: 2000–2001.
44. Moreno A, Ramon y Cajal S, Marazuela M, et al. Sanded nuclei in delta patients. Liver 1989;9:367–371.
45. Nahmias AJ, Roizman B. Infection with herpes-simplex viruses 1 and 2. N Engl J Med 1973;289:667–674.
46. Negro F, Pacchioni D, Shimizu Y, et al. Detection of intrahepatic replication of hepatitis C virus RNA by in situ hybridization and comparison histopathology. Proc Natl Acad Sci U S A 1992;89:2247–2251.
47. Nenert M, Mavier P, Dubuc N, et al. Epstein-Barr virus infection and hepatic fibrin-ring granulomas. Hum Pathol 1988;19:608–610.
48. Nishizawa T, Okamoto H, Konishi K, et al. A novel DNA virus (TTV) associated with elevated transaminase levels in posttransfusion hepatitis of unknown etiology. Biochem Biophys Res Commun 1997;241:92–97.
49. Nuovo GJ, Lidonnici K, MacConnell P, et al. Intracellular localization of polymerase chain reaction (PCR)–amplified hepatitis C cDNA. Am J Surg Pathol 1993;21:37–44.
50. Okamoto H, Nishizawa T, Kato N, et al. Molecular cloning and characterization of a novel DNA virus (TTV) associated with posttransfusion hepatitis of unknown etiology. Hepatology Res 1998;10:1–6.
51. Ottobrelli A, Marzano A, Smedile A, et al. Patterns of hepatitis delta virus reinfection and disease in liver transplantation. Gastroenterology 1991;101:1649–1655.
52. Patti ME, Selvaggi KJ, Kroboth FJ. Varicella hepatitis in the immunocompromised adult: case report and review of the literature. Am J Med 1990;88:77–80.
53. Paya CV, Hermans PE, Wiesner RH, et al. Cytomegalovirus hepatitis in liver transplantation: prospective analysis of 93 consecutive orthotopic liver transplantations. J Infect Dis 1989;160:752–758.
54. Phillips MJ, Blendis LM, Poucell S, et al. Syncytial giant-cell hepatitis. Sporadic hepatitis with distinctive pathological features, a severe clinical course, and paramyxoviral features. N Engl J Med 1991;324:455–460.
55. Ponz E, Garcia-Pagan JC, Bruguera M, et al. Hepatic fibrin-ring granuloma in patient with hepatitis A. Gastroenterology 1991;100:268–270.
56. Popper H, Thung SN, Gerber MA, et al. Histologic studies of severe delta agent infection in Venezuelan Indians. Hepatology 1983;3:906–912.
57. Raga J, Chrystal V, Coovadia HM. Usefulness of clinical features and liver biopsy in diagnosis of disseminated herpes simplex infection. Arch Dis Child 1984;59: 820–824.
58. Ramalingaswami V, Purcell RH. Waterborne non-A, non-B hepatitis. Lancet 1988;1: 571–573.
59. Rippey JJ, Schepers NJ, Gear JHS. The pathology of Marburg virus disease. S Afr Med J 1984;66:50–54.

60. Rizetto M, Chiaberge E, Negro F, et al. Liver transplantation in hepatitis delta virus disease. Lancet 1987;2:469–471.
61. Ross JS, Fanning WL, Beautyman W, et al. Fatal massive hepatic necrosis from varicella-zoster hepatitis. Am J Gastroenterol 1980;74:423–427.
62. Sagnelli E, Felaco FM, Filippini P, et al. Influence of HDV infection on clinical, biochemical and histological presentation of HBsAg positive chronic hepatitis. Liver 1989;9:229–234.
63. Sallie R, Shaw J, Mutimer D. GBV-C virus in fulminant hepatic failure [letter]. Lancet 1996;347:121–122.
64. Scheuer PJ, Maggi G. Hepatic fibrosis and collapse: histological distinction by orcein staining. Histopathology 1980;4:487–490.
65. Sciot R, Van Damme B, Desmet VJ. Cholestatic features in hepatitis A. J Hepatol 1986;3:172–181.
66. Shusterman NH, Frauenhoffer C, Kinsey MD. Fatal massive hepatic necrosis in cytomegalovirus infection. Ann Intern Med 1978;88:810–812.
67. Simmons JN, Leary TP, Dawson GJ, et al. Isolation of novel virus-like sequences associated with human hepatitis. Nat Med 1995;1:564–569.
68. Singer DB. Pathology of neonatal herpes simplex virus infection. Perspect Pediatr Pathol 1981;6:242–278.
69. Skidmore SJ, Yarbough PO, Gabor KA, et al. Imported hepatitis E in UK. Lancet 1991;337:1541.
70. Tam AW, Smith MM, Guerra ME, et al. Hepatitis E virus (HEV): molecular cloning and sequencing of the full length viral genome. Virology 1991;185:120–131.
71. Taylor M, Goldin RD, Ladva S, et al. In situ hybridization studies of hepatitis A viral RNA in patients with acute hepatitis A. J Hepatol 1974;20:380–387.
72. Texeira MR Jr, Weller IVD, Murray AM, et al. The pathology of hepatitis A in man. Liver 1982;2:53–60.
73. Vanstapel M-J, Desmet VJ. Cytomegalovirus hepatitis: a histological and immunohistochemical study. Appl Pathol 1983;1:41–49.
74. Velasquez O, Stetler HC, Avila C, et al. Epidemic transmission of enterically transmitted non-A, non-B hepatitis in Mexico, 1986–1987. JAMA 1990;263:3281–3285.
75. Verme G, Amoroso P, Lettieri G, et al. A histological study of hepatitis delta virus liver disease. Hepatology 1986;6:1303–1307.
76. Vieira W, Gayotto LC, De Lima CP, et al. Histopathology of the human liver in yellow fever with special emphasis on the diagnostic role of the Councilman body. Histopathology 1983;7:195–208.
77. Villamil FG, Hu KQ, Yu CH, et al. Detection of hepatitis C virus with RNA polymerase chain reaction in fulminant hepatic failure. Hepatology 1995;22:1379–1386.
78. Volpes R, van den Oord JJ, Desmet VJ. Memory T cells represent the predominant lymphocytic subset in acute and chronic liver inflammation. Hepatology 1991;13:826–829.
79. Volpes R, van den Oord JJ, Desmet VJ. Vascular adhesion molecules in acute and chronic liver inflammation. Hepatology 1992;15:269–275.
80. White NJ, Juel-Jensen BE. Infectious mononucleosis hepatitis. Semin Liver Dis 1984;4:301–306.
81. Woolf GM, Petrovic LM, Rojter SE, et al. Acute hepatitis associated with the Chinese herbal product jin bu huan. Ann Intern Med 1994;121:729–735.
82. Wright TL, Hsu H, Donegan E, et al. Hepatitis C virus not found in fulminant non-A, non-B hepatitis. Ann Intern Med 1991;115:111–112.
83. Yamada S, Koji T, Nozawa M, et al. Detection of hepatitis C virus (HCV) RNA in paraffin-embedded tissue sections of human liver of non-A, non-B hepatitis patients by in situ hybridization. J Clin Lab Anal 1992;6:40–46.

84. Yoffe B, Burns DK, Bhatt HS, et al. Extrahepatic hepatitis B virus DNA sequences in patients with acute hepatitis B infection. Hepatology 1990;12:187–192.

85. Yoshiba M, Okamoto H, Mishiro S. Detection of the GBV-C hepatitis virus genome in serum from patients with fulminant hepatitis of unknown etiology. Lancet 1995;346: 1131–1132.

86. Zeldis JB, Miller JG, Dienstag JL. Hepatitis in adults with rubella. Am J Med 1985;79: 515–516.

87. Zuckerman AJ. Hepatitis E virus. The main cause of enterically transmitted non-A, non-B hepatitis. Br Med J 1990;300:1475–1476.

9

CHRONIC HEPATITIS (CHRONIC NECROINFLAMMATORY DISEASE OF THE LIVER)—GRADING AND STAGING

Chronic hepatitis is both a clinical term and a pathology term. Clinically, it is a persistent inflammatory reaction of the liver with more than 6 months of clinical signs symptoms and/or biochemical indicators. Various conditions express as the clinical picture of chronic hepatitis (Table 9.1), and biopsy is often, but not always, required for definitive diagnosis. The simplest scheme for the chronic necroinflammatory diseases of the liver is to consider them as (a) chronic hepatitis caused by hepatic viruses, (b) chronic hepatitis caused by autoimmune disorders, and (c) others. In all of these conditions a range of morphologic changes may be seen.

ESTABLISHING THE DIAGNOSIS OF CHRONIC HEPATITIS

Biochemical Studies

Persistent elevation of the transaminase values for more than 6 months is the hallmark of chronic hepatitis (2). Alanine aminotransferase (ALT) is more sensitive for hepatic inflammation than aspartate aminotransferase (AST), and it is generally slightly higher than the AST in patients with chronic hepatitis. In contrast, patients with alcoholic hepatitis have higher AST values.

Other laboratory tests are performed to delineate the cause of chronic hepatitis, including, but not limited to, hepatitis B surface antigen, hepatitis C antibody, autoantibodies (antinuclear, antimitochondrial, anti–smooth muscle), iron studies, ceruloplasmin and copper determinations, and α1-antitrypsin evaluation, in addition to studies to exclude extrahepatic causes (e.g., myositis, thyrotoxicosis, diabetes mellitus) for transaminase elevations.

TABLE 9.1	Etiology Causes of Chronic Necro-inflammatory Disorders of the Liver

Hepatitis virus diseases
  Hepatitis B
  Hepatitis D
  Hepatitis C
Autoimmune disease
  Autoimmune hepatitis
  Autoimmune cholangitis
  Primary biliary cirrhosis
  Primary sclerosing cholangitis
Other conditions
  Chronic drug hepatitis
  Wilson disease
  α1-Antitrypsin deficiency
  Hereditary hemochromatosis
  Alcoholic liver disease
Idiopathic

Liver Biopsy

Although clinical laboratory tests can partially define chronic hepatitis, the liver biopsy remains important. The liver biopsy can (a) confirm the clinical diagnosis and also (b) allows for exclusion of the many diseases that can manifest as "chronic hepatitis" (Table 9.1). The biopsy allows for (c) grading and staging and is necessary to (d) exclude concomitant diseases that can be significant, such as alcoholic liver disease or hemochromatosis, but that may be clinically masked by the principal cause of the chronic hepatitis. In chronic hepatitis C, in particular, the histochemical demonstration of iron pigment in the liver biopsy, whether caused by genetic hemochromatosis or secondary hemosiderosis, is important because the response to interferon therapy can be affected by its presence (30,47). Liver biopsy also allows for (e) monitoring of the effects of specific therapies. In the coming years, liver biopsy will be increasingly used to (f) identify cellular and molecular markers unique for a given patient and his or her disease (personalized medicine), enabling more precise diagnoses and prognoses as well as the most specific therapy.

This chapter will emphasize hepatitis C, since it is the most common necroinflammatory liver disease in North America. Hepatitis C virus (HCV) can be the prototype for a discussion of the morphology of the chronic hepatitides. Other disorders that can result in the histologic picture of a chronic hepatitis will be considered in subsequent chapters.

CHRONIC HEPATITIS C

The cloning and sequencing of HCV and the subsequent development of a clinically useful assay (15,22,37) were major triumphs of the relatively new discipline of molecular biology. An RNA virus related to Flaviviridae and some RNA plant viruses, HCV is a 50- to 60-nm, enveloped, single-stranded, positive-polarity RNA virus. The genome is approximately 10 kb with a single open reading frame. Using the polymerase chain reaction, clinicians can recover hepatitis C from virtually all patients with chronic hepatitis C, including cirrhosis, but not from those with autoimmune hepatitis or cryptogenic cirrhosis (22).

Clinical Features

Chronic HCV infection occurs worldwide and is more common than HBV in North America. Considerable genomic variability exists between strains of HCV from different countries. It is estimated that at least 50% of HCV patients progress to chronic hepatitis and as many as 20% of those patients become cirrhotic (53). HCV is potentially transmitted in blood and blood products and, prior to the widespread serologic testing for hepatitis C, was responsible for most cases of posttransfusion hepatitis. HCV is also common in intravenous drug users and also occurs sporadically. Healthcare workers have a slightly increased risk of developing HCV hepatitis. More than 75,000 cases of HCV hepatitis occur each year in the United States, with at least 6,000 patients developing cirrhosis. Almost all patients undergoing liver transplantation for chronic hepatitis C have recurrence (50). Chapter 8 includes a discussion of acute hepatitis C.

Histopathology

Histopathologic changes potentially seen in the chronic hepatitis liver biopsy are listed in Table 9.2. A series of papers defined the key histologic features of chronic hepatitis C (Table 9.3) (1,6,9,38,43,58), including (a) marked and patchy expansion of portal tracts by predominantly lymphocytic infiltrate with sometimes only minimal spilling over (interface hepatitis) into adjacent lobule (Figs. 9.1, 9.2, e-Figs. 9.1–9.6), often with (b) a well-defined lymphoid aggregate, including true follicle formation with a typical germinal center (e-Fig. 9.6), (c) varying degrees of bile duct damage (e-Fig. 9.5) and, uncommonly, even focal bile duct loss (32), (d) varying degrees of steatosis, including microvesicular and macrovesicular fat, more prominent in genotype 3 (e-Fig. 9.7) (10) and (e) sinusoidal cell hyperplasia. Low-magnification appearance is characteristic: patchy enlargement of portal tracts, often distinctly globular form (e-Fig. 9.1), with partially or well-developed lymphoid follicles (e-Fig. 9.8), usually mild interface hepatitis (e-Fig. 9.2), minimal periportal fibrosis, prominent sinusoidal cells, and mild to moderate steatosis (Fig. 9.3, e-Fig. 9.7).

Interface hepatitis should be considered the *sine qua non* in establishing the diagnosis of chronic hepatitis. Interface hepatitis can be focal

TABLE 9.2 Features of Inflammation/Fibrosis in Chronic Hepatitis Liver Biopsies	
Hepatocyte Changes	**Inflammation**
Ballooning	Portal/periportal distribution/amount
Acidophilic/apoptotic bodies	Lobule distribution/amount
Hepatocyte dropout	Vascular/endothelial
Bridging/confluent necrosis	Kupffer/macrophage (diastase PAS)
"Ground-glass" cells	Granulomas
Mallory hyaline	Biliary changes
Steatosis type/distribution/amount	Bile duct injury
Iron storage—hepatocytes, Kupffer, both	Ductular reaction (proliferation)
Bile stasis—intrahepatic, canalicular, both	Ductopenia
Cholate stasis (feathery)	Fibrosis/septa
Liver plate thickness	Scar or septum or capsule?
	Quantity
	Distribution

TABLE 9.3 Histopathology of Chronic Hepatitis C

Principal histopathologic findings
1. Portal infiltrate (predominantly lymphocytes)
   a. Lymphoid nodules
   b. Germinal center formation
2. Interface hepatitis
3. Bile duct injury (usually mild)
4. Lobular inflammation (usually mild)
5. Macrovesicular steatosis (especially genotype 3)
6. Sinusoidal cell hyperplasia

Variably seen findings
1. Liver cell pleomorphism
   a. Increased binucleate hepatocytes
   b. Multinucleate hepatocytes
2. Histiocytic aggregates
   a. microgranulomas
3. Phlebitis, portal or central or both

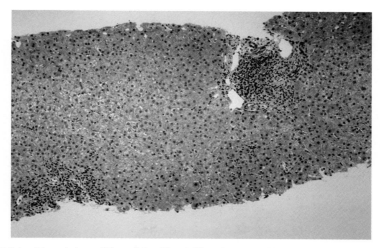

FIGURE 9.1   Chronic hepatitis, mild, without fibrosis, caused by hepatitis C, including mild interface hepatitis and minimal lobular inflammation (Scheuer histologic score: portal/periportal grade 2, lobule grade 1, stage 0). (hematoxylin-eosin, original magnification ×100).

involving only a small portion of the limiting plate of one portal tract. Portal inflammation without interface hepatitis can reflect various conditions and can even be seen in people who have no clinical or biochemical evidence of liver disease (Table 9.4) (70). The amount of inflammation within the confines of the portal tract does not change the grade. The degree of interface hepatitis and lobular inflammation is more important in

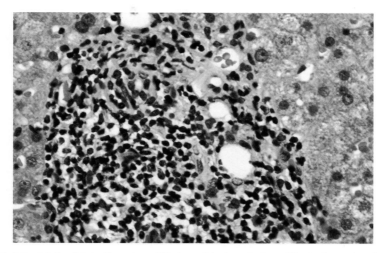

FIGURE 9.2   Minimal interface hepatitis in mild chronic hepatitis C (hematoxylin-eosin, original magnification ×200).

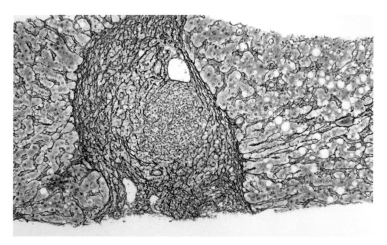

FIGURE 9.3   Minimal portal and periportal fibrosis in chronic hepatitis C, manifesting as delicate extensions from the portal tract seen only with reticulin stain (reticulin stain, original magnification ×200).

terms of both grading and prognosis. It is also important to assess stainable iron. The presence of iron has been shown to correlate with nonresponse to interferon therapy (3).

Less commonly seen features of chronic HCV include (a) mild lobular hepatitis (e-Figs. 9.9, 9.10), (b) liver cell dysplasia, (c) multinucleation, and, rarely, (d) accumulations of Mallory-like material in hepatocytes. Lobular hepatitis can be the presenting histologic feature in hepatitis C recurring after liver transplantation, particularly when it recurs in the first posttransplant year (Figs. 9.4, 9.5, e-Figs. 9.11–9.13). Reticulin stain can be helpful in identifying early hepatocyte loss (Fig. 9.5). Interface hepatitis can be quite prominent (Fig. 9.6) and can progress to bridging inflammation and necrosis (Fig. 9.7). Regenerative nodules can be seen with early bridging fibrosis, before the full appearance of cirrhosis (Fig. 9.8). Cirrhosis typically develops after 10 to 20 years of chronic HCV (e-Figs.

TABLE 9.4	Portal Chronic Inflammation without Interface Hepatitis
	Systemic illnesses
	Adjacency to space-occupying lesions
	Drugs/toxins
	Acute viral hepatitis
	"Normal"

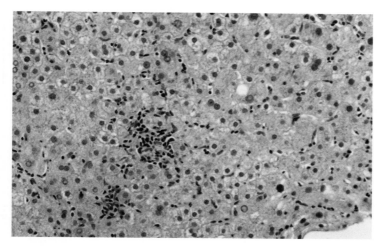

FIGURE 9.4   Lobular hepatitis in recurrent chronic hepatitis, 8 months after orthotopic liver transplantation. Note increased numbers of binucleate hepatocytes, anisocytosis and liver cell dropout with lobular lymphocyte accumulations (hematoxylin-eosin, original magnification ×100).

9.14, 9.15) but can sometimes be the presenting manifestation (e-Figs. 9.16–9.20). Cholestasis is not common in chronic HCV but is seen with cirrhotic decompensation (e-Figs. 9.18–9.20).

These features are not pathognomonic and have been recognized in other forms of chronic hepatitis, including hepatitis B, but they are most

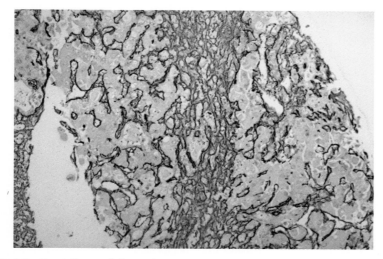

FIGURE 9.5   Focal liver cell loss (dropout) and reticulin collapse in recurrent chronic hepatitis C (reticulin stain, original magnification ×400).

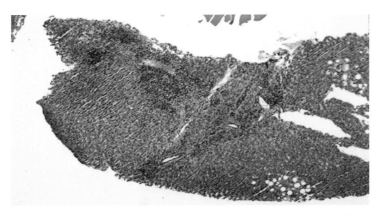

FIGURE 9.6   Chronic hepatitis, moderate, without fibrosis, caused by hepatitis C, showing prominent interface hepatitis with extension into the lobule (Scheuer histologic score: portal/periportal grade 2, lobule grade 2, stage 0) (hematoxylin-eosin, original magnification ×100).

often seen in hepatitis C. The constellation of (a) through (e), not uncommonly seen as a group, is virtually diagnostic.

Various disorders and artifacts can mimic chronic hepatitis C (Table 9.5). Generally, true lymphoid follicles are not seen in those conditions, and other features, such as prominent interface hepatitis, severe lobular necrosis and inflammation, and areas of parenchymal collapse, can be more prominent.

Immunohistochemical methods for demonstration of HCV are not yet widely available. The gold standard for diagnosis has been identification of viral RNA using the polymerase chain reaction. Practically, diagnosis is

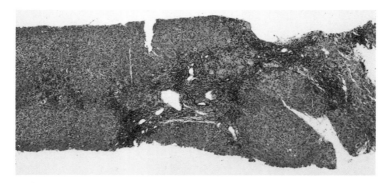

FIGURE 9.7   Marked interface hepatitis and bridging necrosis in chronic hepatitis with periportal but not bridging fibrosis (Scheuer histologic score: portal/periportal grade 3, lobule grade 2, stage 2) (hematoxylin-eosin, original magnification ×100).

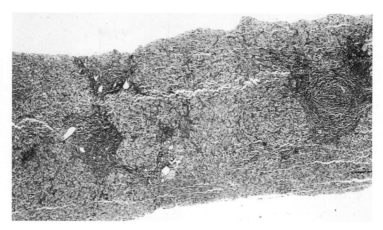

FIGURE 9.8 Focal liver cell regeneration with formation thickened liver plates and early bridging fibrosis in chronic hepatitis C (Scheuer histologic score: portal/periportal grade 2, lobule grade 1, stage 3) (reticulin stain, original magnification ×400).

generally based on the recognition of compatible and characteristic histopathology combined with serologic demonstration of antibody to HCV and/or HCV-RNA quantification. There is concomitant morphologic and clinical exclusion of other liver disorders, although chronic HCV can be seen with alcoholic liver disease, HBV, α1-antitrypsin disease, and some other disorders, and can also occur in the setting of HIV infection (9).

CHRONIC HEPATITIS B

HBV is a partially double-stranded DNA virus that can cause both acute and chronic hepatitis (23). Hepatitis B is discussed in greater detail in Chapter 8.

TABLE 9.5 Some Potential Histologic Mimics of Chronic Hepatitis C
Hepatitis B
Autoimmune hepatitis
Primary sclerosing cholangitis
Primary biliary cirrhosis
Wilson disease
Lymphoma/leukemia
Liver capsule and subcapsular liver parenchyma
Others

Clinical Features

The vast majority of individuals infected with HBV have an acute, self-limited infection. Despite this, as many as 250 million people worldwide, mostly in the Far East, suffer from chronic HBV infection. In the United States, chronic HBV infection is relatively uncommon. There may also be acute exacerbations of disease in the setting of chronic hepatitis B. Clinical manifestations are not specifically diagnostic and are those of a progressive chronic hepatitis. Extrahepatic manifestations, such as glomerulonephritis and arthralgias, are more common in acute viral hepatitis B but can also be seen in the chronic form. Some patients have a hypersensitivity angiitis, resembling polyarteritis nodosa.

Histopathology

A wide spectrum of histologic changes can be seen. One histologic feature, the "ground-glass" hepatocyte, is relatively specific, representing cytoplasmic hepatitis B surface antigen (HBsAg) (e-Figs. 9.21, 9.22). Ground-glass hepatocytes are slightly enlarged cells with cytoplasmic finely granular, pale, eosinophilic material filling the cytoplasm. With formalin fixation HBsAg contracts, leaving a clear halo between the granular cytoplasm and the cell membrane. Ground-glass-like cells can be seen in Lafora disease and, rarely, with some drugs. Hepatitis B surface antigen (HBsAg) accumulates in the replicative stage, demonstrable with immunostain (Fig. 5.6, e-Figs. 9.23, 9.24) or with Victoria blue (e-Figs. 9.25, 9.26), orcein (Shikata), or aldehyde-fuchsin (Gomori) stains.

With active virus replication, inflammation is also seen (68), with portal (e-Figs. 9.27, 9.28) and lobular hepatitis (e-Figs. 9.29, 9.30) of varying degrees. Hepatitis B core antigen (HBcAg) can be demonstrated in hepatocyte nuclei with immunostain (e-Figs. 9.31, 9.32). There is no corresponding histochemical stain. The 25 nm core particles on the surface of or in the nucleus correspond to the inner Dane particle compartment. In acute hepatitis, but also in chronic hepatitis, when core antigen is abundant it is also seen in the cytoplasm. Replication takes place when early antigen is in serum HBV, correlating with the presence of serum HBV-DNA and DNA polymerase and hepatocytes HBcAg. Early antigen expresses in both nucleus and cytoplasm. Portal hepatitis occurs during the phase of low virus replication and can be prominent, although portal or lobular hepatitis may reoccur with either virus reactivation or superinfection with another virus, such as the delta agent (HDV) (e-Fig. 9.33).

In HBsAg carriers, in the absence of active replication, the liver biopsy may have no inflammation or there may be mild portal hepatitis. Ground-glass cells are usually abundant (e-Fig. 9.34). Although most HBV patients recover, progression does occur (e-Figs. 9.35–9.423). When HBV cirrhosis develops, the inflammatory component may disappear, although ground-glass cells containing HBsAg may persist.

CHRONIC HEPATITIS D (DELTA)

HDV is a small, "defective," RNA virus. HDV cannot form its own external envelope and uses HBsAg to form its outer coat, which is required for propagation and infection (16,23,44,55). When infection with HBV and HDV occur at the same time, the patient may have an acute hepatitis, which is sometimes fulminant. Chronic HDV hepatitis occurs in HBsAg carriers who do not have active HBV infection (55). HBV must be present before HDV causes recognizable cell injury and disease (16). Acute hepatitis D is discussed in Chapter 8.

Clinical Features

There are no specific clinical features that identify the patient with chronic HDV (44). HDV should be considered in any HBsAg-positive patients, but especially in those with rapid progression to cirrhosis, in known chronic HBV patients whose clinical course suddenly worsens, and in patients from HDV-prevalent areas (Brazil, Venezuela, southern Italy, the Middle East). HDV occurs only sporadically in North America and mostly in high-risk groups, such as hemodialysis patients, intravenous drug users, hemophiliacs, homosexuals, and prison inmates. HDV is rarely transmitted in blood or blood products used for transfusion, since screening tests almost always detect HBsAg.

Histopathology

When HDV complicates HBV infection, there is always significant histologic injury (39) (e-Fig. 9.33). Although portal hepatitis alone may be seen, the biopsy generally shows more severe inflammation, with severe liver disease, with bridging necrosis and extensive collapse, progressing to either liver failure or cirrhosis. Histologic changes do not differentiate HDV from HBV. A fat-negative foamy cytoplasmic degeneration is indicative of HDV, but this has not proven specific. HDV is identified with a specific immunostain.

CHRONIC HEPATITIS G

Hepatitis G virus is detected in some patients with chronic liver disease, but its relevance remains controversial. In general, it seems that hepatitis G is not in and of itself pathogenic (20) but may accelerate the progress of HBV and HCV (71).

CLASSIFICATION, GRADING, AND STAGING

Chronic hepatitis has been a vexing problem in terms of clinical and therapeutic issues, but also in regard to establishing a histopathologic classification that must deal with multiple causes and considerable morphologic variation while providing a useful prognostic tool. In recent years several semiquantitative numerical grading and staging systems have been proposed. A perfect system does not yet exist, and, in most settings, English language suffices to communicate the information.

Size Matters

Biopsy sample size is critical (6,8,14,25–27,31,42,54,56,67). A 16- or 14-gauge needle should be used whenever possible to obtain satisfactory material. The specimen should be at least 2.0 to 2.5 cm total length with at least 10 portal tracts. This goal can be realized with percutaneous, laparoscopic, and transjugular biopsy, but more than one biopsy pass may be needed. Site of biopsy can also affect interpretation. With increasing age, the left lobe is more fibrotic than the right. Samples obtained close to the liver capsule can be misleading for both fibrosis and inflammation.

Traditional and Now Obsolete Classification

Four decades ago, the terms "chronic persistent hepatitis," "chronic active hepatitis," and "chronic lobular hepatitis" were established (32,33,51). They are now obsolete and should not be used (Table 9.6). Previously, the biopsy "chronic active hepatitis" was thought to have a progressive course, whereas "chronic persistent hepatitis" was considered benign and self-limited. Since the time of publication of those seminal papers it has become known that "chronic persistent" is typical of chronic hepatitis C and that most of these patients, if untreated, progress to chronic liver disease and cirrhosis (10,28,49,53,63). Indeed, the behavior and ultimate prognosis for the patient with "chronic persistent hepatitis" or "chronic lobular hepatitis" may be similar to that for the patient with "chronic active hepatitis."

It is increasingly important for the physician caring for the patient with chronic hepatitis to understand the exact significance of the liver biopsy, and the role of the pathologist in communicating that information is critical.

Portal hepatitis (previously "chronic persistent hepatitis") denotes a biopsy in which hepatic architecture is maintained, with a mononuclear portal tract infiltrate consisting predominantly of lymphocytes, with varying numbers of plasma cells and histiocytes (Fig. 9.1). Eosinophils can also be present. Although the portal tract shows varying degrees of expansion, limiting plate necrosis ("interface hepatitis," "piecemeal necrosis") is often minimal and focal with relatively few cells spilling into the sinusoids

TABLE 9.6	Obsolete and Accepted Nomenclature for Histologic Patterns of Chronic Hepatitis	
Obsolete Term	**Currently Accepted Term**
Chronic persistent hepatitis	Portal hepatitis
Chronic lobular hepatitis	Lobular hepatitis
Chronic active hepatitis	Periportal, or interface, hepatitis

(Fig. 9.2, e-Figs. 9.1, 9.3–9.5). Minimal portal tract fibrosis, including an occasional narrow fibrous extension into the lobule, best visualized with reticulin stain rather than trichrome, is consistent with this diagnosis (Fig. 9.3). This pattern is typical of mild chronic hepatitis C.

The term "chronic lobular hepatitis" was used to describe varying degrees of scattered parenchymal (spotty) necrosis with little or no portal infiltration and no or slight interface hepatitis (Fig. 9.4). The architecture is generally well maintained except for areas of liver cell dropout where liver cells are no longer present. Hepatocyte injury may be seen as individual cell ballooning and acidophilic bodies. Reticulin stain helps demonstrate foci of dropout as well as reticulin collapse (Fig. 9.5). Sinusoidal lining cells are hyperplastic, and Kupffer cells may contain phagocytosed ceroidlike material. Cell loss may be accompanied by focal regenerative activity with thickened liver plates, also best seen with reticulin stain. Histologically, the features can be similar to acute viral hepatitis. The "lobular hepatitis" pattern of inflammation is often seen with recurrent hepatitis C developing relative early after liver transplantation (e-Figs. 9.11–9.13).

Interface hepatitis ("piecemeal necrosis") can be prominent. Inflammatory cells, usually lymphocytes, extend beyond the portal tract with mild destruction of limiting plate hepatocytes and can go farther into the lobule (Fig. 9.6). The term for this histologic picture is *periportal hepatitis* or *interface hepatitis*. Fibroblastic activity, and even collagen, can be seen at this time. Lobular necrosis, which can connect architecturally distinct structures (portal-to-central necrosis, portal-to-portal necrosis; i.e., bridging necrosis), may be apparent (Fig. 9.7, e-Figs. 9.35–9.39) (18,24). Acidophilic bodies are usually easily seen, and sinusoidal cells are prominent. Bile duct injury occurs (e-Fig. 9.5).

Interface hepatitis does not occur uniformly throughout the liver and varies, with some portal tracts not showing this change. Suboptimal biopsies may have unchanged architecture or only minimal portal inflammation although the patient may be quite ill with significant increase of transaminase values. The interface hepatitis activity and the absence or presence of bridging inflammation define chronic hepatitis as mild to severe (13,35,49).

Kupffer cell hyperplasia is usually moderate and less than that seen in acute viral hepatitis. Early fibrosis beginning at the portal tract–lobule interface is seen earliest with reticulin. The evaluation of fibrosis limited to the portal tract only, without even minimal extension into the lobule, is highly inconsistent and should be ignored, except when the portal architecture is clearly altered (e-Fig. 20.14).

Segmental injury of the interlobar bile ducts, manifesting as vacuolization, frank necrosis, and lymphocytic infiltration, is seen in chronic HCV and is distinctly unusual in chronic HBV. Bile duct injury, generally more pronounced, is characteristic of primary biliary cirrhosis and autoimmune cholangitis but can also be seen in autoimmune hepatitis and chronic hepatitis C.

Liver cell regeneration is a characteristic, albeit sometimes subtle without reticulin stain, component of the histologic picture of chronic hepatitis (Fig. 9.8) (29). Liver cell plates can be two or more cells thick. There may be significant nuclear anisocytosis, including many binucleate hepatocytes, and occasionally multinucleate giant hepatocytes. The regenerative activity is irregularly distributed and in some areas can form distinct nodules resembling those of fully developed cirrhosis, but often without fibrosis. The regenerating cells can form acinuslike structures (rosettes). This phenomenon occurs more often in autoimmune hepatitis (e-Fig. 10.4) and is most prominent in the periportal (zone 1) area. Zone 3 (centrolobular) necrosis has been described in patients with chronic hepatitis presumed to be autoimmune after steroid therapy but has not been described in those with chronic viral hepatitis.

Hepatitis C patients likely undergo periodic episodes of lobular necrosis, consistent with recognized biochemical test value fluctuations (8). Sometimes, even with an adequate biopsy, liver cell necrosis may be absent despite documented transaminase value elevations. This sometimes reflects the waxing and waning nature of hepatitis C and the time delay between testing and biopsy. In many cases, PAS with diastase will show prominent Kupffer cells and portal macrophages, evidence of phagocytosis of recently necrotic liver cells.

Systems for Grading and Staging Chronic Hepatitis

Scheuer reviewed the problems with the early chronic hepatitis classifications (58–61). For example, the high virus replicative stage of beginning chronic hepatitis B, when hepatitis B early antigen and high levels of serum hepatitis B virus (HBV) DNA are demonstrable, may vary greatly in histologic appearance; there may be mild "chronic active hepatitis," "chronic lobular hepatitis," or even "chronic persistent hepatitis" (60). In the stage of seroconversion, with anti–hepatitis B early antigen appearing in the serum, severe chronic hepatitis with considerable lobular activity is generally seen, but there may be "chronic active hepatitis" or "chronic persistent hepatitis" with either virus reactivation or superinfection with another virus, such as hepatitis delta virus (HDV). Finally, if cirrhosis develops, the inflammatory component may disappear entirely.

Coupled with the principal responsibility of the pathologist to establish the correct diagnosis is the need for clear communication, wherever possible, of that diagnosis and its significance for prognosis and potential therapy. Various numerical grading and staging systems have been proposed, including Knodell in 1981 (36), Scheuer in 1991 (58), Batts–Ludwig in 1995 (5), Ishak in 1995 (35), and METAVIR in 1996 (7), some relatively complex (Knodell, Ishak), intermediate in difficulty of usage (METAVIR), and relatively simple (Scheuer, Batts–Ludwig) (Table 9.7). In general, complex systems have more interobserver variability (31,46). Several investigators have also proposed using English language principally and scoring systems for research; this is discussed below.

TABLE 9.7	Comparison of Grading and Staging Scores in Various Systems

1. Conventional verbal
2. Knodell—grade 0–18, stage 0, 1, 3, or 4
3. Ishak—grade 0–18, stage 0–6
4. METAVIR—grade 1–3, stage 1–4
5. Scheuer—grade 0–8, stage 0–4
6. Modified Scheuer—portal/periportal grade 0–4, lobular grade 0–4, stage 0–4
7. Batts–Ludwig—grade 0–4, stage 0–4

Summaries of the advantages and disadvantages of the various scoring systems presented are in Table 9.8.

KNODELL CLASSIFICATION. The Knodell classification of 1981 was developed to facilitate a research study and was not primarily intended for clinical use (36). This classification evaluates separately the degree of inflammation,

TABLE 9.8 Comparative Advantages and Disadvantages of Grading/Staging Systems

	Advantages	Disadvantages
Knodell	Detail Excellent for research	Single score can represent varied histopathology Varied reproducibility
Ishak	Detail Excellent for research. Grading fairly reproducible "Confluent necrosis" and "developing cirrhosis" delineated	Scoring can represent varied histopathology Varied reproducibility
Scheuer	Simple, with optimal reproducibility Recognizes importance of interface hepatitis	Staging terminology not completely clear
METAVIR	Relatively simple, with relatively good reproducibility	Gap between stage 3 and 4 as defined Algorithm approach required
Batts–Ludwig	Relatively simple, with good reproducibility Diagrams	Staging terminology not completely clear

necrosis, fibrosis, and architectural distortion in a semiquantitative manner to prepare a histologic activity index for chronic hepatitis. The individual component scores are added to produce the overall activity score, combining necroinflammatory activity parameters (inflammation and necrosis) with the effects of that activity (fibrosis and architectural distortion), and also assesses interface hepatitis (piecemeal necrosis) and bridging necrosis together (6). Two patients can have major differences in histopathology and end up with the same score.

Ishak modified Knodell to develop a histologic activity index with separate scores for interface hepatitis, confluent necrosis, lobular necrosis, and inflammation, as well as portal inflammation, to develop a numeric index (34,35). The system is fairly detailed and potentially allows for increased consistency between observers. Similar to the Knodell system, two patients can vary considerable in histopathology and have similar scores.

Batts–Ludwig (5) is a modification of the Scheuer system (63) using slightly varied definitions. It is relatively straightforward, and the original Batts–Ludwig publication offers diagrams as aids. The METAVIR system (7) is slightly more complicated but has been widely used in clinical trials.

Recommended Approach

There is no universally accepted single system for evaluating chronic hepatitis. Some of the problems with the major systems have been recently reviewed (3,11,12,19,26,38,69). It is still acceptable to use English language terms to convey the key diagnostic message about grade and stage of chronic hepatitis rather than numeric scores, as long as the approach communicates sufficient and appropriate information to the treating physician (Table 9.9). The liver biopsy report should indicate (a) the presence or

TABLE 9.9	Chronic Hepatitis Inflammatory Grade Definitions		
Grade	Interface Hepatitis	Lobular Activity[a]	Overall Activity
Mild	Spotty May be rare, especially in small samples	Spotty, uncommon (<5/low power field[b])	Both interface and lobular activity are mild or less
Moderate	Most portal areas have some, but usually <50% of circumference	5–20/lpf	Either interface or lobular activity is moderate, or both
Marked	>50% circumference of most portal areas	>20/lpf	Either interface hepatitis or lobular activity is marked, or both

[a]Acidophilic (apoptotic) bodies, ballooned cells, inflammatory cell aggregates.
[b]10× objective, 10× ocular.

TABLE 9.10	**Four Elements of Verbal Diagnosis**

1. Diagnosis—i.e., "chronic hepatitis"
2. Grade—mild, moderate, marked inflammation
3. Stage—e.g., "without fibrosis," "with mild portal/periportal fibrosis," "bridging fibrosis," "cirrhosis"
4. Etiology—e.g., "consistent with chronic hepatitis C," "consistent with autoimmune hepatitis," "because of hepatitis B" (when ground-glass cells are present)

absence of chronic hepatitis (i.e., the principal diagnosis of the case), (b) the grade of inflammation, (c) the stage of injury and chronicity, and, wherever possible, (d) the cause (Table 9.10). If a recognized scoring system is used, the definitions should be included in the report for accurate and consistent interpretation.

GRADE. Grade refers to the degree of inflammation. The grade is mild if the histologic picture is that of traditional chronic persistent hepatitis, even if there is some interface hepatitis and lobular inflammation (Fig. 9.2, e-Figs. 9.1–9.4). With more marked interface hepatitis, including extension of the inflammatory process as much as half way into the lobule, the grade is moderate (Fig. 9.6, e-Fig. 9.40). Severe degrees of inflammation, including bridging necrosis, are characterized as severe (Fig. 9.7, e-Fig. 9.37).

STAGE. Stage refers to the degree of fibrosis, which represents relatively permanent architectural injury, potentially reversible with therapy. Early fibrosis is recognized with the reticulin stain. Trichrome or a comparable connective tissue stain, however, is the standard. If fibrosis is determined solely with trichrome method for demonstrating collagen, the stage can be mild, with early fibrosis involving only zone 1 of the acinus (Fig. 9.3); moderate, with fibrosis extending into zone 2 of the lobule; or marked, with fibrosis connecting otherwise separate architectural regions. In practice, moderate fibrosis is rarely recognized and is seen less often than cirrhosis.

We use English language reporting followed by scoring with a modified Scheuer system (Table 9.11). Examples of reports are as follows: "chronic hepatitis, mild inflammatory grade, with minimal portal and periportal fibrosis, consistent with chronic hepatitis C" (Fig. 9.1); "chronic hepatitis, moderate inflammatory grade, with foci of bridging fibrosis, consistent with chronic hepatitis C"; and "chronic hepatitis, severe, with extensive bridging necrosis and moderate portal and periportal fibrosis, caused by hepatitis B, with demonstrable hepatitis B surface and core antigens" (Fig. 9.7).

NONINVASIVE GRADING AND STAGING. Biochemical panels have been developed and imaging methods applied to try to preclude the need for liver

TABLE 9.11	Modified Scheuer Histologic Scoring System			
Grade	Portal/Periportal	Lobule	Stage	Degree
0	None or minimal portal without periportal (interface)	None	0	None
1	Portal inflammation without periportal	Inflammation but no liver cell necrosis	1	Minimal portal fibrosis with extension into lobule seen only with reticulin
2	Mild (spotty) periportal (limiting plate) inflammation	Focal or unicellular necrosis	2	Early periportal fibrosis or rare portal–portal septa with intact architecture
3	Moderate portal/ periportal inflammation, usually <50% of limiting plate	More extensive necrosis, but no or minimal bridging	3	Septal fibrosis with architectural distortion, including nodule formation but not cirrhosis
4	Severe periportal and bridging inflammation	Extensive necrosis including multifocal bridging	4	Probably or definitely cirrhosis

biopsy (40,45,48,52,64,65). In general, these work well when there is cirrhosis but provide lesser accuracy for earlier stages. Further refinements will be necessary before these approaches can replace liver biopsy (59). Table 9.12 lists some considerations in studying the chronic hepatitis liver biopsy.

What histologic information is needed in deciding to treat?

The drugs currently used to treat chronic hepatitis C are α-interferon and ribavirin. Treatment is often applied for 1 to 2 years, is quite expensive, and may have significant detrimental side effects. A full discussion about treatment is beyond the scope of this text, and there are varying guidelines depending on other factors including age and coexisting medical conditions. Sometimes treatment is applied even for patients already cirrhotic to try to slow the progress of disease. As a general statement, however, the decision to treat is often based on whether or not fibrosis is present. Treatment is not applied if there is no fibrosis. The lower the fibrosis score, the better the response. Consequently, of course, accurate staging and

TABLE 9.12	**Chronic Hepatitis Caveats**

1. Adequate tissue is necessary
   a. 14- or 16-gauge needle
   b. ≥2.0 cm
   c. ≥10 complete portal tracts
2. Histology is not always unequivocally diagnostic
   a. Direct communication with clinician is often quite useful for patient, for clinician, and for pathologist
   b. Clinical-pathologic correlation is vital
   c. Sampling variability is common
   d. Interobserver variability is common
3. Portal inflammation, without interface or lobular hepatitis, is not diagnostic of chronic hepatitis if the specimen is adequate (≥10 portal tracts)
   a. The amount of inflammatory cells within the portal tract is not important; interface and lobular hepatitis are more important in the biopsy evaluation
4. Fibrosis/cirrhosis is overinterpreted
   a. Trichrome technique varies and overstaining is common
      i. Reticulin stain
   b. Misinterpreted as cirrhosis
      i. Hepatic vein, in transjugular biopsies, sometimes misinterpreted
      ii. Liver capsule is commonly inadvertently sampled
      iii. Left lobe becomes increasingly fibrotic with age
5. Scoring systems are imperfect
6. If using a scoring system, identify (e.g., Ishak, METAVIR, Scheuer, etc)
7. Non-invasive testing is not yet accurate enough for widespread application

appropriate communication is critical. The histopathologic findings that are associated with more rapid progression to cirrhosis in chronic hepatitis C are bridging necrosis (uncommon in HCV) and fibrosis, even mild, on first biopsy. The significance of interface hepatitis, mild lobular inflammation and necrosis (acidophilic bodies) is less clear.

Should scoring be used for all reports?

Semiquantitative scoring was devised as a research aid. Scoring is particularly useful for evaluation of study material, as in clinical trials, where the METAVIR system is often used. Sometimes scoring is useful when comparing two or more biopsies from the same patient. Scoring is not the standard of care for the general practice of pathology but is most likely used in all larger medical centers. There is both interobserver and intraobserver variability and, ideally, the actual biopsy material should be reviewed by the pathologist most closely working with the responsible clinician, rather than relying on a numerical score.

REFERENCES

1. Bach N, Thung SN, Schaffner F. The histologic features of chronic hepatitis C and autoimmune hepatitis: a comparative analysis. Hepatology 1992;15:572–577.
2. Banner BF, Allan C, Savas L, et al. Inflammatory markers in chronic hepatitis C. Virchows Arch 1997;431:181–187.
3. Banner BF, Barton AL, Cole EE, et al. A detailed analysis of the Knodell score and other histologic parameters as predictors of response to interferon therapy in chronic hepatitis C. Mod Pathol 1995;8:232–238.
4. Barton Al, Banner BF, Cable EE, et al. Distribution of iron in the liver predicts the response of chronic hepatitis C infection to interferon therapy. Am J Clin Pathol 1995; 103:419–424.
5. Batts KP, Ludwig J. Chronic hepatitis. An update in terminology and reporting. Am J Surg Pathol 1995;19:1409–1417.
6. Bedossa P, Bioulac-Sage P, Callard P, et al. Intraobserver and interobserver variations in liver biopsy interpretation in patients with chronic hepatitis C. Hepatology 1994;20: 15–20.
7. Bedossa P, Poynard T. An algorithm for the grading of activity in chronic hepatitis C. Hepatology 1996;24:289–293.
8. Bedossa P, Dargere D, Paradis V. Sampling variability of liver fibrosis in chronic hepatitis C. Hepatology 2003;38:1149–1157.
9. Bierhoff E, Fischer HP, Willsch E, et al. Liver histopathology in patients with concurrent chronic hepatitis C and HIV infection. Virchows Arch 1997;430:271–277.
10. Booth JC, Foster GR, Levine T, et al. The relationship of histology to genotype in chronic HCV infection. Liver 1997;17:144–151.
11. Brunt EM. Grading and staging the histopathological lesions of chronic hepatitis: the Knodell histology activity and beyond. Hepatology 2000;31:241–246.
12. Callea F, Baronchelli C, Rodolfi A, et al. Histopathology of chronic viral hepatitis: guidelines for a revised classification. Ital J Gastroenterol 1995;27:137–140.
13. Chen TJ, Liaw YF. The prognostic significance of bridging hepatic necrosis in chronic type B hepatitis: a histopathologic study. Liver 1988;8:10–16.
14. Cholangitas E, Senzelo M, Standish R, et al. A systematic review of the quality of liver biopsies. Am J Clin Pathol 2006;125:710–721.
15. Choo QL, Kuo G, Weiner AJ, et al. Isolation of a cDNA clone derived from a blood-borne non-A, non-B viral hepatitis genome. Science 1989;244:359–362.
16. Davies SE, Lau JYN, O'Grady JG, et al. Evidence that hepatitis D virus needs hepatitis B virus to cause hepatocellular damage. Am J Clin Pathol 1992;98:554–558.
17. Desmet VJ, Gerber MA, Hoofnagle JH, et al. Classification of chronic hepatitis: diagnosis, grading and staging. Hepatology 1994;9:1513–1520.
18. Dickson RC, Gaffey MJ, Ishitani MB, et al. The international autoimmune hepatitis score in chronic hepatitis C. J Viral Hepatol 1997;4:121–128.
19. Ferrell L. Nomenclature of chronic hepatitis: the new look. In: Fechner RE, Rosen PP, eds. Anatomic Pathology. Chicago: ASCP Press, 1997:21–33.
20. Fong TL, Lee SR, Kim JP, et al. Prevalence of hepatitis C among intravenous drug abusers in Los Angeles. Clin Infect Dis 1997;25:165–166.
21. Fontaine H, Nalpas B, Poulet B, et al. Hepatitis activity index is a key factor in determining the natural history of chronic hepatitis C. Hum Pathol 2001;32:904–909.

22. Geller SA, Nichols WS, Rojter SE, et al. Hepatitis C virus is not recoverable from liver tissue in cryptogenic cirrhosis: failure to identify hepatitis C virus-RNA using reverse transcription–mediated polymerase chain reaction. Hum Pathol 1996;27:1161–1165.

23. Geller SA. Hepatitis B and hepatitis C. Clin Liver Dis 2002;6:317–334.

24. Gerber MA. Chronic hepatitis C: the beginning of the end for a time-honored nomenclature? Hepatology 1992;15:733–734.

25. Goldin RD, Goldin JG, Burt AD, et al. Intra-observer and inter-observer variation in the histopathological assessment of chronic viral hepatitis. J Hepatol 1996;25:649–654.

26. Goodman ZD. Grading and staging system for inflammation and fibrosis in chronic liver disease. J Hepatol 2007;47:598–607.

27. Guido M, Rugge M. Liver biopsy sampling in chronic viral hepatitis. Semin Liv Dis 2004;24:89–97.

28. Hakozaki Y, Shirahama T, Katou M, et al. Long-term prognosis of chronic hepatitis C after treatment with interferon alpha 2b and characterization of incomplete responders. Am J Gastroenterol 1996;91:2144–2149.

29. Hall PDLM. Chronic hepatitis: an update with guidelines for histopathological assessment of liver biopsies. Pathology 1998;30:369–380.

30. Haque S, Chandra B, Gerber MA, et al. Iron overload in patients with chronic hepatitis C: a clinicopathologic study. Hum Pathol 1996;27:1277–1281.

31. Hunt N, Fleming K. Reproducibility of liver biopsy grading and staging. Liver 1999;19: 169–170.

32. International group. A classification of chronic hepatitis. Lancet 1968;2:626–628.

33. International group. Acute and chronic hepatitis revisited. Lancet 1977;2:914–919.

34. Ishak KG. Chronic hepatitis: morphology and nomenclature. Mod Pathol 1994;7:690–713.

35. Ishak KG, Baptista A, Bianchi L, et al. Histological grading and staging of chronic hepatitis. J Hepatol 1995;22:696–699.

36. Knodell RG, Ishak KG, Black WC, et al. Formulation and application of a numerical scoring system for assessing histological activity in asymptomatic chronic active hepatitis. Hepatology 1981;1:431–435.

37. Kuo G, Choo QL, Alter HJ, et al. An assay for circulating antibodies to a major etiologic virus of human non-A, non-B hepatitis. Science 1989;244:362–364.

38. Lefkowitch JH. Liver biopsy assessment in chronic hepatitis. Arh Med Res 2007;38: 634–643.

39. Lok ASK, Lindsay I, Scheuer PJ, et al. Clinical and histological features of delta infection in chronic hepatitis B virus carriers. J Clin Pathol 1985;38:530–535.

40. Lu LG, Zeng AD, Wan MB, et al. Grading and staging of hepatic fibrosis and its relationship with noninvasive diagnostic parameters. World J Gastroenterol 2003;9: 2574–2578.

41. Ludwig J. The nomenclature of chronic active hepatitis: an obituary. Gastroenterology 1993;105:274–278.

42. METAVIR Cooperative Study Group. Intraobserver and interobserver variations in liver biopsy interpretations in patients with chronic hepatitis C. The French METAVIR Cooperative Study Group. Hepatology 1994;20:15–20.

43. Mihm S, Fayyazi A, Hartmann H, et al. Analysis of histopathological manifestations of chronic hepatitis C virus infection with respect to virus genotype. Hepatology 1997;25: 735–739.

44. Monjardina JP, Saldanha JA. Delta hepatitis. Br Med Bull 1990;46:399–407.

45. Morra R, Munteanu M, Bedossa P, et al. Diagnostic value of serum protein profiling by SELDI-TOF ProteinChip compared with a biochemical marker, FibroTest, for the diagnosis of advanced fibrosis in patients with chronic hepatitis C. Aliment Pharmacol Ther 2007;26:847–858.

46. Netto GJ, Watkins DL, Williams JW, et al. Interobserver agreement in hepatitis C grading and staging and in the Banff grading scheme for acute cellular rejection: the "hepatitis C" multi-institutional trial experience. Arch Pathol Lab Med 2006;130:1157–1163.

47. Olynyk JK, Reddy KR, Di Bisceglie AM, et al. Hepatic iron concentration as a predictor of response to interferon alfa therapy in chronic hepatitis C. Gastroenterology 1995; 108:1104–1109.

48. Pan JJ, Yang CF, Chu CJ, et al. Prediction of liver fibrosis in patients with chronic hepatitis B by serum markers. Hepatogastroenterology 2007;54:1503–1506.

49. Paradis V, Mathurin P, Laurent A, et al. Histological features predictive of liver fibrosis in chronic hepatitis C infection. J Clin Pathol 1996;49:998–1004.

50. Petrovic LM, Villamil FG, Vierling JM, et al. Comparison of histopathology in acute allograft rejection and recurrent hepatitis C infection after liver transplantation. Liver Transpl Surg 1997;3:398–406.

51. Popper H. Schaffner F. The vocabulary of chronic hepatitis. N Engl J Med 1971;284: 1154–1156.

52. Poynard T, Munteanu M, Imbert-Bismut F, et al. Prospective analysis of discordant results between biochemical markers and biopsy in patients with chronic hepatitis C. Clin Chem 2004;50:1344–1355.

53. Realdi G, Alberti A, Rugge M, et al. Long-term follow-up of acute and chronic non-A, non-B post-transfusion hepatitis; evidence of progression to liver cirrhosis. Gut 1982;23:270–275.

54. Regev A, Berho M, Jeffers LJ, et al. Sampling error and interobserver variation in liver biopsy in patients with chronic HCV infection. Am J Gastroenterol 2002;97:2614–2618.

55. Rizzetto M. The delta agent. Hepatology 1983;3:729–734.

56. Rousselet MC, Michalak S, Dupré F, et al. Sources of variability in histological scoring or chronic viral hepatitis. Hepatology 2005;4:257–264.

57. Scheuer PJ, Ashrafzadeh P, Sherlock S, et al. The pathology of hepatitis C. Hepatology 1992;15:567–571.

58. Scheuer PJ. Classification of chronic viral hepatitis: a need for reassessment. J Hepatol 1991;13:372–374.

59. Scheuer PJ. The nomenclature of chronic hepatitis: time for a change. J Hepatol 1995;22: 112–114.

60. Scheuer PJ. Histopathological aspects of viral hepatitis. J Viral Hepatol 1996;3:277–283.

61. Scheuer PJ. Scoring of liver biopsies: are we doing it right? Eur J Gastroenterol Hepatol 1996;8:1141–1143.

62. Scheuer PJ. Chronic hepatitis: what is activity and how should it be assessed? Histopathology 1997;30:103–105.

63. Scheuer PJ, Krawczynski K, Dhillon AP. Histopathology and detection of hepatitis C virus in liver. Springer Semin Immunopathol 1997;19:27–45.

64. Schiavon LL, Schiavon JL, Filho RJ, et al. Simple blood tests as noninvasive makers of liver fibrosis in hemodialysis patients with chronic hepatitis C infection. Hepatology 2007;46:307–314.

65. Scripenova S, Trainer TD, Krawitt El, et al. Diagnostic value of serum markers of connective tissue turnover for predicting histology staging and grading in patients with chronic hepatitis C. J Clin Pathol 2007;60:321–324.

66. Shaheen AA, Wan AF, Meuers RP. FibroTest and FibroScan for the prediction of hepatitis C-related fibrosis: a systematic review of diagnostic test accuracy. Am J Gastroenterol 2007;102:2589–2600.

67. Sherman KE, Goodman ZD, Sullivan ST, et al. Liver biopsy in cirrhotic patients. Am J Gastroenterol 2007;102:789–793.

68. Suzuki K, Uchida T, Shikata T. Histopathological analysis of chronic hepatitis B virus (HBV) infection in relation to HBV replication. Liver 1987;7:260–270.

69. Theise ND. Liver biopsy assessment in chronic viral hepatitis: a personal, practical approach. Mod Pathol 2007;20:S3–S14.

70. Tran TT, Changsri C, Shackleton CR, et al. Living donor liver transplantation: histological abnormalities found on liver biopsies of apparently healthy potential donors. J Gastroenterol Hepatol 2006;21:381–383.

71. Yang JF, Dai CY, Chuang WL, et al. Prevalence and clinical significance of HGV/GBV-C infection in patients with chronic hepatitis B or C. Jpn J Infect Dis 2006;59:25–30.

10

AUTOIMMUNE HEPATITIS AND RELATED DISORDERS

The syndrome of autoimmune hepatitis (AIH) (Table 10.1) was recognized in the 1950s in young women, with hypergammaglobulinemia, acnelike skin rashes, myalgia, amenorrhea, liver disease (including hepatomegaly and splenomegaly), and a fluctuating course (13,26,33). The term "lupoid hepatitis" was adopted to distinguish AIH from systemic lupus erythematosus (LE) because some patients had circulating LE cells (25), antinuclear antibodies (ANAs) in the sera, and other serologic abnormalities, including the presence of antibodies directed against smooth muscle antibody (SMA). However, the term has appropriately been abandoned because an LE test is positive in fewer than 20% of patients and because liver involvement is distinctly unusual in classical systemic lupus erythematosus.

Autoimmune mechanisms contribute to injury in many liver diseases (47), including acute and chronic hepatitis caused by hepatitis A, B, and C viruses, primary biliary cirrhosis (PBC), primary sclerosing cholangitis (PSC), and drug-induced chronic hepatitis (6,41,44), but also in alcoholic liver disease, Wilson disease, and perhaps α1-antitrypsin deficiency. However, the autoimmune liver diseases are principally thought of as (a) AIH (e-Figs. 10.1–10.16), (b) primary biliary cirrhosis (PBC), (c) primary sclerosing cholangitis (PSC), (d) drug-induced/associated autoimmune hepatitis (e-Figs. 10.17–10.20), and, in recent years, (e) autoimmune cholangiopathy (e-Figs. 10.21–10.29). In addition, some patients have (f) "overlap syndrome," with combined clinical and/or serologic features of AIH and one of the cholangiopathies (e-Figs. 10.30–10.32) (4,58). AIH can recur after transplantation (e-Figs. 10.33–10.36). In recent years the development of AIH has been recognized in individuals who had undergone liver transplantation for other reasons ("de novo autoimmune hepatitis") (e-Fig. 10.37–10.41) (26).

AUTOIMMUNE HEPATITIS

The term "autoimmune chronic active hepatitis" is no longer used because "autoimmune" and "chronic" are redundant terms and, more important,

TABLE 10.1	Synonyms for Autoimmune Hepatitis
Lupoid hepatitis	
Plasma cell hepatitis	
Active chronic hepatitis	
Chronic liver disease in young women	
Active juvenile cirrhosis	
Dysproteinemic cirrhosis of unknown origin in young women	
Autoimmune chronic hepatitis	
Autoimmune chronic active hepatitis	

because AIH may present as an acute, or occasionally fulminant, disorder difficult to distinguish from acute viral hepatitis (3,8,16,17,27). Also, biopsy does not always show typical features of chronic active hepatitis (3).

The usual patient is a young woman, 15 to 35, or perimenopausal. Men and children of both sexes may be affected (9,26). More than 50% of patients present with episodic jaundice, anorexia, and fatigue, and premenopausal women are often amenorrheic. Epistaxis, bleeding gums, and easy bruisability, as well as right upper quadrant abdominal pain and tenderness occur. As many as 20% are febrile. Many patients present with advanced disease, including cirrhosis and portal hypertension. Rarely, AIH may be asymptomatic at discovery. Various extrahepatic manifestations (e.g., thyroiditis, vasculitis, uveitis, ulcerative colitis (26,41), arthritis, Coombs-positive hemolytic anemia, glomerulonephritis, neuropathy, vitiligo (43), alopecia (43), mixed connective tissue disorders, and pneumonitis are seen. An international panel established diagnostic criteria (Table 10.2) (1,25).

AIH is fatal if untreated. The typical patient responds to corticosteroid therapy, with improvement in symptoms and normalization of laboratory test results, but often, the histologic picture may not change and the disease may progress. Fibrosis can decrease (44). With treatment, the 5-year survival is approximately 85%. Patients with liver–kidney microsomal (LKM) antibody–positive disease may have a somewhat poorer prognosis (23). Death is generally due to cirrhotic hepatocellular failure with bleeding esophageal varices or end stage liver disease. Rarely death may follow a fulminant hepatitis–like course. Other causes of death include sepsis and hepatocellular carcinoma. AIH may recur after liver transplantation (14,38) and may also occur in patients who have been transplanted for other diseases (de novo AIH) (26,58).

Genetics

There is a relationship between AIH and certain human leukocyte antigens (HLAs) (12,13). HLA A1-B8-DR3 and DR4 have strong, and probably independent, associations (18,23,36,61). Familial occurrence is distinctly

TABLE 10.2	International Autoimmune Hepatitis Group Scoring (Modified)
Positive Weighting	**Negative Weighting**
Low alkaline phosphatase (ALP): AST (or ALT) ratio	High ALP:AST (or ALT) ratio
Hypergammaglobulinemia	Anti–mitochondrial antibody (AMA)[+]
Autoantibody[a]	—
Negative viral serology	Positive viral serology
Negative drug history	Positive drug history[a]
Low alcohol consumption	High alcohol consumption
Interface hepatitis on biopsy	Bile duct damage on biopsy[b]
Concurrent immunologic disorders, patient or family	Incompatible histopathologic changes
Positive for relevant HLA haplotypes	
Positive treatment response	

[a]AIH can develop after use of some medications.
[b]Mild bile duct injury can be seen in AIH.

unusual (9,22). However, first-degree relatives may demonstrate circulating ANAs, SMAs, and antimitochondrial antibodies (AMAs). An increased familial incidence of C4 deficiency in relatives of children with AIH has been shown and a familial reduction in suppressor T-cell activity in AIH patients who express the HLA B8-DR3 haplotype.

Mechanisms of Injury

Predominantly an antibody-dependent cytotoxic cellular reaction, the immune response is most likely activated by helper T lymphocytes and mediated by K lymphocytes elaborating an antibody directed against antigens at the hepatocyte surface, with the probable involvement of cytokines, including tumor necrosis factor (TNF) and interferon-g (24). The lymphocytes may directly stimulate the production of autoantibodies (30). Cell injury could also be independent of antigen-specific mechanisms, as a kind of defective immune response to the hepatocyte that is triggered by various infections. For example, P450IID6, the putative antigen against which LKM-1 antibody is thought to act, is not on the surface of the hepatocyte and consequently is not exposed to possible antibody-mediated cell lysis. Infectious agents implicated as potential initiators of the defective immune response have been enterobacteria, rubeola, rubella, and cytomegalovirus, in addition to hepatitis C virus (HCV). Medications have also been associated (44).

Laboratory Tests

The serum levels of transaminases, aspartate aminotransferase (AST), and alanine aminotransferase (ALT) are generally moderately elevated, with

AST values generally between 200 and 1,000 U. Bilirubin and alkaline phosphatase values may also be moderately elevated. Most patients demonstrate polyclonal hypergammaglobulinemia, with levels as high as 50 to 70 g/L, as well as abnormal serum copper and ceruloplasmin values.

Autoantibodies

Various circulating autoantibodies have been found (1,16,26). The identification of specific antibodies has led to the recognition of clinically, as well as serologically, distinct groups. The most intensely studied autoantibodies are listed in Table 10.3. The demonstration of SMAs (70%) and/or ANAs (50%) is classic in AIH. Fewer than 20% have AMAs, many (? all) of these as overlap. These intracellular target antigens may not be exposed to the immune effector mechanisms thought responsible for AIH. Antibodies react with P450IID6 (19,36,46,60), and LKM-2 with P450IIC11. Thus far, there is no conclusive evidence that any AIH-associated autoantibodies directly contribute to the development of AIH. Antibodies directed against gastric parietal cells and against thyroid may also be found in AIH patients.

TABLE 10.3	Autoantibodies Described in Association with Autoimmune Hepatitis
Antibody	**Target or Putative Target**
Organ nonspecific	
Anti-LKM	Liver–kidney microsomes
Anti-LP	Liver–pancreas antigen
Antimitochondrial (AMA)	Mitochondria
Antinuclear (ANA)	Nuclei
Antineutrophil cytoplasmic (ANCA)	Neutrophil cytoplasmic antigens
Smooth muscle (SMA)	Smooth muscle
Organ specific	
Anti-ASGP-R	Hepatic asialoglycoprotein receptor
Anti-GOR	Fusion protein expressed by a cDNA clone of hepatitis C virus
Anti-HHPM	Human hepatocyte plasma membrane antigen
Anti-LC1	Liver cytosolic antigen 1
Anti-LSP	Liver-specific membrane lipoprotein
Anti-SLA	Soluble liver antigen (cytokeratins 8 and 18)
HMA	Hepatocyte membrane

Antineutrophil cytoplasmic antibodies (ANCAs), autoantibodies reacting with neutrophil cytoplasmic antigens, are demonstrable in AIH and PSC, but not PBC, chronic hepatitis as a result of HBV or HCV, or other liver disorders (20,28). Various "liver-specific" antibodies have been evaluated, the most important of which are those directed against liver and kidney microsomes, including variants against different cytochrome P450 components in smooth endoplasmic reticulum, with at least five related antibodies (54). Some AIH patients have anti-LKM-1 (16), the most widely studied of the LKM antibodies, which is directed against cytochrome P450s from the IID subfamily (35). It is also in sera of HCV-infected patients (43), but the antigenic sites recognized by the sera from patients with HCV differ from those recognized by sera from patients with AIH (61).

Classification

Four AIH subgroups can be distinguished (16,26,38) (Table 10.4).

Type 1 is the classical and most common form (e-Figs. 10.1–10.16) (25), characterized by the demonstration of SMA and ANA in the serum.

Type 2 AIH patients have LKM antibodies but not ANAs. LKM-associated AIH is uncommon in the United States (e-Fig. 10.42–10.44). Two subgroups have been recognized (Table 10.5). One resembles type 1 AIH, with typical histologic findings. A more common subgroup also has antibodies to HCV, as well as antibodies to GOR, suggesting previous infection with HCV (16). HCV may induce autoimmune antibodies to both GOR and LKM-1 usually in Mediterranean men. Liver biopsy findings resemble those of hepatitis C.

Two other AIH subtypes are rare. Patients with type 3 have antibodies against soluble liver antigens (SLAs) and AMAs, and sometimes SMAs (40). Type 4 occurs principally in children who demonstrate high SMA titers, but without SLA or AMA (38).

TABLE 10.4	Classification of Autoimmune Hepatitis			
Antibody	Type I	Type II	Type III	Type IV
ANA	+	−	−	−
SMA	+	−	+/−	+
AMA	−	−	+	−
LKM	−	+[a]	−	−
SLA	+	+	+	−
anti-LC1	−	+	−	−
anti-GOR	−	+[a]	−	−

[a]Possibly induced by prior infection with hepatitis C virus.
ANA, antinuclear antibody; SMA, smooth muscle antibody; AMA, antimitochondrial antibody; LKM, liver–kidney microsomal (antibody); SLA, soluble liver antibody; LC1, liver cytosolic antigen 1.

TABLE 10.5	**LKM-Positive Autoimmune Hepatitis**		
Group	Characteristics	Geography	Biopsy
1	Young	England	Plasma cells
	Women		Rosettes
	Other immune disorders		Interface hepatitis
	Steroid responsive		Bridging necrosis
2	Older	Mediterranean	Interlobular infiltrate
	Male > female		Lymphoid aggregates
	Low titers of anti-LKM		Fat
	Anti-GOR positive		Bile duct lesions
	HCV-RIBA positive		—
	? response to interferon-α		—

LKM, liver–kidney microsomal (antibody); HCV, hepatitis C virus; RIBA, recombinant immunoblot assay.

Pathology

AIH is a progressive disease (Fig. 10.1, e-Figs. 10.4–10.9) that, if untreated, progresses inexorably from the early, inflammatory stages to cirrhosis.

Liver biopsy findings are not specifically diagnostic. In spite of this, liver biopsy can be useful in cases in which the diagnosis has not been clinically established. In general, the biopsy shows the picture of chronic hepatitis and other causes for this pattern, such as chronic viral hepatitis, Wilson disease, α1-antitrypsin deficiency, and drug-associated chronic hepatitis, should be considered and clinically or morphologically excluded (3,27). Typically, the biopsy shows an irregularly distributed relatively heavy portal infiltrate, with periportal or paraseptal interface hepatitis (Figs. 10.1B, 10.2, e-Figs. 10.4, 10.5, 10.10), with increased numbers of plasma cells and eosinophils in addition to lymphocytes (Fig. 10.2). Interface hepatitis is usually quite prominent, and there may also be portal-to-portal or portal-to-central bridging necrosis (e-Figs. 10.10, 10.11, 10.15, 10.16), also with plasma cells. Early in the development of AIH, there may be zone 3 necrosis (63).

Lobular hepatitis is often seen, especially when there is an acute clinical relapse (25). With significant lobular involvement, which affects zone 1 (periportal) hepatocytes predominantly, there is pseudoacinar (rosette) formation (e-Figs. 10.4–10.6), generally without obvious lumen formation (Figs. 10.2, 10.3). This pattern is typical of AIH, as is the presence of increased numbers of plasma cells. However, these features are not pathognomonic and are not seen in every biopsy from an AIH patient.

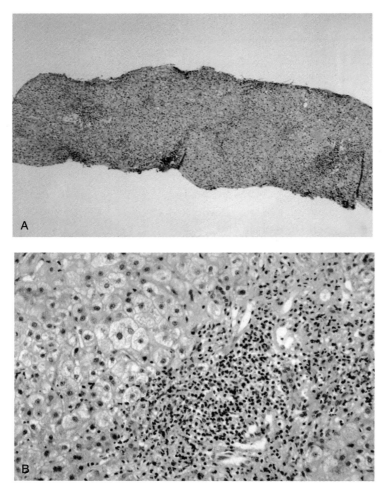

FIGURE 10.1   The progressive course of autoimmune hepatitis. A 52-year-old woman pre-sented with anorexia, easy fatigability, and mild jaundice, with elevated levels of antinuclear antibodies. Liver biopsy, obtained approximately 2 years after presentation (**A, B**), showed portal tracts expanded by a chronic inflammatory cell infiltrate composed of approximately equal numbers of plasma cells and lymphocytes, with scattered eosinophils and histiocytic cells, with interface hepatitis and scattered foci of lobular inflammation. Four years later (**C, D**) the biopsy showed definite but incomplete nodularity with interface hepatitis, bridging fibrosis and inflammation, and a portal infiltrate consisting mostly of lymphocytes, with scattered plasma cells and only rare eosinophils. Four years after the second biopsy, and almost 10 years after the onset of symptoms, the patient underwent orthotopic liver trans-plantation. The explant was a cirrhotic, predominantly macronodular liver, with areas of col-lapse and a few macroregenerative nodules (hematoxylin-eosin; **A**, original magnification ×200; **B**, ×400; **C**, ×40; **D**, ×400).

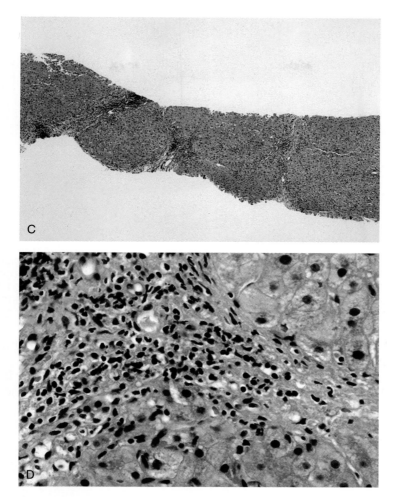

FIGURE 10.1. **(Continued)**

Both rosettes and increased numbers of plasma cells can be seen in association with chronic hepatitis as a result of other causes. In some patients with AIH, giant cell transformation ("giant cell hepatitis") may be seen.

Features to distinguish AIH from chronic hepatitis C include a more severe degree of lobular inflammation and necrosis, greater numbers of plasma cells, more marked interface hepatitis, and broad areas of parenchymal collapse (Table 10.6). Biliary changes are uncommon in AIH, and their presence may be indicative of some other disorder, such as PBC, PSC, or, to a lesser degree, HCV. In a patient in whom ANAs are demonstrable, bile duct injury should suggest the diagnosis of autoimmune cholangiopathy, discussed below. In chronic HBV, plasma cells may also be prominent. Histologic diagnosis for these three entities has high specificity and

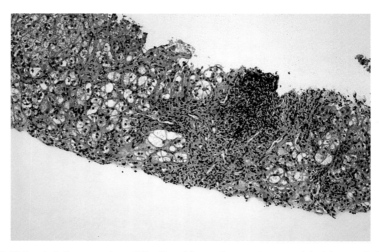

FIGURE 10.2 Autoimmune hepatitis. Liver biopsy from a 14-year-old with easy fatigability and malaise. Both antinuclear antibodies and anti–smooth muscle antibodies were demonstrable. The biopsy demonstrates a severe inflammatory process with almost complete effacement of the portal tract structure and with bridging inflammation and rosette formation (hematoxylin-eosin, original magnification ×40).

predictability but relatively low sensitivity. Acute hepatitis A, rarely biopsied, can be indistinguishable from AIH, with many plasma cells.

The biopsy in LKM-associated AIH is similar to that of other forms (Fig. 10.4, e-Figs. 10.42–10.44). There are no known light microscopic

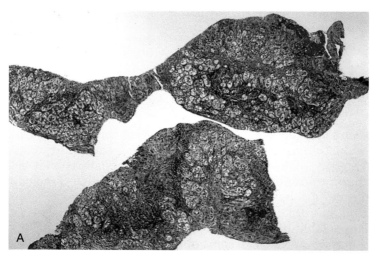

FIGURE 10.3 Autoimmune hepatitis. Liver biopsy from a 19-year-old man with a history of approximately 4 years of clinical liver disease and high levels of antinuclear antibodies, showing portal and periportal fibrosis, with prominent rosette formation and moderate portal and lobular inflammation (Masson trichrome; **A**, original magnification ×40; **B**, ×200). (See Color Figure 10.3A following page 129.)

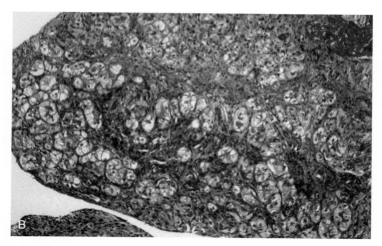

FIGURE 10.3. **(Continued)**

correlates for the various autoantibodies. Fulminant hepatitis in AIH is indistinguishable from other forms of massive and submassive necrosis.

The cirrhotic stage usually shows a greater degree of inflammation than cirrhosis arising from other causes. Septa are easily recognized, with obvious areas of prior parenchymal collapse, separating nodules of varying size (Fig. 10.1C,D). There may be dysplastic (macroregenerative) nodules and small hepatocellular carcinomas.

Immunohistochemical Studies

The great majority of portal tract lymphocytes are T cells, and CD4 cells predominate (21,29,49). In contrast, the T lymphocytes in the area of interface hepatitis are mostly CD8 antigen–positive and CD11b antigen–negative and

TABLE 10.6	Histologic Features Most Useful in Differentiating Autoimmune Hepatitis from Chronic Hepatitis C		
		AIH	**HCV**
Lobular inflammation/necrosis		+−+++	+/−
Plasma cells		+−+++	0−+
Interface hepatitis ("piecemeal necrosis")		+−+++	0−++
Parenchymal collapse		+−+++	0
Steatosis		0−+	+−++++[a]
Portal lymphoid aggregates		0−+	+−+++
Germinal center formation in lymphoid aggregates		0	0−++
Bile duct injury[b]		0−+	+−++

[a]Steatosis is particularly seen with genotype 3 HCV.
[b]Can sometimes be seen in AIH and is characteristic of AIC.

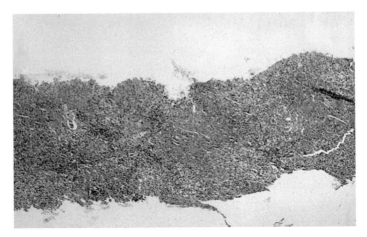

FIGURE 10.4   Liver–kidney microsomal (LKM) autoimmune hepatitis. Photomicrographs of biopsy from a 48-year-old man with chronic hepatitis. Antinuclear antibodies were not demonstrable, but his serum showed elevated titers of anti-LKM antibodies. There is extensive interface hepatitis with bridging and lobular inflammation (hematoxylin-eosin, original magnification ×40).

therefore are phenotypically cytotoxic T cells. Regulatory T cells (Tregs) are typically deficient in AIH (32).

Class I and class II antigens of the major histocompatibility complex have a major role in the induction and modulation of the immune response (48). Most hepatocytes are class II reacting cells.

What is the Relationship of Hepatitis C to Autoimmune Hepatitis?

An etiopathogenic relationship has been suggested for HCV and AIH (14,31,40). This seems unlikely (31,50). The association of LKM-1 with HCV is mostly in southern European countries, with much less evidence for this in the United States, western Europe, or Australia (27).

Key features of AIH are listed in Table 10.7.

AUTOIMMUNE CHOLANGIOPATHY

Autoimmune cholangiopathy is a variant of AIH. It is serologically indistinguishable from type 1, often with high ANA titers, and can show clinical, biochemical, and histologic features (Fig. 10.5) of PBC, but without demonstrable AMAs (7,22,37,56). Liver biopsies show the bile duct damage characteristic of PBC (e-Figs. 10-21–10.29) and may also show granuloma formation. Patients with this condition have previously been designated as having atypical PBC or AMA-negative PBC; it may be that they represent a unique entity, although there is not complete agreement on this (18,57). Response to corticosteroid therapy has not been uniformly

TABLE 10.7	Key Features of Autoimmune Hepatitis

1. Disease of young and middle-aged women
2. Antinuclear antibodies and/or anti–smooth muscle antibodies usually demonstrable
3. Chronic hepatic disease, progressive and ultimately fatal
4. Steroid therapy often leads to symptomatic improvement but generally does not prevent progression
5. May present as acute, fulminant liver failure
6. Strong association with HLA A1-B8-DR3 and DR4
7. Biopsy shows moderate to severe necroinflammatory process, with prominent portal infiltration, many plasma cells, interface hepatitis (piecemeal necrosis), and acinar transformation of hepatocytes (rosettes)
8. Autoimmune cholangiopathy is a distinct disorder, histologically resembling primary biliary cirrhosis but without antimitochondrial antibodies in serum and with antinuclear antibodies
9. Autoimmune liver disease variants may show features of more than one immune disorder (overlap syndromes) (Table 10.8)

HLA, human leukocyte antigen.

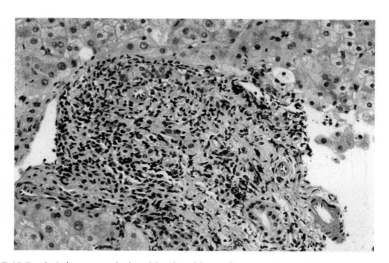

FIGURE 10.5   Autoimmune cholangitis. Liver biopsy from a 66-year-old woman with clinical and laboratory evidence of chronic hepatitis. Transaminase levels were approximately 200 U, and the alkaline phosphatase determination was >1,600 U. Antimitochondrial antibodies were not demonstrable on at least three occasions. The biopsy shows markedly expanded portal tracts with minimal piecemeal necrosis. The inflammatory cell infiltrate consists mostly of lymphocytes, with significant numbers of plasma cells. A bile duct (*upper left*) shows epithelial cell variation and infiltration by lymphocytes. The bile duct adjacent to the small artery (*center*) is almost completely destroyed (hematoxylin-eosin, original magnification ×200).

TABLE 10.8 Autoimmune Disease Variants		
Overlap Syndromes	Outlier Syndrome	Sequential Syndromes
AIH + PBC	AIC	AIH<---->PBC
AIH + PSC		AIH<---->PSC
AIH + AIC		

AIH, autoimmune hepatitis, AIC, autoimmune cholangitis, PBC, primary biliary cirrhosis, PSC, primary sclerosing cholangitis.

confirmed (66). Extrahepatic manifestations may be seen (2). This histologic picture has also been described in association with drug sensitivity (42). Bile duct injury can also be seen in AIH (3,11).

OVERLAP SYNDROMES

Table 10.8 lists overlap syndromes. Some patients have mixed clinical and/or histologic features, and definitive diagnosis may be difficult to establish, usually requiring correlation of signs and symptoms, laboratory test results, and histopathology.

REFERENCES

1. Alvarez F, Berg PA, Bianchi FB, et al. International Autoimmune Hepatitis Group Report: a review of criteria for diagnosis of autoimmune hepatitis. J Hepatol 1999;31: 929–938.
2. Archimandritis A, Tjivras M, Tsirantonaki M, et al. Sjogren's syndrome with antimitochondrial-negative primary biliary cirrhosis: a case of autoimmune cholangitis. J Clin Gastroenterol 1995;20:268–270.
3. Bach N, Thung SN, Schaffner F. The histological features of chronic hepatitis C and autoimmune chronic hepatitis: a comparative analysis. Hepatology 1992;15:572–577.
4. Ben-Ari Z, Czaga AJ. Autoimmune hepatitis and its variant syndromes. Gut 2001;49: 589–594.
5. Beuers U, Rust C. Overlap syndromes. Semin Liv Dis 2005;25:311–320.
6. Bourdi M, Larrey D, Nataf J, et al. Anti–liver endoplasmic reticulum autoantibodies are directed against human cytochrome P-450IA2: a specific marker for dihydralazine-induced hepatitis. J Clin Invest 1990;85:1967–1973.
7. Corte G, Kaplan M, Olivera M, et al. Prevalence of antinuclear antibodies (ANA) in patients with negative antimitochondrial antibodies (AMA) primary biliary cirrhosis (PBC). Hepatology 1992;16:189A.
8. Crapper RM, Bhathal PS, Mackay IR, et al. "Acute" autoimmune hepatitis. Digestion 1986;34:216–225.
9. Czaja AJ. Natural history, clinical features, and treatment of autoimmune hepatitis. Semin Liv Dis 1984;4:1–12.
10. Czaja AJ, Carpenter HA, Santrach PJ, et al. Genetic predisposition for the immunological features of chronic active hepatitis. Hepatology 1993;18:816–822.
11. Czaja AJ, Carpenter HA. Autoimmune hepatitis with incidental histologic features of bile duct injury. Hepatology 2001;34:659–665.

12. Donaldson PT, Doherty DG, Hayllar K, et al. Susceptibility of autoimmune chronic active hepatitis: human leukocyte antigens DR4 and A1-B8-DR3 are independent risk factors. Hepatology 1991;13:701–706.

13. Eddleston AL, Donaldson PT, Hegarty JE, et al. Immunological aspects of liver disease. Gut 1991(Suppl):S40–S46.

14. Fried MW, Draguesku JO, Shindo M, et al. Clinical and serological differentiation of autoimmune and hepatitis C virus–related chronic hepatitis. Dig Dis Sci 1993;38:631–636.

15. Frust TW. Recurrent primary biliary cirrhosis, primary sclerosing cholangitis, and autoimmune hepatitis after transplantation. Liver Transpl 2000;7(11 Suppl 1):S99–S108.

16. Geller SA. Autoimmune hepatitis. Pathol: State of the Art Rev 1994;3:57–76.

17. Gish RG, Mason A. Autoimmune liver disease. Current standards, future direction. Clin Liver Dis 2001;5:287–314.

18. Goodman Z, McHally PR, Davis D, et al. "Autoimmune cholangitis": a variant of primary biliary cirrhosis. Dig Dis Sci 1995;40:1232–1242.

19. Gueguen M, Boniface O, Bernard O, et al. Identification of the main epitope on human cytochrome P450 IID6 recognized by anti–liver kidney microsome antibody. J Autoimmun 1991;4:607–615.

20. Hardarson S, Labrecque DR, Mitros FA, et al. Antineutrophilic cytoplasmic antibody in inflammatory bowel and hepatobiliary diseases. High prevalence in ulcerative colitis, primary sclerosing cholangitis, and autoimmune hepatitis. Am J Clin Pathol 1993;99:277–281.

21. Hashimoto E, Lindor KD, Homburger HA, et al. Immunohistochemical characterization of hepatic lymphocytes in primary biliary cirrhosis in comparison with primary sclerosing cholangitis and autoimmune chronic active hepatitis. Mayo Clin Proc 1993;68:1049–1055.

22. Hatzis GS, Vassiliou VA, Delladetsima JK. Overlay syndrome of primary sclerosing cholangitis and autoimmune hepatitis. Eur J Gastroenterol Hepatol 2001;13:203–206.

23. Homberg JC, Abuaf N, Bernard O, et al. Chronic active hepatitis associated with anti-liver/kidney microsome antibody type 1: a second type of "autoimmune hepatitis." Hepatology 1987;7:1333–1339.

24. Hussain MJ, Mustafa A, Mowat AP. Immunohistochemical detection of TNF-a and IFN-g in the liver of children with autoimmune chronic active hepatitis and primary cholangitis. J Hepatol 1992;16:S59.

25. Johnson PJ, McFarlane IG. Meeting report: International Autoimmune Hepatitis Group. Hepatology 1993;18:998–1005.

26. Krawitt El. Autoimmune hepatitis. N Engl J Med 2006;354:54–66.

27. Lenzi M, Johnson PJ, McFarlane BM, et al. Antibodies to hepatitis C virus in autoimmune liver disease: evidence for geographical heterogeneity. Lancet 1991;338:277–280.

28. Lo SK, Chapman RWG, Cheeseman P, et al. Antineutrophil antibody: a test for immune primary sclerosing cholangitis in childhood? Gut 1993;34:199–202.

29. Lohr H, Manns M, Kyriatsoulis A, et al. Clonal analysis of liver-infiltrating T cells in patients with LKM-1 antibody–positive autoimmune chronic active hepatitis. Clin Exp Immunol 1991;84:297–302.

30. Lohr H, Treichel U, Poralla T, et al. Liver-infiltrating T helper cells in autoimmune chronic active hepatitis stimulate the production of autoantibodies against the human asialoglycoprotein receptor in vitro. Clin Exp Immunol 1992;88:45–49.

31. Lohse AW, Gerken G, Mohr H, et al. Relation between autoimmune liver diseases and viral hepatitis: clinical and serological characteristics in 859 patients. Z Gastroenterol 1995;33:527–533.

32. Longhi MS, Hussain MJ, Mitry RR, et al. Functional study of CD4+CD25+ regulatory T cells in health and autoimmune hepatitis. J Immuno 2006;176:4484–4491.

33. Lunel F, Abuaf N, Franguel L, et al. Liver/kidney microsome antibody type 1 and hepatitis C virus infection. Hepatology 1992;16:630–636.

34. Magrin S, Craxi A, Fiorentino G, et al. Is autoimmune chronic active hepatitis a HCV-related disease? J Hepatol 1991;13:56–60.

35. Manns MP, Johnson EF, Griffen KJ, et al. Major antigen of liver kidney microsomal autoantibodies in idiopathic autoimmune hepatitis is cytochrome P450 db1. J Clin Invest 1989;83:1066–1072.

36. Manns MP, Griffin KJ, Sullivan KF, et al. LKM-1 autoantibodies recognize a short linear sequence in P450IID6, a cytochrome P450 monooxygenase. J Clin Invest 1991;88:1370–1378.

37. Michieletti P, Wanless IR, Katz A, et al. Antimitochondrial antibody negative primary biliary cirrhosis: a distinct syndrome of autoimmune cholangitis. Gut 1994;35:260–265.

38. Odievre M, Maggiore G, Homberg JC, et al. Seroimmunologic classification of chronic hepatitis in 57 children. Hepatology 1983;3:407–409.

39. Oo JH, Neuberger J. Recurrence of nonviral diseases. Clin Liv Dis 2007;11:377–395.

40. Pawlotsky J-M, Deforges L, Bretagne S, et al. Hepatitis C virus infection can mimic type 1 (antinuclear antibody positive) autoimmune chronic active hepatitis. Gut 1993;(Suppl):S66–S68.

41. Rabinovitz M, Demetris AJ, Bou-Abboud CF, et al. Simultaneous occurrence of primary sclerosing cholangitis and autoimmune chronic active hepatitis in a patient with ulcerative colitis. Dig Dis Sci 1992;37:1606–1611.

42. Ryley NG, Fleming KA, Chapman RW. Focal destructive cholangiopathy associated with amoxycillin/clabulanic acid (Augmentin). J Hepatol 1995;23:278–282.

43. Sacher M, Blumel P, Thaler H, et al. Chronic active hepatitis associated with vitiligo, nail dystrophy, alopecia and a new variant of LKM antibodies. J Hepatol 1990;10:364–369.

44. Schvarcz R, Glaumann H, Weiland O. Survival and histological resolution of fibrosis in patients with autoimmune chronic active hepatitis. J Hepatol 1983;18:15–23.

45. Scully LJ, Clarke D, Barr RJ. Diclofenac induced hepatitis. Dig Dis 1993;38:744–761.

46. Seelig R, Renz M, Bunger G, et al. Anti-LKM-1 antibodies determined by use of recombinant P450 2D6 in ELISA and Western blot and their association with anti-HCV and HCV-RNA. Clin Exp Immunol 1993;92:373–380.

47. Seki T, Kiyosawa K, Inoko H, et al. Association of autoimmune hepatitis with HLA-Bw54 and DR4 in Japanese patients. Hepatology 1990;12:1300–1304.

48. Senaldi G, Lobo-Yeo A, Mowat AP, et al. Class I and class II major histocompatability complex antigens on hepatocytes: importance of the method of detection and expression in histologically normal and diseased livers. J Clin Pathol 1991;44:107–114.

49. Senaldi G, Portmann B, Mowat AP, et al. Immunohistochemical features of the portal tract mononuclear cell infiltrate in chronic aggressive hepatitis. Arch Dis Child 1992;67:1447–1453.

50. Strassburg CP, Obermayer-Straum P, Manns MP. Autoimmunity in hepatitis C and D virus infection. J Viral Hepatitis 1996;3:49–59.

51. Talwalker JA, Keach JC, Angulo P, et al. Overlap of autoimmune hepatitis and primary biliary cirrhosis: an evaluation of a modified scoring system. Am J Gastroenterol 2002;97:1191–1197.

52. Taylor SL, Dena PJ, Riely CA. Primary autoimmune cholangitis. Am J Surg Pathol 1994;18:91–99.

53. Thung SN, Bach N, Fasy TM, et al. Hepatocellular carcinoma associated with autoimmune chronic active hepatitis. Mt Sinai J Med 1990;57:165–168.

54. Todros L, Touscoz G, D'Urso N, et al. Hepatitis C virus–related chronic liver disease with autoantibodies to liver-kidney microsomes (LKM). Clinical characterization from idiopathic LKM-positive disorders. J Hepatol 1991;13:128–131.

55. Tomsic M, Ferlan-Marolt V, Kveder T, et al. Mixed connective tissue disease associated with autoimmune hepatitis and thyroiditis. Ann Rheum Dis 1992;51:544–546.

56. Vierling JM. Autoimmune cholangiopathy. Clin Liver Dis 1999;3:571–584.
57. Washington K. Autoimmune cholangitis: not just AMA-negative primary biliary cirrhosis. Adv Anat Pathol 2002;9:244–250.
58. Washington K. Autoimmune liver disease: overlap and outliers. Mod Pathol 2007;20(Suppl 1): S15–30.
59. Yabe H, Noma K, Tada N, et al. A case of CREST syndrome with rapidly progressive liver damage. Intern Med 1992;31:69–73.
60. Yamamoto AM, Mura C, Morales MG, et al. Study of CYP2D6 gene in children with autoimmune hepatitis and P450 IID6 autoantibodies. Clin Exp Immunol 1992;87: 251–255.
61. Yamamoto AM, Cresteil D, Homberg JC, et al. Characterization of anti-liver-kidney microsome antibody (anti-LKM1) from hepatitis C virus–positive and –negative sera. Gastroenterology 1993;104:1762–1767.
62. Yousuf M, Kiyosawa K, Sodeyama T, et al. Development of hepatocellular carcinoma in a man with auto-immune chronic active hepatitis. J Gastroenterol Hepatol 1992;7:66–69.
63. Zen Y, Notsumata K, Tanak N, et al. Hepatic centrilobular zone necrosis with positive antinuclear antibody: a unique subtype or early disease of autoimmune hepatitis. Hum Pathol 2007;38:1669–1675.

11

EFFECTS OF DRUGS AND TOXINS ON THE LIVER

This chapter summarizes some major aspects of hepatotoxicity (80). Many examples of response to drug or toxic injury are shown in the electronic figures. They are listed alphabetically for easy reference. Most are also cited in the text.

Drug-induced liver injury (DILI) encompasses a wide spectrum of clinicopathologic alterations ranging from mild biochemical abnormalities to acute liver failure. There are two broad categories: intrinsic and idiosyncratic hepatotoxicity.

INTRINSIC TOXICITY

Intrinsic toxicity refers to drugs that have a high incidence of predictable hepatotoxicity and that are dose dependent. Their effects can be induced in experimental animals (64). There are two groups: direct and indirect hepatotoxic effect. Both cause cytotoxic and cholestatic liver injury.

In direct cytotoxicity, liver cell injury occurs at the subcellular level, affecting various organelles with subsequent steatosis, necrosis, or both. An example is carbon tetrachloride poisoning (71). Another example is phosphorus poisoning, now only of historical significance (27). Paraquat causes cholestatic direct hepatotoxic injury, with biliary epithelium as the primary target of injury (56).

Indirect toxicity refers to cell injury caused by alterations of various metabolic pathways or selective effects on membrane cell receptors, DNA and RNA molecules, either within the nuclei or in the cytosol. Many drugs cause indirect cytotoxic injury, leading to steatosis or hepatocellular necrosis, including phalloidin, dimethylnitrosamine, acetaminophen, aflatoxin B, pyrrolizidine alkaloids, tetracycline, galactosamine, and inorganic arsenic (19,62). Some of the effects of alcohol are also reflections of altered metabolic pathways. Drugs that cause cholestatic indirect toxic injury by selective interference with bile excretion and uptake from the blood include contraceptive steroids, C17 alkylated anabolic steroids, and lithocholic acid.

IDIOSYNCRATIC HEPATOTOXICITY

Idiosyncratic drug-induced liver injury (DILI) (also termed "immune-mediated" and "immunogenetic") can have various systemic reactions, including fever, rash, and peripheral eosinophilia. Symptoms usually develop weeks following exposure, and, more important, symptoms recur with re-exposure. Effects are not experimentally demonstrable (65).

Although drug-associated acute liver failure is uncommon, as many as 15% of all acute liver failure cases are attributed to idiosyncratic drug reactions (e-Figs. 11.1–11.9, 11.18, 11.19, 11.35, 11.36, 11.44). Chronic disease occurs in up to 6%, even after withdrawal of the offending drug. Antibiotics and NSAIDs are the most common causes of DILI acute liver failure.

The mechanisms of DILI are complex and multifactorial. They involve a complex interplay between intracellular stress and tumor necrosis factor (TNF)-alpha-activated apoptosis/necrosis, coupled with proinflammatory responses of the innate and adaptive immune systems. Risk factors include age, sex, and genetic polymorphisms of drug-metabolizing enzymes such as cytochrome P450.

Many drugs produce DILI by interfering with metabolism and by producing toxic metabolites. Examples are halothane (e-Figs. 11.40–11.44), phenytoin (e-Fig. 11.29), paraaminosalicylic acid (e-Fig. 11.61), sulfonamides, phenylbutazone (e-Fig. 11.62), valproic acid (e-Fig. 11.96), isoniazid (e-Figs. 11.45–11.48), and chlorpromazine (e-Fig. 11.21) (8,23,34,49, 57,70). A wide range of morphologic responses that mimic many hepatic disorders can be induced (Table 11.1).

TABLE 11.1 Morphologic Lesions in the Liver Associated with Drug-Induced Injury

1. Steatosis (macrovesicular, microvesicular, zonal distribution)
2. Necrosis
   a. Zonal
   b. Focal (acute, chronic hepatitis)
   c. Diffuse, massive
3. Cholestasis
4. Granulomas
5. Fibrosis (portal, pericellular), cirrhosis
6. Vascular changes
7. Neoplasms
   a. Hepatocellular adenoma
   b. Hepatocellular carcinoma
   c. Cholangiocarcinoma
   d. Angiosarcoma
8. Cellular inclusions and pigments

STEATOSIS

Drugs and toxins produce variable degrees of macrovesicular or microvesicular steatosis or both. The zonal distribution is generally not prominent except in phosphorus poisoning, in which steatosis is predominantly in zone 1 (periportal), and tetracycline-induced toxicity, in which steatosis is predominantly in zone 3 (perivenular) (21,62) (Fig. 11.1). Alcohol, at first, shows zonal distribution, initially in zone 3.

Macrovesicular steatosis is common in alcoholic liver disease after total parenteral nutrition (TPN) (e-Figs. 11.92–11.95) (4,5) and methotrexate therapy (e-Figs. 11.49–11.53) (2,49,68). Focal microvesicular steatosis may occur with macrovesicular steatosis, however, and so-called foam cells may be present.

Steatosis and necrosis occur concomitantly with carbon tetrachloride– (e-Figs. 11.18, 11.19), tannic acid–, and amanitin-induced injury, but in the latter, steatosis predominates (71).

Microvesicular steatosis is common in tetracycline-induced toxic injury (62), Reye syndrome, acute fatty liver of pregnancy, and after use of valproic acid (23), salicylates (73,79), and cocaine (40).

Steatosis mostly affects hepatocytes. Perisinusoidal stellate (Ito) cells can also contain significant numbers of fat droplets, particularly in hypervitaminosis A (e-Figs. 11.102–11.104) (Table 11.2) (28,30,38,53).

Phospholipidosis is a special form of drug-induced steatosis, first described in patients given coronary vasodilator medications, such as perhexiline maleate (61) and after amiodarone (e-Fig. 11.11) (Table 11.2) (31,39). Hepatocytes contain many small fat droplets (foam cells), and electron microscopy shows lamellar or crystalloid cytoplasmic inclusions, identical to those seen in metabolic types of phospholipidosis. Kupffer cells may also be affected (Fig. 11.2). Cirrhosis can result.

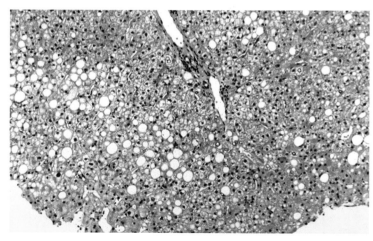

FIGURE 11.1 Predominantly macrovesicular steatosis in a patient treated with methotrexate for rheumatoid arthritis (hematoxylin-eosin, original magnification ×100).

TABLE 11.2	Medications Associated with the Picture of Steatosis and Steatohepatitis

A. Predominantly macrovesicular
   Alcohol
   Corticosteroids
   Methotrexate
   Carbon tetrachloride
   Total parenteral nutrition
B. Predominantly microvesicular
   Valproic acid
   Parenteral tetracycline
   Salicylate intoxication
C. Steatohepatitis
   Alcohol
   Amiodarone
   Perhexiline maleate
   Synthetic estrogens
   Long-term corticosteroids
D. Phospholipidosis
   Amiodarone
   Perhexiline maleate
   Synthetic estrogens
   Total parenteral nutrition

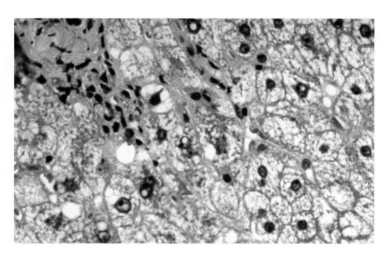

FIGURE 11.2 Microvesicular steatosis, focal nonalcoholic hepatitis, and Mallory material in a patient treated with amiodarone (hematoxylin-eosin, original magnification ×200).

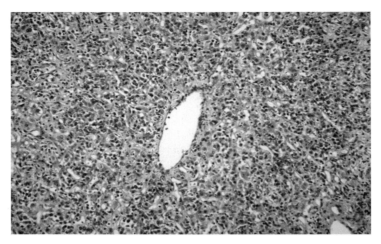

FIGURE 11.3   Perivenular and submassive necrosis in acetaminophen toxicity (hematoxylin-eosin, original magnification ×100).

NECROSIS

Perivenular (zone 3) liver cell necrosis is typical of toxicity induced by the poison mushroom *Amanita phalloides* (e-Figs. 11.56), paracetamol, halothane (e-Figs. 11.40–11.44), and, well shown experimentally, carbon tetrachloride (e-Figs. 11.18, 11.19). Perivenular hemorrhagic necrosis is associated with pyrrolizidine alkaloids and aflatoxin B (27,50,66) (Fig. 11.3). Periportal (zone 1) liver cell necrosis is commonly associated with phosphorus poisoning and ferrous sulfate toxicity. Necrosis limited to zone 2 has not been described with drug-induced injury. Extensive zonal necrosis may lead to diffuse and/or massive necrosis, as in some cases of phenytoin toxicity (69).

ACUTE AND CHRONIC HEPATITISLIKE PICTURE

Many drugs cause histopathologic changes of DILI indistinguishable from acute or chronic viral hepatitis (e-Figs. 11.22, 11.23, 11.38, 11.39, 11.45, 11.48, 11.54, 11.55, 11.59–11.61, 11.88–11.91, 11.97–11.101), including halothane, a-methyldopa, indomethacin, isoniazid, nitrofurantoin, and the recently reported anticholesterol drug ezetimibe (3,7,11,37,49, 55,60,67). Nitrofurantoin-induced hepatitis usually affects females, often with autoimmune serologic markers, making it difficult to differentiate from autoimmune hepatitis. Furthermore, nitrofurantoin-induced chronic hepatitis may progress to fibrosis/cirrhosis.

CHOLESTASIS

Cholestatic injury can follow use of chlorpromazine, anabolic and contraceptive steroids, antibiotics, and paraquat (1,18,35,36,51,56) (Fig. 11.4, e-Figs. 11.14–11.16, 11.21–11.23, 11.64, 11.69, 11.75–11.79 (Table 11.3).

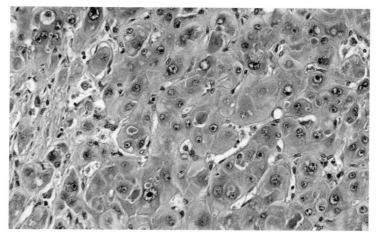

FIGURE 11.4 Canalicular cholestasis in a patient on long-term oral contraceptives (hematoxylin-eosin, original magnification ×200).

In chlorpromazine-induced injury (e-Fig. 11.21), in addition to canalicular cholestasis, there is an associated portal tract inflammatory reaction of variable degree, sometimes with many eosinophils. This type of injury, with both cholestatic and inflammatory components, has been described as hypersensitivity cholestasis or hepatocanalicular cholestasis (35) (Figs. 11.5, 11.6).

In contrast, cholestasis induced by steroids, both anabolic and contraceptive, usually shows little, if any, portal inflammation and has been described as bland or canalicular (36). When bile duct injury predominates, as in paraquat toxicity or with the no-longer used ajmaline (e-Fig. 11.10), the cholestasis is described as ductal or cholangiodestructive (56). Bile duct loss (vanishing bile duct syndrome) can rarely be seen (e-Figs. 11.79–11.82).

Cholestatic drug injuries generally have a short, acute, and self-limited course but can sometimes lead to chronic liver disease, similar to primary biliary cirrhosis or drug-induced secondary sclerosing cholangitis (12,13,22,48). Mixed forms, including cholestatic and parenchymal

TABLE 11.3	Medications Associated with a Cholestasis Picture
Steroids (estrogenic and androgenic)	
Phenothiazine (chlorpromazine)	
Erythromycin	
Phenylbutazone	

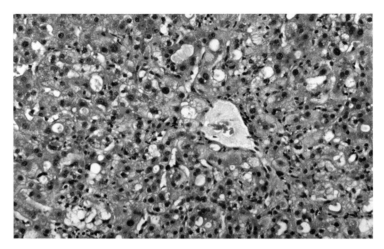

FIGURE 11.5 Severe cholestasis in a patient treated with chlorpromazine (hematoxylin-eosin, original magnification ×100).

damage, can be seen with phenytoin (69) and amoxicillin/clavulanic acid preparations.

GRANULOMAS

Granulomas may be one of the manifestations of DILI (52). This can be isolated or associated with other features, including portal tract inflammatory reaction and cholestasis. As many as 30% of granulomas in liver biopsies are attributed to approximately 60 drugs, including allopurinol (75),

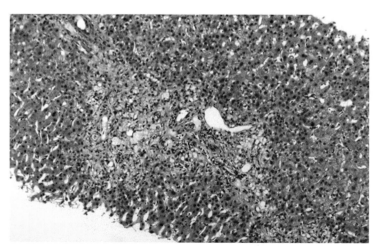

FIGURE 11.6 Ductopenic reaction in the same patient (hematoxylin-eosin, original magnification ×200).

TABLE 11.4	Medications Causing Hepatic Granulomas
	Allopurinol
	Phenylbutazone
	Sulfonamide
	Carbamazepine

aspirin, carbamazepine (46), cephalexin, chlorpromazine, dapsone (37), diazepam, gold, halothane, isoniazid (11), nitrofurantoin, oxacillin, phenylbutazone (8), procainamide (69), quinidine (17), sulfadiazine, sulfasalazine, tolbutamide, and others. There is no zonal predilection (Table 11.4). Allopurinol granulomas can resemble fibrin ring–type granulomas typically seen in Q fever (Fig. 11.7). Granulomas may resolve completely without sequelae after the drug has been discontinued.

FIBROSIS AND CIRRHOSIS

Fibrosis develops in patients treated with high doses of methotrexate for various indications (e-Fig. 11.53) (2,10,29,59,68), with variable periportal/pericellular fibrosis. In early methotrexate-induced toxicity, macrovesicular steatosis alone may be present (e-Figs. 11.49–11.51). Portal and focal pericellular fibrosis is also seen in chronic hypervitaminosis A (30,43). Drug-induced fibrosis occurs after exposure to arsenic and vinyl chloride (64). Fibrosis develops in various drug/toxin settings, including nonalcoholic

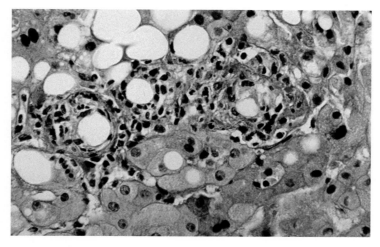

FIGURE 11.7 So-called fibrin-ring granulomas in allopurinol toxicity (Masson trichrome, original magnification ×200).

steatohepatitis, phospholipidosis, and after drug-induced chronic hepatitis (e.g., nitrofurantoin) (60).

VASCULAR LESIONS

Venous outflow obstruction (hepatic vein thrombosis or Budd–Chiari syndrome) occurs in patients using oral contraceptives (47) (Table 11.5). Venoocclusive disease (VOD) (e-Figs. 11.102–11.104) can be caused by pyrrolizidine alkaloids, alcohol, azathioprine (20,58), thioguanine, and irradiation therapy.

Peliosis hepatis (e-Figs. 11.12, 11.13, 11.27, 11.28), pseudocystic (lake-like) transformation of sinusoids, occurs in patients taking anabolic steroids, azathioprine, contraceptive pills, and tamoxifen (12,20,35,58,72). Sinusoidal dilatation and peliosis may occur together (e-Figs. 11.24–11.28) (2,35).

Striking regenerative activity in liver cells and liver nuclei can be seen in patients taking oral contraceptives for only a few months, highlighted by strong reactivity of liver cells with proliferating cell nuclear antibody (Fig. 11.8). Chapter 19 contains a more detailed discussion of hepatic vascular disorders.

TABLE 11.5 Medications Causing Vascular Lesions
A. Venoocclusive disease
Pyrrolizidine alkaloids
Immunosuppressive agents (e.g., azathioprine)
Antineoplastic agents (mitomycin C, fluorodeoxyuridine)
B. Budd–Chiari syndrome
Oral contraceptives
Antineoplastic agents (vincristine, cyclophosphamide)
C. Sinusoidal dilatation
Oral contraceptives
Azathioprine
Vitamin A
D. Peliosis hepatitis
Androgenic steroids
Corticosteroids
Tamoxifen
Vitamin A
Thorotrast
Vinyl chloride

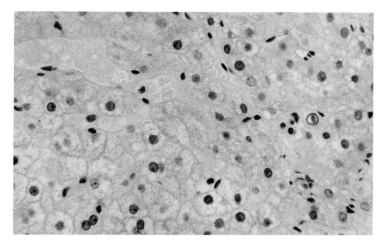

FIGURE 11.8 Striking regenerative and proliferative nuclear activity in a patient on oral contraceptives (antibody for proliferative cell nuclear antigen, immunoperoxidase avidin-biotin-peroxidase complex, original magnification ×100).

NEOPLASMS

Both benign and malignant neoplasms, as well as nonneoplastic proliferating lesions, have been described in association with various drugs and toxic agents (Table 11.1).

Liver cell adenoma was exceedingly rare before the introduction of oral contraceptives. This tumor is no longer rare, particularly in women taking oral contraceptives (35). Adenoma can regress when contraceptives are discontinued. Adenoma also develops after treatment with danazol and testosterone enanthate (15,24). An association between oral contraceptives and focal nodular hyperplasia remains controversial.

Malignant tumors, including hepatocellular carcinoma and cholangiocarcinoma, have been associated with thorium dioxide (Thorotrast) exposure (36) (Fig. 11.9). Hepatocellular carcinoma has been described in patients on long-term anabolic steroid and contraceptive steroid therapy (26).

Occupational exposure to vinyl chloride, long-term exposure to inorganic arsenic, and injection of thorium dioxide are associated with primary angiosarcoma of the liver (e-Figs. 11.85–11.87), an otherwise rare neoplasm (64).

As one example of a proliferative lesion, nodular hyperplasia can be seen in association with 6-thioguanine therapy for inflammatory bowel diseases (e-Figs. 11.70–11.74)

CELLULAR INCLUSIONS

Hepatocytes can undergo various adaptive changes after exposure to various drugs.

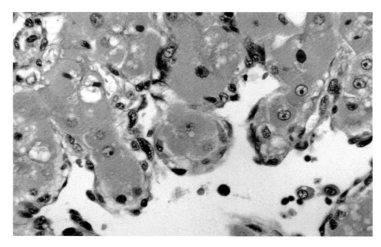

FIGURE 11.9   Angiosarcoma of the liver in a patient previously exposed to vinyl chloride (hematoxylin-eosin, original magnification ×100).

"Ground-glass" hepatocytes are enlarged hepatocytes with pale eosinophilic cytoplasm similar to ground-glass hepatocytes containing hepatitis B surface antigen. Drug-induced ground-glass hepatocytes have hyperplastic and dilated smooth endoplastic reticulum. These cells are diastase resistant and paraaminosalicylic acid positive; they also resemble the cells seen in glycogenosis IV. In contrast to both hepatitis B and glycogenosis, drug-induced ground-glass cells are in zone 1 rather than scattered. Drug-induced ground-glass cells occur with chlorpromazine, barbiturates, and after long-term therapy with steroids, azathioprine, and phenytoin (e-Fig. 11.29) (20,55,70). Ground-glass cells are particularly prominent in patients treated with cyanamide and disulfiram (6,14).

Mallory material, typically associated with alcoholic liver disease, can be seen in amiodarone toxicity (39).

PIGMENTS

Pigments associated with drugs and toxins may be endogenous (e.g., hemosiderin, copper, bilirubin) or exogenous (e.g., gold, thorium dioxide, titanium).

Hemosiderin is often seen with alcoholic liver disease, primarily in sinusoidal cells. Hepatocyte deposition can be prominent, and iron analysis may be necessary to exclude hereditary hemochromatosis. Hemosiderin is also found with alcohol-induced porphyria cutanea tarda. Patients on long-term hemodialysis have hemosiderosis to varying degrees. Copper and copper-binding protein can accumulate in hepatocytes in long-standing cholestasis, including primary biliary diseases such as primary biliary cirrhosis and primary sclerosing cholangitis. Copper is also found in Kupffer cells after occupational exposure to copper salts. Thorium dioxide (Thorotrast), with a half-life of decades to years, is found in the liver long after exposure, recognized as granular, somewhat refractile gray-brown material, either in single or in clustered histiocytic cells (e-Figs. 11.83–11.85) (36). Gold can be demonstrated in patients with rheumatoid arthritis treated with gold salts. The fine black granules of gold in Kupffer cells show golden birefringence with polarized light (24). Titanium accumulates in intravenous drug abusers.

IMMUNOSUPPRESSIVE DRUGS AND THEIR EFFECT ON THE LIVER

Immunosuppressive drugs administered after solid organ transplantation, particularly liver transplantation (LT), include cyclosporine, azathioprine, corticosteroids, antilymphocytic preparations (OKT3), tacrolimus (FK-506), RS-61443, and rapamycin. In addition, patients may receive various antiviral and antifungal medications, including trimethoprim/sulfamethoxazole, cephalosporins, amphotericin, ketoconazole, fluconazole, isoniazid, ganciclovir, hyperalimentation preparations, interferon-a, and, more recently, lamivudine for recurrent forms of hepatitis B and C (20,41,42,74). Some antirejection drugs, such as cyclosporine, OKT3, and tacrolimus cause relatively mild histopathologic changes and only rarely cause significant hepatotoxicity (16,20, 41,43,74,75).

DILI should be considered in the differential diagnosis whenever the histopathologic features of the liver biopsy after transplantation appear unusual. Both TPN and azathioprine can induce cholestatic hepatitis, and both are used in liver transplantation patients. Cyclosporine causes cholestasis, without other changes. Corticosteroids cause sinusoidal dilatation and a variable steatosis. There has been no evidence of hepatotoxicity with tacrolimus (74) or mycophenolate mofetil (43). Antiretroviral drugs used for treatment of HIV-positive patients can cause various changes ranging from mild nonspecific changes, nonalcoholic fatty liver disease (NAFLD), cholestasis, to acute liver failure (44,63).

TOTAL PARENTERAL NUTRITION

The spectrum of histopathologic findings associated with TPN includes cholestasis, cholestatic hepatitis, steatosis, steatohepatitis, phospholipidosis, fibrosis, and cirrhosis (4,5,13).

Cholestasis is common, especially in children. Canalicular cholestasis may be accompanied by cholestatic hepatitis. Giant cells may be seen. Portal tracts usually contain an inflammatory infiltrate composed of lymphocytes and histiocytes, often with eosinophils. Kupffer cells are prominent. After long-term TPN treatment, fibrosis and biliary cirrhosis may develop (e-Figs. 11.92–11.95) (4,5,13).

In adults, steatosis, initially zone 1, is the first and predominant feature, developing in the first weeks of treatment. Cholestasis is often present, and features mimicking bile duct obstruction may develop, including bile ductular reaction (proliferation), fibrosis, and biliary cirrhosis (4,5,13).

In TPN-induced phospholipidosis, the histopathologic changes are similar to those seen in amiodarone-induced phospholipidosis.

ACUTE HEPATITIS ASSOCIATED WITH HERBAL PRODUCTS

Herbal products, popular in North America as potential remedies for various conditions, can be hepatotoxic. Patients develop acute hepatitis as early as 2 weeks and as long as a year after ingestion (77,78), with fatigue, hepatomegaly, nausea, abdominal pain, jaundice, vomiting, peripheral eosinophilia, and pruritus. Children can have central nervous system and respiratory depression along with bradycardia. Symptoms resolve within 2 to 30 weeks, but reuse of the product causes recurrence (78). Hypersensitivity reaction, direct hepatotoxic effect, and an idiosyncratic reaction have all been individually or synergistically implicated.

Many "natural" herbal products, including germander, chaparral, senna, mistletoe, skullcap, comfrey, crotalaria, and various herbal teas, are hepatotoxic (9,32,33,42,45,54,77). Their effect is focal lobular necrosis, with variable numbers of eosinophils (Figs. 11.10, 11.11). Focal steatosis may be present.

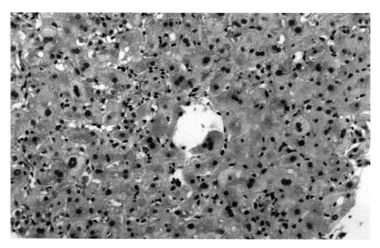

FIGURE 11.10   Acute hepatitis in a patient taking herbal product (jin bu huan) (hematoxylin-eosin, original magnification ×100).

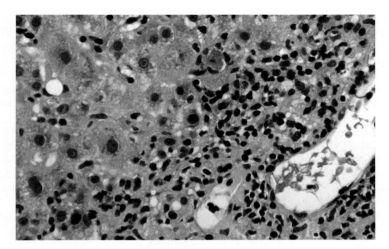

FIGURE 11.11   Portal inflammation in the same patient (hematoxylin-eosin, original magnification ×200).

REFERENCES

1. Ammann R, Neftel K, Hardmeier T, et al. Cephalosporin-induced cholestatic jaundice. Lancet 1982;2:336–337.
2. Aponte J, Petrelli M. Histopathologic findings in the liver of rheumatoid arthritis patients treated with long-term bolus methotrexate. Arthritis Rheum 1988;31:1457–1461.
3. Arranto AJ, Sotaniemi EA. Morphologic alterations in patients with alpha-methyldopa-induced liver damage after short- and long-term exposure. Scand J Gastroenterol 1981;16:853–863.
4. Baker AL, Rosenberg IH. Hepatic complications of total parenteral nutrition. Am J Med 1990;82:489–497.
5. Balistreri WF, Bove KE. Hepatobiliary consequences of parenteral alimentation. Prog Liver Dis 1990;9:567–601.
6. Bartle WR, Fisher MM, Kerenyi N. Disulfiram-induced hepatitis: report of two cases and review of the literature. Dig Dis Sci 1985;30:834–837.
7. Benjamin SB, Goodman ZD, Ishak KG. The morphologic spectrum of halothane-induced hepatic injury. Hepatology 1985;5:1163–1171.
8. Benjamin SB, Ishak KG, Zimmerman H, et al. Phenylbutazone liver injury: a clinical-pathologic survey of 23 cases and review of the literature. Hepatology 1981;1:255–263.
9. Beuers U, Spengler U, Pape GR. Hepatitis after chronic abuse of senna [letter]. Lancet 1991;337:372–373.
10. Bjorkman DJ, Hammond EH, Lee RG, et al. Hepatic ultrastructure after methotrexate therapy for rheumatoid arthritis. Arthritis Rheum 1988;31:1465–1472.
11. Black M, Mitchell JR, Zimmerman HJ, et al. Isoniazid-associated hepatitis in 114 patients. Gastroenterology 1975;69:289–374.
12. Blackburn AM, Amiel SA, Mills RR, et al. Tamoxifen and liver damage. Br Med J 1984;289:288.
13. Body JJ, Bleiberg H, Bron D, et al. Total parenteral nutrition–induced cholestasis mimicking large bile duct obstruction. Histopathology 1982;6:787–792.
14. Bruguera M, Pares A, Heredia D, et al. Cyanamide hepatotoxicity. Incidence and clinical-pathological features. Liver 1987;7:216–222.

15. Carrasco D, Prieto M, Pallardo L, et al. Multiple hepatic adenomas after long-term therapy with testosterone enanthate. Review of the literature. J Hepatol 1985;1:573–578.

16. Carrier M, Jenicek M, Pelletier L. Value of monoclonal antibodies (OKT3) in solid organ transplantation—a meta analysis. Transplant Proc 1992;24:2586–2591.

17. Chajek T. Quinidine and granulomatous hepatitis [letter]. Ann Intern Med 1975;82:282.

18. Davies MH, Harrison RF, Elias E, et al. Antibiotic-associated acute vanishing bile duct syndrome: a pattern associated with severe, prolonged, intrahepatic cholestasis. J Hepatol 1994;20:112–116.

19. Decker K, Keppler D. Galactosamine induced liver injury. Prog Liver Dis 1972;4:183–199.

20. De Pinho R, Goldberg CS, Lefkowitch JH. Azathioprine and the liver. Evidence favoring idiosyncratic mixed cholestatic-hepatocellular injury in humans. Gastroenterology 1984;86:162–165.

21. Diaz-Rivera RS, Collazo PJ, Pons ER, et al. Acute phosphorus poisoning in men: a study of 56 cases. Medicine 1950;29:269–298.

22. Doria MI, Shepard KV, Levin B, et al. Liver pathology following hepatic arterial infusion chemotherapy. Cancer 1986;58:855–861.

23. Eadie MJ, Hooper WD, Dickinson RG. Valproate-associated hepatotoxicity and its biochemical mechanisms. Med Toxicol 1988;3:85–106.

24. Fermand JP, Levy Y, Bouscary D, et al. Danazol-induced hepatocellular adenoma. Am J Med 1990;88:529–530.

25. Fleishner GM, Morecki I, Manaichi T, et al. Light and electron microscopical study of a case of gold salt induced hepatotoxicity. Hepatology 1991;14:422–425.

26. Forman D, Vincent TJ, Doll R. Cancer of the liver and use of oral contraceptives. Br Med J 1986;292:1357–1361.

27. Galler GW, Weisenberg E, Brasitus TA. Mushroom poisoning: the role of orthotopic liver transplantation. J Clin Gastroenterol 1992;15:229–232.

28. Geubel AP, DeGalocsy C, Alves N, et al. Liver damage caused by therapeutic vitamin A administration: estimate of dose-related toxicity in 41 cases. Gastroenterology 1991;100:1701–1709.

29. Gilbert SC, Klinmalm G, Menter A, et al. Methotrexate-induced cirrhosis requiring liver transplantation in three patients with psoriasis. A word of caution in light of the expanding use of this "steroid-sparing" agent. Ann Intern Med 1990;150:889–891.

30. Gurascio P, Portmann B, Visco G, et al. Liver damage with reversible portal hypertension from vitamin A intoxication: demonstration of Ito cells. J Clin Pathol 1983;36:759–771.

31. Harrison RF, Elias E. Amiodarone-associated cirrhosis with hepatic and lymph node granulomas. Histopathology 22:80–82.

32. Harvey J, Colin-Jones DG. Mistletoe hepatitis. Br Med J (Clin Res Ed) 1981;282:186–187.

33. Huxtable RJ, Luthy J, Zweifel U. Toxicity of comfrey-pepsin preparations [letter]. N Engl J Med 1986;315:1095.

34. Ishak KG, Irey NS. Hepatic injury associated with phenothiazines. Clinicopathologic and follow-up study of 36 patients. Arch Pathol 1972;49:630–648.

35. Ishak KG, Zimmerman HJ. Hepatotoxic effects of the anabolic/androgenic steroids. Semin Liver Dis 1987;7:230–236.

36. Ito Y, Kojiro, Nakashima T, et al. Pathomorphologic characteristics of 102 cases of thorotrast-related hepatocellular carcinoma, cholangiocarcinoma and hepatic angiosarcoma. Cancer 1982;62:1153–1162.

37. Jayalakshmi P, Ting HC. Dapsone-induced liver necrosis. Histopathology 1990;17:89–91.

38. Jorens PG, Michielsen PP, Pelckmans PA, et al. Vitamin A abuse: development of cirrhosis despite cessation of vitamin A. A six-year clinical and pathological follow-up. Liver 1992;12:381–386.

39. Kalantzis N, Gabriel P, Mouzas J, et al. Acute amiodarone-induced hepatitis. Hepatogastroenterology 1991;38:71–74.

40. Kanel GC, Cassidy W, Shuster L, et al. Cocaine-induced liver cell injury: comparison of morphological features in man and experimental models. Hepatology 1990;11:646–651.

41. Kassianides C, Nussenblatt R, Palestine AG, et al. Liver injury from cyclosporine A. Dig Dis Sci 1990;35:693–697.

42. Katz M, Saibil F. Herbal hepatitis: subacute hepatic necrosis secondary to chaparral leaf. J Clin Gastroenterol 1990;12:203–206.

43. Klintmalm GB, Ascher NL, Busuttil R, et al. RS-61443 for treatment of resistant human liver rejection. Transplant Proc 1993;25:697.

44. Lai KK, Gang DL, Zawacki JK, et al. Fulminant hepatic failure associated with 2′,3′-dideoxyuridine (ddI). Ann Intern Med 1991;115:283–284.

45. Larrey D, Vial T, Pauwels A, et al. Hepatitis after germander (*Teucrium chamaedrys*) administration: another instance of herbal medicine hepatotoxicity. Ann Intern Med 1992;117:129–132.

46. Levy M, Goodman MW, Van Dyne BJ, et al. Granulomatous hepatitis secondary to carbamazepine. Ann Intern Med 1981;95:64–65.

47. Lewis JH, Tice H, Zimmerman HJ. Budd-Chiari syndrome associated with oral contraceptive steroids. Review of treatment of 47 cases. Dig Dis Sci 1983;28:673–683.

48. Ludwig J, Kim CH, Wiesner RH, et al. Floxuridine-induced sclerosing cholangitis: an ischemic cholangiopathy? Hepatology 1989;9:215–218.

49. Maddrey WC. Isoniazid-induced liver disease. Semin Liver Dis 1981;1:129–133.

50. Maddrey WC. Hepatic effects of acetaminophen. Enhanced toxicity in alcoholics. J Clin Gastroenterol 1987;9:180–185.

51. Mallat A, Dhumeaux D. Cocaine and the liver. J Hepatol 1991;12:275–278.

52. Mc Master KR, Hennigar GR. Drug-induced granulomatous hepatitis. Lab Invest 1981; 44:61–73.

53. Minuk GY, Kelly JK, Hwang W-S. Vitamin A hepatotoxicity in multiple family members. Hepatology 1988;8:272–275.

54. Mostefa-Kara N, Pauwels A, Pines E, et al. Fatal hepatitis after herbal tea. Lancet 340:674.

55. Mullick FG, Ishak KG. Hepatic injury associated with diphenylhydantoin therapy. A clinicopathologic study of 20 cases. Am J Clin Pathol 1980;74:442–452.

56. Mullick FG, Ishak KG, Mahabir R, et al. Hepatic injury associated with paraquat toxicity in humans. Liver 1981;1:209–221.

57. Munoz SJ, Martinez-Hernandez A, Maddrey WC. Intrahepatic cholestasis and phospholipidosis associated with the use of trimethoprim-sulfamethoxazole. Hepatology 1990;12: 342–347.

58. Nadell J, Kosek J. Peliosis hepatis. Twelve cases associated with oral androgen therapy. Arch Pathol Lab Med 1977;101:405–410.

59. Newman M, Auerbach R, Feiner H, et al. The role of liver biopsies in psoriatic patients receiving long-term methotrexate treatment. Improvement in liver abnormalities after cessation of treatment. Arch Dermatol 1989;125:1218–1224.

60. Paiva LA, Wright PJ, Koff RS. Long-term hepatic memory for hypersensitivity to nitrofurantoin. Am J Gastroenterol 1992;87:891–893.

61. Paliard P, Vitrey D, Fournier G, et al. Perhexiline maleate-induced hepatitis. Digestion 1978;17:419–427.

62. Peters RL, Edmondson HA, Mikkelsen W, et al. Tetracycline induced fatty liver in nonpregnant patients. Am J Surg 1972;113:622–632.

63. Petrovic LM. HIV/HCV co-infection: histopathologic findings, natural history, fibrosis, and impact of antiretroviral treatment: a review article. Liver Int 2007;27(5):598–606.

64. Popper H, Thomas LB. Alterations of liver and spleen among workers exposed to vinyl chloride. Ann NY Acad Sci 1975;246:172–194.
65. Popper H, Geller SA. Pathogenetic considerations in the histologic diagnosis of drug-induced liver injury. Prog Surg Pathol 1981;2:233–246.
66. Portmann B, Talbot IC, Day DW, et al. Histopathological changes in the liver following paracetamol overdose: correlation with clinical and biochemical parameters. J Pathol 1975;117:169–181.
67. Qiang L, Tobias H, Petrovic LM. Drug-induced hepatitis caused by ezetimibe therapy. Dig Dis Sci 2007;52(2):602–605.
68. Rabinowitz M, Van Thiel DH. Hepatotoxicity of nonsteroidal anti-inflammatory drugs. Am J Gastroenterol 1992,87:1696–1704.
69. Rollins BJ. Hepatic veno-occlusive disease. Am J Med 1986;81:297–306.
70. Rotmensch HH, Yust I, Siegman-Igra Y, et al. Granulomatous hepatitis: a hypersensitivity response to procainamide. Ann Intern Med 1978;89:646–647.
71. Roy AK, Mahoney HC, Levine RA. Phenytoin-induced chronic hepatitis. Dig Dis Sci 1993;38:740–743.
72. Ruprah M, Mant TGK, Flanagan RJ. Acute carbon tetrachloride poisoning in 19 patients: implications for diagnosis and treatment. Lancet 1985;1:1027–1029.
73. Shepherd P, Harrison DJ. Idiopathic portal hypertension associated with cytotoxic drugs. J Clin Pathol 1990;43:206–210.
74. Starko KM, Mullick FG. Hepatic and cerebral pathology findings in children with fatal salicylate intoxication: further evidence for a causal relationship between salicylate and Reye's syndrome. Lancet 1983;1:326–329.
75. Sterncek M, Wiesner R, Ascher N, et al. Azathioprine hepatotoxicity after liver transplantation. Hepatology 1991;14:465–471.
76. United States Multicenter FK 506 Liver Study Group. Use of FK 506 for the prevention of recurrent allograft rejection after successful conversion from cyclosporine for refractory rejection. Transplant Proc 1993;25:635–637.
77. Verhamme M, Ramboer C, Van de Bruaene P, et al. Cholestatic hepatitis due to amoxycillin/clavulanic acid preparation. J Hepatol 1989;9:260–264.
78. Woolf GM, Petrovic LM, Rojter SE, et al. Acute hepatitis associated with the Chinese herbal product jin bu huan. Ann Int Med 1994;121:729–735.
79. Zafrani ES, Pinaudeau Y, Dhumeaux D. Drug-induced vascular lesions of the liver. Arch Intern Med 1983;143:495–502.
80. Zimmerman HJ, Ishak KG. Valproate-induced hepatic injury: analysis of 23 fatal cases. Hepatology 1982;2:591–597.

12

GRANULOMAS

Granulomas are found in as many as 10% of liver biopsies, often unexpectedly encountered in biopsies performed for various indications. There are many identifiable causes, including infections and parasitic infestations (4, 7–10, 14,16,26,27,30,35,38,44,55,58,59), immune responses (3,7,11,17,41), foreign materials, and reactions to many drugs (22,23,33,43,45,54,61) (Table 12.1). In as many as one third of cases, the cause may not be determined even when all clinical data are examined and all histologic methods are applied (e-Figs. 12.1–12.4) (1,2,15,18,19,25,28,32,56,57,67). Even after applying special techniques, histologic and immunohistochemical, the cause will still be undetermined in as many as half of the cases studied. Molecular approaches, including polymerase chain reaction (PCR) to identify organisms (e.g., *Histoplasma* (10)), *Mycobacteria* (e-Figs. 12.5, 12.6) are useful but not yet widely applied.

TYPES OF GRANULOMAS

Liver granulomas resemble those seen in other organs. Nonnecrotizing, noncaseating epithelioid and giant cell granulomas are characteristically seen in association with sarcoidosis (Fig. 12.1, e-Figs. 12.7–12.15) (13,28,29) and drug reactions, as well as immune responses, although the sarcoid granulomas may sometimes show slight central necrosis with polymorphonuclear leukocytic infiltration. Older sarcoid lesions show varying degrees of hyalinization and may even disappear to be replaced by collagenous scars (e-Figs. 12.13, 12.14). Sarcoidosis typically has clusters of granulomas (e-Figs. 12.13, 12.14) in the portal and periportal region with eventual fibrosis. The granulomas of drug reaction and primary biliary cirrhosis (PBC) are sarcoid-type but, unlike sarcoid, are sporadic and, often, individual. PBC granulomas tend to be in portal tracts close to the bile duct. Drug-induced granulomas can involve any area of the liver. Many cases reported as "granulomatous hepatitis consistent with sarcoidosis" are actually instances of drug-induced granulomatous disease. The natural history of drug-induced granulomas is not known. Granulomas, without necrosis, are seen in some viral disorders, including hepatitis C (16,65).

Granulomas with necrosis suggest, but do not prove, infectious cause. The prototype, of course, is tuberculosis, with typical central caseation. In early tuberculosis, including miliary, there may be little or no

TABLE 12.1	Causes of Hepatic Granulomas
	1. Undetermined (idiopathic)
	2. Infections
	3. Immunologic
	4. Drugs
	5. Chemicals
	6. Foreign bodies
	7. Neoplasia
	8. Other

necrosis (e-Figs. 12.5, 12.6) and, instead, a polymorphonuclear response may be prominent. Other organisms, including bacteria, fungi, and protozoa, also cause necrotizing granulomas. Patients treated for malignancy with bacillus Calmette-Guérin (bCG) also have necrotizing granulomas (3). In chronic granulomatous disease (CGD) of childhood, granulomas contain homogeneous eosinophilic material, necrotic debris, or typical acute inflammatory exudate (28,47). CGD portal tracts show chronic inflammation and fibrosis, as well as ceroid-type pigment. Specific organisms can sometimes be demonstrated with special stains.

Foreign body granulomas sometimes include recognizable material, such as talc, silicon, or suture material, and can also be seen with specific organisms, such as schistosomiasis (e-Fig. 12.16) (1,51,56).

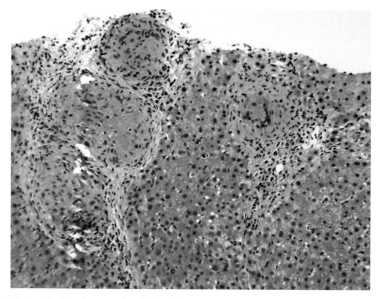

FIGURE 12.1 Photomicrograph of liver biopsy from a patient with sarcoidosis showing multiple noncaseating epithelioid and giant cell granulomas in the portal tract and periportal (zone 1) portion of the liver (hematoxylin-eosin, original magnification ×100).

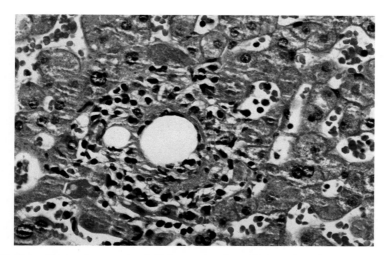

FIGURE 12.2 Photomicrograph of Q fever, showing characteristic, but not pathogno-monic, fibrin ring granuloma (hematoxylin-eosin, original magnification ×400).

Lipogranuloma is a special form of granuloma developing in various conditions (5,40,63) after rupture of steatotic hepatocytes or when excess lipid enters the liver from abdominal and mesenteric sites. They are most often seen in alcoholic liver disease. The usual lipogranuloma consists of focal accumulations of macrophages, which may be epithelioid (e-Fig. 12.17). Alternatively, leukocytes, including polymorphonuclear forms, are seen without epithelioid or giant cell clusters. Lipogranulomas can be indistinguishable from other granulomas since their lipid component is irregularly distributed and not seen in every level of sectioning. Lipogranulomas ultimately become fibrotic. At one time, mineral oil ingestion was considered the principal cause of lipogranuloma, but this is unlikely.

Fibrin-ring granulomas are distinctive, but not etiologically specific (Fig. 12.2) (28,39,46). Previously considered diagnostic for Q fever (e-Figs. 12.18–12.23) (21,49,51,60), they are recognized in other conditions, including cytomegalovirus (37), Epstein-Barr infection (48), hepatitis A (53,66), leishmaniasis (45), allopurinol hypersensitivity (62), and others (21,39,46).

Incomplete (poorly formed) granulomas are seen in patients with acquired immune deficiency syndrome (e-Figs. 12.24, 12.25) (28,64). These generally consist of small clusters of epithelioid cells, without giant cells and generally without necrosis. Despite their relatively modest appearance, they may contain innumerable *Mycobacterium avium-intracellulare* complex (MAI) acid-fast bacilli (Fig. 12.3, e-Fig. 12.26).

DISTRIBUTION OF GRANULOMAS

In some disorders the granulomas almost always occur in a specific area, whereas in other disorders they may be randomly distributed (Table 12.2).

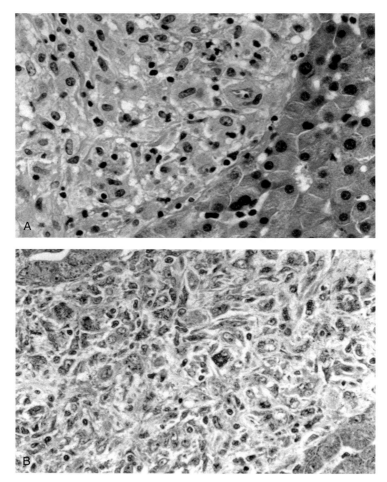

FIGURE 12.3 Photomicrograph of poorly formed (incomplete) granuloma from a patient with acquired immunodeficiency syndrome, with innumerable acid-fast bacilli of *Mycobacterium avium-intracellulare* complex (MAI). (**A.** Hematoxylin-eosin, original magnification ×400; **B.** Ziehl-Neelsen, ×400).

For example, sarcoid-like PBC granulomas are portal, usually close to the bile duct (Fig. 12.4), and are distinctly unusual in the lobule. In sarcoidosis, granulomas are usually portal or periportal (Fig. 12.1).

Infectious disorders generally do not display a particular geographic preference. The granulomas of tuberculosis and fungal or bacterial disorders may be distributed throughout the liver. Similarly, drug-associated granulomas may be anywhere in the liver. Drug-induced granulomas, as well as those with parasitic disorders, can show many eosinophils in addition to the usual lymphocytes and monocytes.

TABLE 12.2	**Examples of Distribution Patterns of Hepatic Granulomas**
Portal	Primary biliary cirrhosis
	Sarcoid
	Schistosomiasis
Portal/periportal	Sarcoid
Portal and/or central	Lipogranulomas
Random	Tuberculosis
	Drug
	Q fever
	Cytomegalovirus
	Chronic granulomatous disease of childhood

IDENTIFYING THE CAUSE OF THE GRANULOMA

Hepatic granulomas can be considered to belong to one of four groups (12): (i) the cause is obvious on the initial liver biopsy specimen; (ii) the cause is determined with special histochemical or immunohistochemical methods, or with supporting clinical information; (iii) the cause remains unproven but is strongly favored by histologic findings; and (iv) the cause cannot be established. Some examples of these are the following:

1. A granuloma whose cause is obvious with hematoxylin-eosin is schistosomiasis (42) (Fig. 12.5, e-Fig. 12.16).

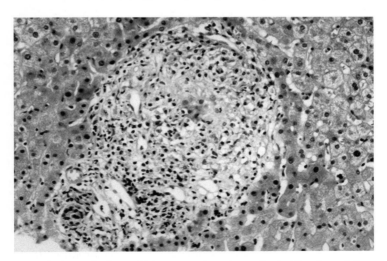

FIGURE 12.4   Photograph of sarcoid-type granuloma in a patient with primary biliary cirrhosis, showing close proximity to injured bile duct (hematoxylin-eosin, original magnification ×200).

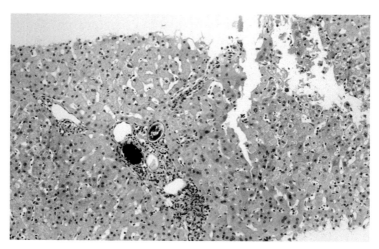

FIGURE 12.5 Photomicrograph of portal tract granuloma showing partially digested shells of *Schistosoma mansoni* (hematoxylin-eosin, original magnification ×200).

2. Special histochemical or immunohistochemical methods may be required to identify tuberculosis and other infectious disorders. In situ hybridization can confirm cytomegalovirus in the immunosuppressed liver transplantation patient (Fig. 12.6). Simple polarizing lenses can demonstrate foreign material. In PBC, the typical clinical presentation of granuloma, characteristic laboratory findings, including elevated titers of antimitochondrial antibodies, coupled with bile duct injury explains the nature of the characteristic granuloma. In drug-induced

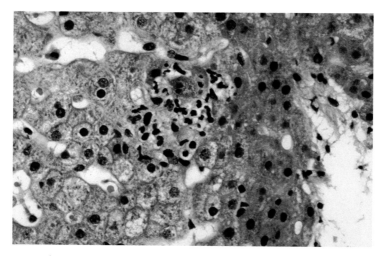

FIGURE 12.6 Photomicrograph of liver biopsy showing a poorly formed granuloma with cytomegalovirus in a patient 8 days after orthotopic liver transplantation (hematoxylin-eosin, original magnification ×400).

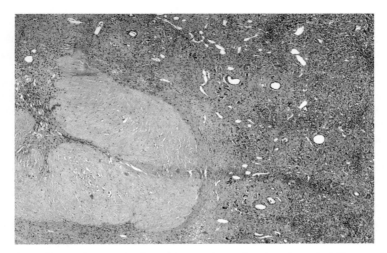

FIGURE 12.7 Photomicrograph of autopsy specimen showing characteristic granuloma of syphilis (gumma) (hematoxylin-eosin, original magnification ×100).

granulomas, eosinophils are often prominent, and when this etiology is suggested, a detailed history may suggest a likely cause (28).

3. Some granulomas, such as the fibrin-ring granuloma of Q fever (Fig. 12.6, e-Figs. 12.18–12.23) or the gumma of syphilis (Fig. 12.7), can help direct the clinical studies that establish cause. The clustering of epithelioid granulomas in sarcoid, although not specific, is strongly suggestive of that diagnosis (Fig. 12.1, e-Figs. 12.14, 12.15).

4. In many instances a diagnosis cannot be established (e-Figs. 12.1–12.4). In these cases, drug reaction or exposure to toxin is generally suspected, but the possibility of a remote neoplasm, including lymphoma (31,50), should be considered.

Key features are summarized in Table 12.3.

TABLE 12.3   **Key Features of Hepatic Granulomas**
1. Any type of granuloma seen in other parts of the body can be seen in the liver.
2. The cause of the granuloma is rarely apparent.
3. The type of granuloma will suggest certain diagnoses.
4. The location of the granuloma will suggest certain diagnoses.
5. Special techniques and historical data may not be helpful, and diagnosis may be impossible in one third of cases.

REFERENCES

1. Alexander JF, Galambos JT. Granulomatous hepatitis. Am J Gastroenterol 1973;59:23–30.
2. Anderson CS, Nicholls J, Rowland R, et al. Hepatic granulomas: a 15-year experience in the Royal Adelaide Hospital. Med J Aust 1988;148:71–74.
3. Artz, MR, Forouhar F. Granulomatous hepatitis as a complication of intravesical bacillus Calmette–Guérin therapy for bladder carcinoma. Ann Clin Lab Sci 1995;25:409–413.
4. Bach N, Thiese ND, Schaffner F. Hepatic histopathology in the acquired immunodeficiency syndrome. Semin Liv Dis 1992;12:205–212.
5. Baptista A, Bianchi L, Groote J, et al. Alcoholic liver disease: morphological manifestations. Lancet 1981;1:707–711.
6. Cathebras PJ, Mosnier JF, Gouilloud S, et al. Hepatic granulomatosis in a patient with Graves' disease. Eur J Gastroenterol Hepatol 1995;7:905–908.
7. Chavenet P, Dillon D, Lancon JP, et al. Granulomatous hepatitis associated with Lyme disease. Lancet 1987;2:623–624.
8. Chien RN, Liu NJ, Lin PY, et al. Granulomatous hepatitis associated with scrub typhus. J Gastroenterol Hepatol 1995;10:484–487.
9. Chien RN, Lin PY, Liaw YF. Hepatic tuberculosis: comparison of miliary and local form. Infection 1995;23:5–8.
10. Collins MH, Jiang B, Croffie JM, et al. Hepatic granulomas in children. A clinicopathologic analysis of 23 cases including polymerase chain reaction for *Histoplasma*. Am J Surg Pathol 1996;20:332–338.
11. de Bayser L, Roblot P, Ramassamy A, et al. hepatic fibrin-ring granulomas in giant cell arteritis. Gastroenterology 1993;105:272–273.
12. Denk H, Scheuer PJ, Baptista A, et al. Guidelines for the diagnosis and interpretation of hepatic granulomas. Histopathology 1993;25:209–218.
13. Devaney K, Goodman, ZD, Epstein MS, et al. Hepatic sarcoidosis. Clinicopathologic features in 100 patients. Am J Surg Pathol 1993;17:1272–1280.
14. De Vega T, Echevarria S, Crespo J, et al. Acute hepatitis by *Listeria monocytogenes* in an HIV patient with chronic HBV hepatitis. J Clin Gastroenterol 1992;15:251–255.
15. Drebber U, Kasper HU, Ratering J, et al. Hepatic granulomas: histological and molecular pathological approach to differential diagnosis – a study of 442 cases. Liver Int 2008;28(6):828–834. 2008 Feb 26 [Epub ahead of print].
16. Emile JF, Sebagh M, Feray C, et al. The presence of epithelioid granulomas in hepatitis C virus–related cirrhosis. Hum Pathol 1993;24:1095–1097.
17. Everett GD, Mitros FA. Eosinophilic gastroenteritis with hepatic eosinophilic granulomas. Am J Gastroenterol 1980;74:519–521.
18. Fauci AS, Wolff SM. Granulomatous hepatitis. In: Popper H, Schaffner F, eds. Progress in Liver Diseases, vol. 5. New York: Grune & Stratton, 1976:609–621.
19. Ferrell LD. Hepatic granulomas: a morphologic approach to diagnosis. Surg Pathol 1990;3:87–106.
20. Ferrell LD, Lee R, Brixco C, et al. Hepatic granulomas following liver transplantation. Clinicopathologic features in 42 patients. Transplantation 1995;60:926–933.
21. Font J, Bruguera M, Perez-Villa F, et al.. Hepatic fibrin-ring granulomas caused by *Staphylococcus epidermidis* generalized infection. Gastroenterology 1987;93:1449–1451.
22. Habior A, Walewska-Zielecka B, Butruk E. Hepatocellular-cholestatic liver injury due to amoxycillin-clavulanic acid combination. Clin Invest 1994;72:616–618.
23. Harrison RF, Elias E. Amiodarone-associated cirrhosis with hepatic and lymph node granulomas. Histopathology 1993;22:80–82.
24. Hofmann CE, Heaton JW Jr. Q fever hepatitis: clinical manifestations and pathologic findings. Gastroenterology 1982;83:474–479.

25. Holtz T, Mosely RH, Scheiman JM. Liver biopsy in fever of unknown origin. J Clin Gastroenterol 1993;17:29–32.

26. Ishibashi H, Shimamura R, Hirata Y, et al. Hepatic granuloma in toxocaral infection: role of ultrasonography in hypereosinophilia. J Clin Ultrasound 1992;20:204–210.

27. Jain R, Sawhney S, Bhargava DK, et al. Hepatic granulomas due to visceral larva migrans in adults: appearance on US and MRI. Abdom Imaging 1994;19:253–256.

28. James DG, Scheuer PJ. Hepatic granulomas. In: Bircher J, Benhamou J-P, McIntyre N, et al., eds. Oxford Textbook of Clinical Hepatology. Oxford: Oxford University Press, 1999: 1099–1108.

29. James DG, Sherlock S. Sarcoidosis of the liver. Sarcoidosis 1994;11:2–6.

30. Johnson TL, Barnett JL, Appelman HD, et al. Candida hepatitis: histopathologic diagnosis. Am J Surg Pathol 1988;12:716–720.

31. Kadin ME, Donaldson SS, Dorfman RF. Isolated granulomas in Hodgkin's disease. N Engl J Med 1970;283:859–861.

32. Kurumaya H, Kono N, Makanuma Y, et al. Hepatic granulomata in long-term hemodialysis patients with hyperalbuminemia. Arch Pathol Lab Med 1989;113: 1132–1134.

33. Larrey D, Vial T, Micaleff A, et al. Hepatitis associated with amoxycillin-clavulanic acid combination; report of 15 cases. Gut 1992;33:368–371.

34. Le Bail B, Jouhanole H, Deugnier Y, et al. Liver adenomatosis with granulomas in two patients on long-term oral contraceptives. Am J Surg Pathol 1992;16:982–987.

35. Lee JD, Kim PG, Jo HJ, et al. A case of primary hepatic actinomycosis. J Korean Med Sci 1993;8:385–389.

36. Liaw YF, Huang MJ, Fan KD, et al. Hepatic injury during propylthiouracil therapy in patients with hyperthyroidism. A cohort study. Ann Intern Med 1993;118:424–428.

37. Lobdell DH. "Ring" granulomas in cytomegalovirus hepatitis. Arch Pathol Lab Med 1987;111:881–882.

38. Malatack JJ, Jaffe R. Granulomatous hepatitis in three children due to cat-scratch disease without peripheral adenopathy. Am J Dis Child 1993;147:949–953.

39. Marazuela M, Moreno A, Yebra M, et al. Hepatic fibrin-ring granulomas: a clinicopathologic study of 23 patients. Hum Pathol 1991;22:607–613.

40. Markin RS, Wisecarver JL, Radio SJ, et al. Frozen section evaluation of donor livers before transplantation. Transplantation 1993;56:1403–1409.

41. Mauer LH, Hughes RW, Folley JH, et al. Granulomatous hepatitis associated with regional enteritis. Gastroenterology 1967;53:301–305.

42. McKerrow JH, Sun E. Hepatic schistosomiasis. Prog Liver Dis 1994;12:121–135.

43. Mirada Canals A, Monteagudo Jiminez M, Sole Villa J, et al. Methyldopa-induced granulomatous hepatitis. DICP 1991;25:1269–1270.

44. Mondou EN, Gnepp DR. Hepatic granuloma resulting from *Enterobius vermicularis*. Am J Clin Pathol 1989;91:97–100.

45. Moreno A, Marazuela M, Yebra M, et al. Hepatic fibrin-ring granulomas in visceral leishmaniasis. Gastroenterology 1988;95:1123–1126.

46. Murphy E, Griffiths MR, Hunter JA, et al. Fibrin-ring granulomas: a non-specific reaction to liver injury? Histopathology 1991;19:91–93.

47. Nakhleh RE, Glock M, Snover DC. Hepatic pathology of chronic granulomatous disease of childhood. Arch Pathol Lab Med 1992;116:71–75.

48. Nevert M, Mavier P, Dubuc N, et al. Epstein–Barr virus infection and hepatic fibrin-ring granulomas. Hum Pathol 1988;19:608–610.

49. Qizilbash AH. The pathology of Q fever as seen on liver biopsy. Arch Pathol Lab Med 1983;107:364–367.

50. Pak HY, Friedman NB. Pseudosarcoid granulomas in Hodgkin's disease. Hum Pathol 1981;12:832–837.

51. Pelligrin M, Delsol G, Auvergnat JC, et al. Granulomatous hepatitis in Q fever. Hum Pathol 1980;11:51–57.

52. Roberts-Thomson IC, Anders RF, Bhathal PS. Granulomatous hepatitis and cholangitis associated with giardiasis. Gastroenterology 1982;83:480–483.

53. Ruel M, Sevestre H, Henry-Biabaud E, et al. Fibrin ring granulomas in hepatitis A. Dig Dis Sci 1992;37:1915–1917.

54. Ruiz-Valverde P, Zafon C, Segarra A, et al. Ticlopidine-induced granulomatous hepatitis. Ann Pharmacother 1995;29:633–634.

55. Saint-Marc Girardin MF, Zafrani ES, Chaumette MT, et al. Hepatic granulomas in Whipple's disease. Gastroenterology 1984;86:753–756.

56. Sartin JS, Walker RC. Granulomatous hepatitis: a retrospective review of 88 cases at the Mayo Clinic. Mayo Clin Proc 1991;66:914–918.

57. Simon HB, Wolff SM. Granulomatous hepatitis and prolonged fever of unknown origin. A study of 13 patients. Medicine 1973;52:1–21, 1973.

58. Smith JW, Utz JP. Progressive disseminated histoplasmosis. Ann Intern Med 1972;76: 557–565.

59. Stjernberg V, Silseth C, Ritland S. Granulomatous hepatitis in Yersinia enterocolitica infection. Hepatogastroenterology 1987;34:56–57.

60. Thung SN, Gerber MA, Lebovics E, et al. Granulomatous hepatitis in Q fever. Mt Sinai J Med 1986;53:283–286.

61. Toft E, Vyberg M, Therkelsen K. Diltiazem-induced granulomatous hepatitis. Histopathology 1991;18:474–475.

62. Vanderstigel M, Zafrani ES, Lejonc JL, et al. Allopurinol hypersensitivity syndrome as a cause of hepatic fibrin-ring granulomas. Gastroenterology 1986;90:188–190.

63. Weitberg AB, Alper JC, Diamond I, et al. Acute granulomatous hepatitis in the course of acquired toxoplasmosis. N Engl J Med 1979;300:1093–1096.

64. Wilkins MJ, Lindley R, Dourakis SP, et al. Surgical pathology of the liver in HIV infection. Histopathology 1991;18:459–464.

65. Yamamoto S, Iguchi Y, Ohomoto K, et al. Epithelioid granuloma formation in type C chronic hepatitis: report of two cases. Hepatogastroenterology 1995;42:291–293.

66. Yamamoto T, Ishii M, Nagura H, et al. Transient hepatic fibrin-ring granulomas in a patient with acute hepatitis A. Liver 1995;15:276–279.

67. Zoutman DE, Ralph ED, Frei JV. Granulomatous hepatitis and fever of unknown origin. J Clin Gastroenterol 1991;13:69–75.

13

ALCOHOLIC LIVER DISEASE

Alcohol-related liver diseases (ALD) are among the earliest recognized and most frequently documented of human disorders (23,30). Alcohol hepatotoxicity is well established and generally relates to amount and duration of excess consumption (26,30,36,43). Genetic polymorphism of both liver alcohol and aldehyde dehydrogenases may predispose to liver injury (28,38). Genetic differences affect individual susceptibility and degrees of dependence and addiction (46). Women have greater susceptibility (26,44,58).

The contribution to susceptibility of additional factors, such as malnutrition, remains controversial. Susceptibility might also be modified by malabsorption, impaired carbohydrate metabolism, and concurrent diseases–associated impaired hepatic metabolism, so-called alcoholic secondary malnutrition, despite adequate diet (33,64).

Three pathways of alcohol metabolism are recognized: the alcohol dehydrogenase (ADH) system, peroxisomal catalase pathways, and, most recently, the microsomal ethanol-oxidizing system (MEOS), a cytochrome p450-dependent pathway (41,43) principally responsible for accelerated clearance of alcohol from blood and also for tolerance (32,41,56). MEOS activity is increased by prolonged and excessive alcohol consumption. In nonalcoholic fatty liver disease (NAFLD), in contrast, insulin resistance and mitochondrial abnormalities have a major role in pathogenesis.

SPECTRUM OF PATHOLOGIC CHANGES IN ALCOHOLIC LIVER DISEASE

A range of clinical liver diseases and morphologic changes is seen in patients with alcoholism (Table 13.1). Several other conditions are also seen (Table 13.2).

Alcoholic Steatosis (Fatty Change)

Patients may be asymptomatic or have mild nonspecific, mostly gastrointestinal, symptoms. Uncommonly, liver failure develops (23,52). Patients often present with hepatomegaly, have elevated serum aminotransferase and α-glutamyl transpeptidase values.

TABLE 13.1	Spectrum of Hepatic Morphologic Changes in Alcoholic Liver Disease

A. Alcoholic steatosis (fatty liver)
  1. Macrovesicular steatosis
  2. Microvesicular steatosis
  3. Mixed, microvesicular and macrovesicular steatosis
  4. Fat granulomas (lipogranulomas)
  5. Alcoholic foamy degeneration
B. Alcoholic steatohepatitis
  1. Ballooning
  2. Steatosis
  3. Inflammation
  4. Perivenular fibrosis (with or without pericellular fibrosis)
  5. Venous occlusion
C. Hemosiderosis, often mimicking hemochromatosis
D. Cirrhosis
  1. Micronodular (Laennec) progressing to macronodular
E. Hepatocellular carcinoma

TABLE 13.2	Other Conditions That May Be Associated with Alcoholic Liver Disease

A. Pancreatitis (acute and chronic)
B. Sepsis
C. Cholestasis
D. Hepatitis C virus infection
E. Porphyria cutanea tarda
F. Zieve syndrome (alcoholic steatosis, jaundice, hyperlipidemia, hemolytic anemia)
G. Fetal alcohol syndrome
H. Drug and toxin interactions
I. Alcoholic cardiomyopathy (usually seen independently of alcoholic liver disease)
J. Alcoholic myopathy (can be seen with or independently of alcoholic liver disease)

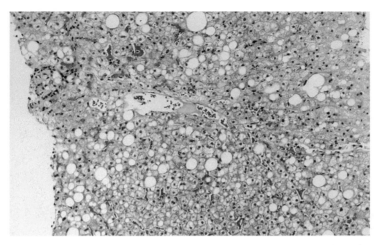

FIGURE 13.1 Macrovesicular steatosis with zonal distribution (zone 3 of the acinus). Large fat droplets replace the liver cell nuclei to the periphery of the cell (hematoxylin-eosin, original magnification ×100).

Alcoholic steatosis is the most common histopathologic feature of chronic ALD. It is the first manifestation of excessive alcohol consumption to appear and the first to resolve, usually within 4 to 6 weeks following abstinence. Steatosis is almost always predominantly macrovesicular with fat droplets (vacuoles) displacing liver cell nuclei to the cell periphery (Fig. 13.1). "Steatosis" and "steatohepatitis" are sometimes used interchangeably. However, "pure" alcohol-induced steatosis, without any inflammatory component, occurs. Patients can also have acute alcohol-induced hepatitis superimposed on steatosis (19,68).

ZONAL DISTRIBUTION OF STEATOSIS. Steatosis is distinctly zonal, initially zone 3 and then zone 2 of the acinus. In severe diffuse steatosis, the entire acinus is involved (Fig. 13.2). This zonal pattern can also be seen in obesity, diabetes mellitus, and after corticosteroid therapy (Table 13.3). In contrast, zone 1 (periportal) steatosis is more often seen in acquired immune deficiency syndrome (AIDS), after total parenteral nutrition (TPN), and in kwashiorkor (36,71). Variable macrovesicular steatosis without zonality is seen with hepatitis C virus infection. Nonspecific mild focal macrovesicular steatosis is also seen.

Early, microvesicular steatosis predominates, with multiple tiny fat droplets surrounding the central nucleus (Fig. 13.3, e-Fig. 13.1). Initially membrane-bound small droplets enlarge and coalesce forming macrovesicles (e-Figs. 13.2, 13.3) with nuclear compression against the cell membrane. Distended hepatocytes can rupture to release their fat and trigger a local inflammatory reaction, with lymphocytes and histiocytes forming a fat granuloma (lipogranuloma) (13) (Fig. 13.4). Lipogranulomas are

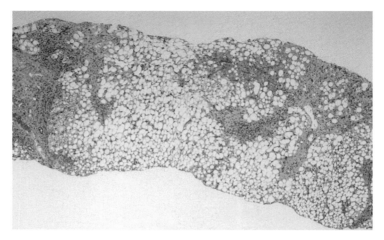

FIGURE 13.2 Diffuse macrovesicular steatosis (hematoxylin-eosin, original magnification ×100).

usually in zones 2 and 3 but also in portal tracts. They may resolve or persist indefinitely, sometimes with minimal scarring. Uncommonly, there is little or no fat (e-Figs. 13.4, 13.5).

Alcoholic Foamy Degeneration

Alcoholic foamy degeneration, also seen in nonalcoholics with liver failure (64), can be transient. Jaundice, hepatomegaly and marked elevations of serum transaminase, alkaline phosphatase, and bilirubin values mimic the clinical picture of large bile duct obstruction (1,16,63).

In addition to macrovesicular steatosis, zone 3 (perivenular) hepatocytes contain numerous tiny fat droplets, giving the cytoplasm a distinctly foamy appearance (Fig. 13.5, e-Fig. 13.1). Intracanalicular cholestasis, focal zone 3 pericellular collagen deposition, and giant mitochondria may

TABLE 13.3	Zonal Distribution of Macrovesicular Steatosis	
Zones 3 and 2	**Zone 1**	**Haphazard, Focal, or Diffuse**
Alcohol	AIDS	Chronic hepatitis C
Diabetes mellitus (NAFLD)	Malnutrition	
Obesity (NAFLD)	Kwashiorkor	
Corticosteroids		
Jejunal bypass		

NAFLD, nonalcoholic fatty liver disease.

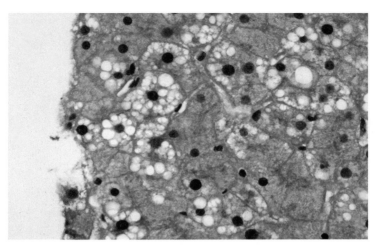

FIGURE 13.3　Microvesicular steatosis. Small fat droplets are clustered around the centrally located nucleus (hematoxylin-eosin, original magnification ×200).

be associated (8,20) (e-Figs. 13.6, 13.7). Mallory material is usually not prominent, and other histopathologic features of acute alcoholic hepatitis are not seen.

Intracytoplasmic Material

Mallory material (Mallory body, Mallory hyline, alcoholic hyalin) (Figs. 13.6, 13.7, 13.11, e-Figs. 13.8–13.12) is somewhat amorphous, eosinophilic or

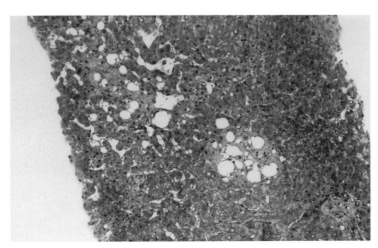

FIGURE 13.4　Lipogranuloma (fat granuloma). Large fat droplets are surrounded by histiocytic and lymphocytic inflammatory cells (hematoxylin-eosin, original magnification ×200).

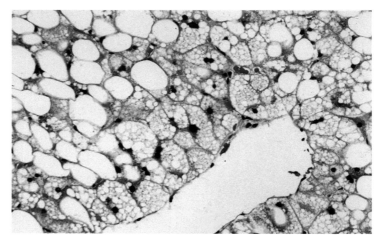

FIGURE 13.5 Foamy degeneration. Numerous small fat droplets in the cytoplasm give the cytoplasm a foamy appearance (hematoxylin-eosin, original magnification ×200).

amphophilic, clumped (ropy) intracytoplasmic material, often surrounding the nucleus as a slightly irregular ring (circular hyaline) (Table 13.4). Mallory material can be irregularly coiled or randomly dispersed in the cytoplasm. Red-purple with Masson trichrome stain, it is blue or red with chromotrope–aniline blue. Usually seen in ballooned hepatocytes, Mallory can also occasionally be in bile duct epithelium. It occurs in all forms of ALD but is in approximately 80% of cases of acute alcoholic hepatitis (6,15,20,21,70).

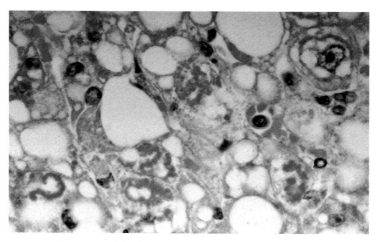

FIGURE 13.6 Mallory material, circular, perinuclear form (hematoxylin-eosin, original magnification ×400).

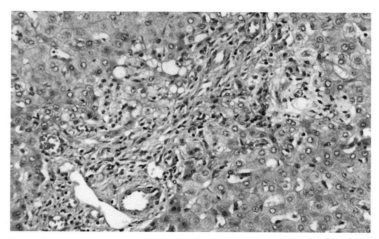

FIGURE 13.7 Mallory material associated with prolonged cholestasis is typically present in the zone 1 (periportal) of the acinus (hematoxylin-eosin, original magnification ×200).

Mallory material represents disrupted cytoskeleton prekeratin and keratin intermediate filaments. Immunostains for both low (CAM 5.2) and high (AE 1/3) molecular weight keratin confirm its cytoskeletal nature. Ubiquitin immunostain particularly highlights Mallory material (14). Hepatocytes with Mallory material can lose cytoplasmic components, primarily cytokeratin (empty cells). The light microscopic appearance of Mallory material reflects three different ultrastructural patterns (65,70).

Mallory material is not specifically diagnostic, but its zonal distribution and association with other histologic features help establish the ALD diagnosis. Other settings are prolonged cholestasis (Fig. 13.7), amiodarone-induced phospholipidosis (53), nonalcoholic steatohepatitis (NASH) (51,54), and Wilson disease (Table 13.5) (35,65,70).

TABLE 13.4 Cytoplasmic Changes in Alcoholic Liver Disease
Ballooning
Steatosis (macrovesicular, microvesicular, mixed)
Foamy steatosis
Mallory material
Giant mitochondria (megamitochondria)
Oncocytic change

TABLE 13.5	Conditions Associated with Mallory Material
1. Alcoholic liver disease	
2. Prolonged cholestasis	
3. Drug-induced (e.g., amiodarone) phospholipidosis	
4. Nonalcoholic steatohepatitis (NASH, NAFLD)	
5. Wilson disease	

NASH, nonalcoholic steatohepatitis; NAFLD, nonalcoholic fatty liver disease.

Mallory material is typically found in zone 3 (centrolobular) in ALD (particularly alcoholic hepatitis), as well as in nonalcoholic fatty diseases (NASH, NAFLD) associated with morbid obesity, diabetes mellitus, and jejunoileal bypass. In chronic cholestasis and Wilson disease, Mallory is usually in zone 1. Mallory material generally disappears approximately 3 months after alcohol use discontinuation.

Giant mitochondria (megamitochondria) are sometimes seen in chronic ALD and as many as 20% of alcoholic steatohepatitis (ASH) cases (9,10). Generally round, sometimes spindle-shaped, these eosinophilic cytoplasmic inclusions (Fig. 13.8, e-Figs. 13.7, 13.8) are not easily seen with hematoxylin, but are bright red with trichrome. Not specific for ALD, they may represent chronic disease or more recent drinking (9,10,29). Numerous giant mitochondria can be seen in zone 3 hepatocytes with foamy degeneration (29).

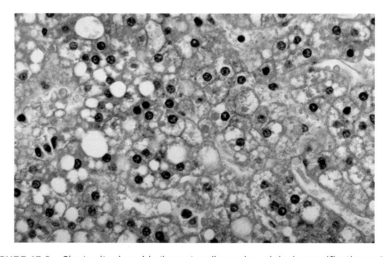

FIGURE 13.8   Giant mitochondria (hematoxylin-eosin, original magnification ×400).

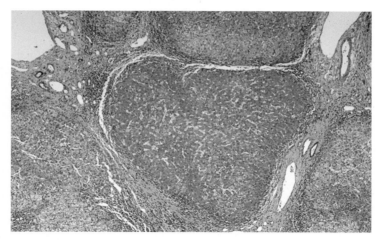

FIGURE 13.9   Oncocytic (oxyphilic) change. The cells have finely granular and glassy, eosinophilic cytoplasm (hematoxylin-eosin, original magnification ×100).

Oncocytic hepatocytes are also seen, most often in already developed cirrhosis from many causes (Fig. 13.9). They have dense, eosinophilic, finely granular, or glassy-appearing cytoplasm, packed with mitochondria. Their significance is not entirely clear (37).

Hemosiderin is often present in hepatocytes, in relatively small quantities in ALD livers (27,39,65). It can also be in sinusoidal endothelial cells (Fig. 13.10, e-Fig. 13.13) and bile duct epithelium (65), and can mimic hereditary hemochromatosis (HH) (see Chapter 15). As in HH, hemosiderin

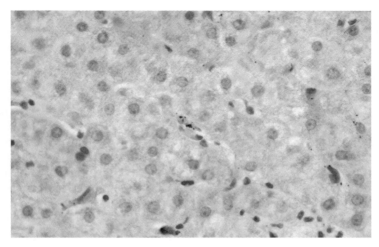

FIGURE 13.10   Hemosiderin is present in sinusoidal endothelial cells (Perls reaction, original magnification ×400).

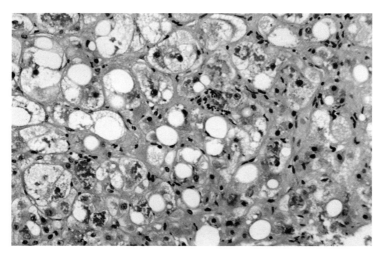

FIGURE 13.11 Acute steatohepatitis (alcoholic). Liver cells with ballooned cytoplasm, Mallory material, surrounded by inflammatory cells (hematoxylin-eosin, original magnification ×200).

initially concentrates in zone 1 hepatocytes. Sometimes it can be difficult to differentiate between ALD hemosiderosis and HH, and quantitative tissue iron and hepatic iron index determination may be necessary (39).

Immunohistochemically demonstrable deposition of sinusoidal immunoglobulin A (IgA) is relatively common in ALD but is not specific. The deposits are a result of impaired IgA intrahepatic transport and metabolism. There is no correlation between the amount of IgA and the severity of histopathologic change (3). Deposits are linear in contrast to the irregular granular pattern seen in other forms of steatohepatitis.

Alcoholic steatohepatitis (ASH), an acute necroinflammatory liver disease usually, but not always, occurs with marked alcoholic intake (binge drinking) (5,6,19,62). The classic histologic triad includes (a) ballooned, distended hepatocytes with (b) Mallory material, and (c) surrounded by clusters of polymorphonuclear leukocytes (Fig. 13.11, e-Figs. 13.2–13.5, 13.9, 13.10), most prominent in zone 3. Macrovesicular steatosis is prominent. These changes involve most of the acinus, as well as multiple acini, forming true bridging necrosis with subsequent bridging/septal fibrosis. If steatosis is scanty, diagnosis is difficult. Mallory material and megamitochondria can also be seen in hepatocytes that do not undergo necrosis (47).

Intrahepatic gene expression in alcoholic steatosis (AS) differs from that of ASH (60). AS-associated genes mostly affect transport biosynthesis, and fatty acid and lipid metabolism. In ASH, genes are involved in many processes including cell adhesion, acute phase response, carbohydrate and cholesterol metabolism, cytoskeleton organization, and immune and inflammatory response. Some genes affect fibrogenesis and ductular reaction.

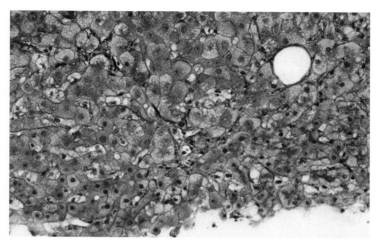

FIGURE 13.12 Perivenular sclerosis (central hyaline sclerosis) (Masson trichrome, original magnification ×100).

Although fibrosis is often seen and is an important feature, its role in the progression of the disease and transition to cirrhosis remains controversial (47,62,67,68). Zone 3 fibrosis (central hyalin sclerosis) (Fig. 13.12, e-Figs. 13.11, 13.15) is typical, resulting from local liver cell destruction and is seen as thick collagen bands around terminal hepatic venules or, characteristically, as stellate distinctive pericellular (perisinusoidal "chicken wire") pattern, well seen with trichrome (Fig. 13.13, e-Figs. 13.16–13.18) (47,61,66,68).

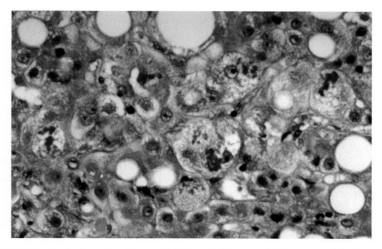

FIGURE 13.13 Pericellular/perisinusoidal fibrosis (Masson trichrome, original magnification ×400).

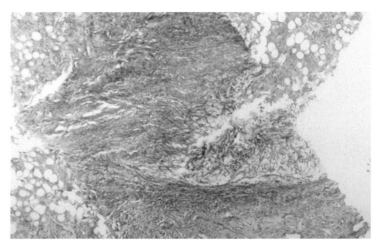

FIGURE 13.14 Venoocclusive disease associated with excess alcohol intake (Masson trichrome, original magnification ×100).

Fibrosis in ASH contributes to narrowing or complete occlusion of terminal hepatic venules, resembling veno-occlusive disease (16,18,53). Not always obvious on needle biopsy, it should be carefully sought for with trichrome stain (Fig. 13.14). There may be no clinical manifestations of venous outflow obstruction. Pericellular fibrosis can also be seen in hypervitaminosis A and after long-term methotrexate therapy, although methotrexate-associated fibrosis is predominantly periportal (24,34,53).

Perivenular cholestasis, intracellular and intracanalicular, is relatively common in ASH and, when severe, is a poor prognostic sign. If there is significant ductular reaction and portal tract edema, large duct obstruction (Fig. 13.15, e-Fig. 13.10) or alcohol-induced acute and chronic pancreatitis should be considered (1,62). Alcoholics can also be septic, also contributing to cholestasis (see Chapter 21). Kupffer cells may be prominent (51).

Differentiating alcoholic hepatitis from viral hepatitis is usually not difficult. Steatosis and ballooning of the hepatocytes with Mallory material surrounded by polymorphonuclear leukocytes contribute to the diagnosis of ASH. Perivenular fibrosis is generally not seen in viral hepatitis. In contrast to ASH, confluent viral hepatitis necrosis leads to collapse of underlying reticulin network. The infiltrate in viral hepatitis is almost invariably lymphocytes, whereas polymorphonuclear cells usually predominate in alcoholic hepatitis. Alcoholics can have other liver diseases, and there is a greater prevalance of both hepatitis B (HBV) and hepatitis C (HCV) (45,50,51,54,57,61).

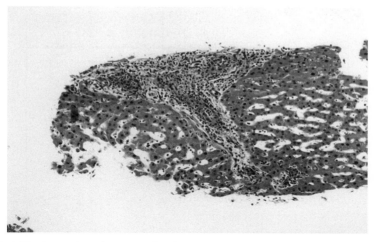

FIGURE 13.15   Secondary changes reflecting chronic pancreatitis and mimicking large bile duct obstruction. Expanded edematous portal tracts with bile ductular proliferation and polymorphonuclear leukocytes (hematoxylin-eosin, original magnification ×100).

DIFFERENTIAL DIAGNOSIS

Differentiating between ASH and NASH/NAFLD (Chapter 21) can be diffi-cult. Histopathologic features can be indistinguishable (2,4,16,25,35,42, 46,48,55), and clinical history is vital (17,47). NASH and NAFLD are asso-ciated with many conditions including diabetes mellitus, morbid obesity, and jejunoileal bypass, as well as various medications such as perhexiline maleate or amiodarone. Subtle histopathologic differences described in NASH (NAFLD) associated with diabetes mellitus include pale Mallory material, mixed and often patchy microvesicular and macrovesicular steato-sis, and more abundant portal lymphoplasmocytic infiltrate (12,25,34,54). Prominence of Mallory material and fat in zone 1 hepatocytes, often with many glycogenated nuclei, is more suggestive of NASH (NAFLD). Recently, several grading and staging systems for NASH/ NAFLD have been proposed (Table 13.6) (7,23). Biopsies in Wilson disease, as well as Indian childhood cirrhosis, can also have features indistinguishable from alcoholic steatohep-atitis with hyaline sclerosis. NASH is also seen in patients with abetal-ipoproteinemia and Weber-Christian disease (31).

CIRRHOSIS WITH ALCOHOLIC CAUSE

Although alcoholic cirrhosis (Laennec cirrhosis) was grossly recognized more than two centuries ago, its pathogenesis remains unclear. Cirrhosis can be preceded by acute alcoholic hepatitis with fibrosis. However, cirrhosis

TABLE 13.6	Histologic Scoring System for NAFLD (Brunt et al. (7), Kliner et al. (23))

Steatosis (0–3)
1 = <33% hepatocytes involved
2 = 33%–66% hepatocytes involved
3 = >66% hepatocytes involved

Hepatocyte ballooning (0–2)
1 = few ballooned cells
2 = many ballooned hepatocytes

Lobular inflammation (0–3)
1 = <2 foci per ×200 field
2 = 2–4 foci per ×200 field
3 = >4 foci per ×200 field

Fibrosis stage
1 Perisinusoidal or portal/periportal
   1A Mild perisinusoidal, zone 3
   1B Moderate perisinusoidal, zone 3
   1C Portal/periportal fibrosis only
2 Perisinusoidal and portal/periportal
3 Bridging fibrosis
4 Cirrhosis

manifests with esophageal varices and/or ascites in many patients lacking clinical or morphologic evidence of liver injury.

Alcoholic cirrhosis, classically micronodular (see Chapter 20), has regenerative nodules less than 0.3 cm in diameter. Delicate fibrous septa connect perivenular areas with portal tracts (Fig. 13.16). Other features of ALD, such as steatosis, Mallory material, and giant mitochondria, may be evident but become less obvious as cirrhosis progresses (6,9, 11,18,19,53,62) (e-Figs. 13.14, 13.16–13.19). Other conditions, such as viral hepatitis, also contribute to the development and progression of cirrhosis.

Regenerative nodules tend to progressively grow, and the micronodular pattern may not persist. Also coexisting liver disorders, such as viral hepatitis, α1-antitrypsin deficiency, and hemosiderin deposition can lead to a mixed micronodular and macronodular pattern of cirrhosis. Cirrhosis generally develops sooner in hepatitis B surface antigen–positive patients who also consume alcohol (50,59). The cirrhosis of

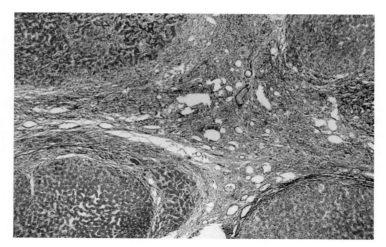

FIGURE 13.16 Alcoholic cirrhosis. Note that the fibrous septa are often paucicellular with numerous newly formed thin-walled vascular channels (hematoxylin-eosin, original magnification ×100).

hereditary hemochromatosis (HH) is also often initially micronodular. Consequently, the cause of cirrhosis cannot always be determined solely based on the pattern of nodularity. Cirrhotics also have disorders that contribute to liver changes, including sepsis, pancreatitis, granulomas, both infectious and drug-associated, and acute hepatitis.

ASSOCIATED DISEASES

Chronic Alcoholic Pancreatitis

Associated hepatic changes resemble those seen at large bile duct obstruction, sometimes with acute ascending cholangitis. There may be marginal bile ductular proliferation and portal and periportal fibrosis (1,62,69). Cholestasis, mostly canalicular and zone 3, may be the first sign of acute or chronic recurrent pancreatitis.

Fetal Alcohol Syndrome

Fetal alcohol syndrome is seen in children of alcoholic mothers. The changes are similar to those of adult alcoholic liver disease, including fatty liver, as well as portal and perisinusoidal (pericellular) fibrosis.

Alcohol-Induced Porphyria Cutanea Tarda

In patients with alcohol-induced porphyria cutanea tarda, the liver biopsy shows steatosis. The Kupffer cells also contain fat droplets and hemosiderin (27).

Hepatitis C Virus

Patients with hepatitis C virus infection generally have more severe disease as well as a higher risk of developing hepatocellular carcinoma (45,69).

Drug and Toxin Interactions

Alcohol potentiates acute liver injury caused by various drugs, including acetaminophen (30,42,49,59). Since zone 3 hepatocytes contain the greatest amount of smooth endoplasmic reticulum and the greatest concentration of P450 cytochromes, the effects of drug or toxin interactions in the setting of alcohol are often most evident in this part of the acinus.

REFERENCES

1. Afroudakis A, Kaplowitz N. Liver histopathology in chronic common bile duct stenosis due to chronic alcoholic pancreatitis. Hepatology 1981;1:65–72.
2. Angulo P. Nonalcoholic fatty liver disease. N Engl J Med 2002;346:1221–1231.
3. Batman PA, Scheuer PJ. Diabetic hepatitis preceding the onset of glucose intolerance. Histopathology 1985;9:237–243.
4. Bird GLA, Sheron N, Goka AKJ, et al. Increased tumor necrosis factor in severe alcoholic hepatitis. Ann Intern Med 1990;112:917–920.
5. Birschbach HR, Harinasuta U, Zimmerman HJ. Alcoholic steatonecrosis. II. Prospective study of prevalence of Mallory bodies in biopsy specimen and comparison of severity of hepatic disease in patients with and without this histological feature. Gastroenterology 1974;66:1195–1202.
6. Bruguera M, Bertran A, Bombi JA, et al. Giant mitochondria in hepatocytes: a diagnostic hint for alcoholic liver disease. Gastroenterology 1977;73:1383–1387.
7. Brunt EM, Janney CG, Di Bisceglie AM, et al. Nonalcoholic steatohepatitis: a proposal for grading and staging the histological lesions. Am J Gastroenterol 1999;94:2467–2474.
8. Chedid A, Mendenhall CL, Tosch T, et al. Significance of megamitochondria in alcoholic liver disease. Gastroenterology 1986;90:1858–1864.
9. Chedid A, Mendenhall CL, Moritz TE, et al. Cell-mediated hepatic injury in alcoholic liver disease. Gastroenterology 1993;105:254–266.
10. Clain DJ, Lefkowitch JH. Fatty liver disease in morbid obesity. Gastroenterol Clin North Am 1987;16:239–252.
11. DiBisceglie AM, Paterson AC, Segal I. The liver in biliary obstruction due to chronic pancreatitis. Liver 1985;5:189–195.
12. Diehl AM, Goodman Z, Ishak KG. Alcohol-like liver disease in nonalcoholics. A clinical and histologic comparison with alcohol-induced liver injury. Gastroenterology 1988; 20:594–598.
13. Falchuk KR, Fiske SC, Haggit RC, et al. Pericentral hepatic fibrosis. Gastroenterology 1980;78:535–541.
14. French SW, Nash J, Shibata P, et al. Pathology of alcoholic liver disease. Semin Liver Dis 1993;13:154–169.
15. Goldberg SJ, Mendenhall CL, Connell AM, et al."Nonalcoholic" chronic hepatitis in the alcoholic. Gastroenterology 1977;72:598–604.
16. Goodman ZD, Ishak KG. Occlusive venous lesions in alcoholic liver disease. A study of 200 cases. Gastroenterology 1982;83:786–796.
17. Hall P de M. Genetic and acquired factors that influence individual susceptibility to alcohol-associated liver disease. J Gastroenterol Hepatol 1992;7:417–426.

18. Jakobovits AW, Morgan MY, Sherlock S. Hepatic siderosis in alcoholics. Dig Dis 1979;24:305–310.

19. Johnson RD, Williams R. Genetic and environmental factors in individual susceptibility to the development of alcoholic liver disease. Alcohol Alcohol 1985;20:137–160.

20. Junge J, Horn T, Christofferson P. Megamitochondria as a diagnostic marker for alcohol induced centrolobular and periportal fibrosis. Virchows Arch APathol Anat Histopathol 1987;410:553–558.

21. Keller M. A historical overview of alcohol and alcoholism. Cancer Res 1979;39: 2822–2829.

22. Kliner DH, Brunt EM, Van Natta M, et al. Design and validation of a histologic scoring system for nonalcoholic fatty liver disease. Hepatology 2005;41:1313–1321.

23. Lane BP, Lieber CS. Ultrastructural alterations in human hepatocytes following ingestion of ethanol with adequate diets. Am J Pathol 1966;49:593–603.

24. Latry P, Bioulac-Sage P, Echinard E, et al. Perisinusoidal fibrosis and basement-like material in the livers of diabetic patients. Hum Pathol 1987;18:775–780.

25. Lee RG. Nonalcoholic steatohepatitis: a study of 49 patients. Hum Pathol 1989;20: 594–598.

26. Lelbach WK. Cirrhosis in the alcoholic and its relation to the volume of alcohol abuse. Ann NY Acad Sci 1975;252:85–105.

27. Le Sage GD, Baldus WP, Fairbanks VF, et al. Hemochromatosis: genetic or alcohol-induced? Gastroenterology 1983;84:1471–1477.

28. Lewis D, Wainwright HC, Kew MC, et al. Liver damage associated with perhexiline maleate. Gut 1979;20:186–189.

29. Lieber CS, Lasker JM, Alderman J, et al. The microsomal ethanol oxidizing systems and its interactions with other drugs, carcinogens and vitamins. Ann NY Acad Sci 1987; 492:11–23.

30. Lieber CS. Metabolic effects of ethanol and its interaction with other drugs, hepatotoxic agents, vitamins and carcinogens: a 1988 update. Semin Liver Dis 1988;8:47–68.

31. Lieber CS. Metabolism of ethanol and associated hepatotoxicity. Drug Alcohol Rev 1991;10:175–202.

32. Loft S, Olesen K-L, Dossing M. Increased susceptibility to liver disease in relation to alcohol consumption in women. Scand J Gastroenterol 1987;10:1251–1256.

33. Lucey MR, Merion RM, Henley KS, et al. Selection for and outcome of liver transplantation in alcoholic liver disease. Gastroenterology 1992;102:1736–1741.

34. Ludwig J, Viggiano TR, McGill DB, et al. Nonalcoholic steatohepatitis: Mayo Clinic experiences with hitherto unnamed disease. Mayo Clin Proc 1980;55:434–438.

35. Maddrey WC. Alcoholic hepatitis: clinicopathologic features and therapy. Semin Liver Dis 1988;8:91–102.

36. McClain CJ, Kromhout JP, Peterson FJ, et al. Potentiation of acetaminophen hepatotoxicity by alcohol. JAMA 1980;244:251–253.

37. Mendenhall CL, Seeff L, Diehl AM, et al. Antibodies to hepatitis B and hepatitis C virus in alcoholic hepatitis and cirrhosis; the prevalence and clinical relevance. Hepatology 1991;14:581–589.

38. Mills LR, Scheuer PJ. Hepatic sinusoidal macrophages in alcoholic liver disease. J Pathol 1985;147:127–132.

39. Morgan MY, Sherlock S, Scheuer PJ. Portal fibrosis in the livers of alcoholic patients. Gut 1978;19:1015–1021.

40. Nakano M, Worner TM, Lieber CS. Perivenular fibrosis in alcoholic liver injury: ultrastructure and histologic progression. Gastroenterology 1982;83:777–785.

41. Nalpos B, Thiers V, Pol S, et al. Hepatitis C viremia and anti-HCV antibodies in alcoholics. J Hepatol 1992;14:381–384.

42. Nasrallah SM, Wills CE Jr, Galambos JT. Hepatic morphology in obesity. Dig Dis Sci 1981;26:325–327.

43. Nebert DW, Adesnick M, Coon MJ, et al. The P-450 gene superfamily: recommended nomenclature. DNA 1987;6:1–11.

44. Nishiguchi S, Kuroki T, Yabusako T, et al. Detection of hepatitis C virus antibodies and hepatitis C virus RNA in patients with alcoholic liver disease. Hepatology 1991;14: 985–989.

45. Norton R, Batey R, Dwyer T, et al. Alcohol consumption and the risk of alcohol related cirrhosis in women. Br Med J 1987;2:80–82.

46. Ohnishi K, Iida S, Iwama S, et al. The effect of chronic habitual alcohol intake on the development of liver cirrhosis and hepatocellular carcinoma: relation to hepatitis B surface antigen carriage. Cancer 1982;49:672–677.

47. Orrego H, Blake JE, Blendis LM, et al. Prognosis of alcoholic hepatitis in the presence and absence of alcoholic hepatitis. Gastroenterology 1987;92:208–214.

48. Pares A, Barrera JM, Caballeria J, et al. Hepatitis C virus antibodies in chronic alcoholic patients: association with severity of liver injury. Hepatology 1990;12:1295–1299.

49. Patek AJ. Alcohol, malnutrition and alcoholic cirrhosis. Am J Clin Nutr 1979;32: 1304–1312.

50. Petrovic LM, Burroughs A, Scheuer PJ. Hepatic sinusoidal endothelium: Ulex binding. Histopathology 1989;14:233–234.

51. Peura DA, Stromeyer FW, Johnson LF. Liver injury with alcoholic hyaline after intestinal resection. Gastroenterology 1980;79:128–130.

52. Popper H, Thung S, Gerber MA. Pathology of alcoholic liver disease. Semin Liver Dis 1981;1:203–216.

53. Poucell S, Ireton J, Valencia-Mayoral P, et al. Amiodarone-associated phospholipidosis and fibrosis of the liver. Light, immunohistochemical and electron microscopic studies. Gastroenterology 1984;86:926–936.

54. Powel EE, Cooksley GE, Hanson R, et al. The natural history of nonalcoholic steatohepatitis: a follow-up study of forty two patients for up to 21 years. Hepatology 1990;11:74–80.

55. Quigley EMM, Marsh MN, Shaffer JL, et al. Hepatobiliary complications of total parenteral nutrition. Gastroenterology 1993;104:286–301.

56. Rigas B, Rosenfeld LE, Barwick KW, et al. Amiodarone hepatotoxicity. A clinicopathologic study of five patients. Ann Intern Med 1986;104:348–351.

57. Rosman AS, Paronnetto F, Galvin K, et al. Hepatitis C virus antibody in alcoholic patients. Association with the presence of portal/or lobular hepatitis. Arch Intern Med 1993;153:965–969.

58. Rubin E, Lieber CS. Fatty liver, alcoholic hepatitis and cirrhosis produced by alcohol in primates. N Engl J Med 1974;290:128–135.

59. Seeff LB, Cuccherini BA, Zimmerman HJ, et al. Acetaminophen hepatotoxicity in alcoholics: a therapeutic misadventure. Ann Intern Med 1986;104:399–404.

60. Seth D, Gorrell MD, Cordoba S, et al. Intrahepatic gene expression in human alcoholic hepatitis. J Hepatol 2006;45(2):306–320.

61. Shimizu S, Kiyusawa K, Sodeyama T, et al. High prevalence of antibody to hepatitis C virus in heavy drinkers with chronic liver disease in Japan. J Gastroenterol Hepatol 1992;7:30–35.

62. Takase S, Takada N, Enomoto N, et al. Different types of chronic hepatitis in alcoholic patients: does chronic hepatitis induced by alcohol exist? Hepatology 1991;13:876–881.

63. Uchida T, Peters RL. The nature and origin of proliferated bile ductules in alcoholic liver disease. Am J Clin Pathol 1983;79:326–333.

64. Uchida T, Kao H, Quispe-Sjogren M, et al. Alcoholic foamy degeneration: a pattern of acute alcoholic liver injury of the liver. Gastroenterology 1983;84:683–692.

65. Uchida T, Kronborg I, Peters RL. Alcoholic hyalin–containing hepatocytes: a characteristic morphologic appearance. Liver 1984;4:233–243.

66. Van Waes L, Lieber CS. Early perivenular sclerosis in alcoholic fatty liver: an index of progressive liver injury. Gastroenterology 1977;73:646–650.

67. Wanless IR, Lentz JS. Fatty liver hepatitis (steatohepatitis) and obesity: an autopsy study with analysis of risk factors. Hepatology 1990;12:1106–1110.

68. Worner TM, Lieber CS. Perivenular fibrosis as precursor lesion of cirrhosis. JAMA 1985;253:627–630.

69. Yamauchi M, Nakahara M, Maezawa Y, et al. Prevalence of hepatocellular carcinoma in patients with alcoholic cirrhosis and prior exposure to hepatitis C. Am J Gastroenterol 1993;88:39–43.

70. Yokoo H, Minick OT, Batti F, et al. Morphologic variants of alcoholic hyalin. Am J Pathol 1972;69:25–40.

71. Zacharie H, Kragballe S, Sogaard H. Methotrexate induced liver cirrhosis. Br J Dermatol 1980;102:407–512.

14

METABOLIC DISORDERS

This chapter will emphasize the most important or most commonly encountered metabolic disorders, highlighting the principal liver biopsy features (Table 14.1).

DISORDERS OF CARBOHYDRATE METABOLISM

Glycogenoses

At least nine metabolic diseases are associated with variably impaired or defective enzymes of glycogen metabolism (61,74,134).

TYPE 1 GLYCOGENOSIS (VON GIERKE DISEASE). Type 1a glycogenosis results from deficiency of glucose-6-phosphatase. In type 1b, enzyme levels are normal but transmembrane transport protein translocase 1 is ineffective. Excess glycogen accumulates in the liver and kidney, and these organs enlarge (61,94). Neonates present with hypoglycemic convulsions and hepatomegaly, obesity, and slow growth. Although compatible with long-term survival, children with type 1a usually die from recurrent infections, complications of gout, or hepatic neoplasms. Definitive treatment is liver transplantation (89).

Pathology. Hepatocytes are enlarged, pale, and distended with glycogen, compressing sinusoids and giving a uniform mosaic pattern (94) (Fig. 14.1, e-Fig. 14.1). Intracellular glycogen is demonstrated with periodic acid–Schiff (PAS) reaction, slightly resistant to diastase digestion, or Best carmine. Optimal glycogen preservation is obtained with alcohol fixation. Glycogenated nuclei are mostly seen in acinus zone 1. Mallory hyalin can be present.

Hepatocellular adenoma, multiple adenomas (Fig. 14.2), macroregenerative nodules, hepatocellular carcinoma (HCC), and hepatoblastoma can be seen (27,28,71,134).

TYPE 2 GLYCOGENOSIS (POMPE DISEASE). Type 2 glycogenosis results from deficiency of lysosomal acid maltase. There are three forms: infantile, childhood, and adult (56,61,94). Infants present with hypotonia, firm

Disorder	Cells Affected	Special Studies
α-Antitrypsin deficiency	Hepatocytes	1) PAS-positive, diastase-resistant globules 2) Specific antibody for α1-antitrypsin 3) EM (granular material in RER)
Fibrinogen storage disease	Hepatocytes	1) Specific antibody for fibrinogen 2) EM (amorphous, granular material in RER, fingerprint pattern)
Gaucher disease	Kupffer cells	1) EM (lysosomal tubular disease, portal macrophages, inclusions)
Glycogenosis IV	Hepatocytes	1) PAS-positive, partially digested with diastase 2) EM (non-membrane-bound filamentous material)
Lafora disease	Hepatocytes	1) PAS-, PAS/D-positive inclusions 2) EM (non-membrane-bound filaments)
Mucopoly-saccharidosis	Hepatocytes, Kupffer cells	1) Colloidal iron–positive 2) EM (lysosomes with stellate [Ito] cells, flocculent material)

TABLE 14.1 Metabolic Disorders with Diagnostic Histopathologic and Ultrastructural Features

PAS, periodic acid–Schiff; EM, electron microscopy; RER, rough endoplasmic reticulum.

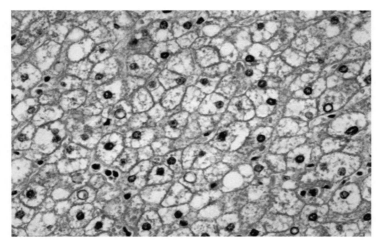

FIGURE 14.1 Glycogenosis I. Note the hepatocytes with pale, glycogen-rich cytoplasm (hematoxylin-eosin, original magnification ×200).

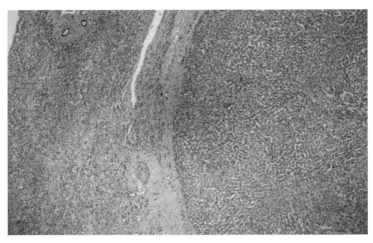

FIGURE 14.2 Hepatic adenoma in glycogenosis I. One of the multiple adenomas that developed in association with this metabolic disorder. The patient subsequently underwent liver transplantation (hematoxylin-eosin, original magnification ×100).

skeletal musculature, respiratory distress, significant cardiomegaly, and mild hepatomegaly. Hypoglycemia and liver dysfunction are not seen, and death results from heart and respiratory failure during the first year of life.

The childhood form is clinically similar to muscular dystrophy, with glycogen accumulation in the muscle. Liver and muscles are deficient in acid maltase, but glycogen characteristically accumulates only in muscle. Adults present in the third or forth decade with muscle weakness without evidence of liver and heart involvement.

Pathology. The liver findings may be nonspecific. Ultrastructurally, glycogen is seen in the lysosomes of many cells, including hepatocytes (74).

TYPE 3 GLYCOGENOSIS (FORBES DISEASE, CORI DISEASE). Type 3 glycogenosis results from a deficiency of debrancher enzyme (amylo-1,6-glucosidase) (14,61,74). The liver and smooth muscle are variably affected, and a spectrum of diseases is seen. Usually manifesting by age 5, there is hypoglycemia, ketoacidosis, glucagon unresponsiveness after fasting, recurrent infections, and significant hepatomegaly.

Pathology. Similar to type 1, abundant glycogen is in hepatocytes, smooth muscle, heart, and peripheral blood leukocytes (e-Figs. 14.2–14.4). Fibrosis and cirrhosis may occur. Ultrastructurally, lipid droplets are also seen (74).

TYPE 4 GLYCOGENOSIS (BRANCHER DEFICIENCY, AMYLOPECTINOSIS, ANDERSON DISEASE). Fewer than 20 cases have been described (62). The brancher enzyme deficit causes deposition of abnormal amylopectin-type glycogen (70,118). Patients present with hepatomegaly and failure to thrive. Cirrhosis usually

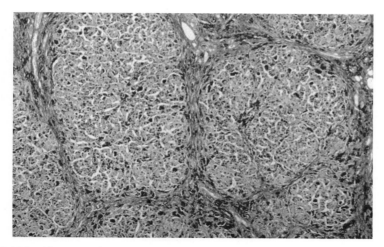

FIGURE 14.3   Glycogenosis IV. Note numerous hepatocytes containing abnormal glycogen amylopectin (hematoxylin-eosin, original magnification ×200).

develops within the first few years of life, and death is often due to heart failure. The only curative treatment is liver transplantation. Deposition of abnormal glycogen in the heart can lead to death from heart failure despite liver transplantation.

Pathology. The histopathology is characteristic. Enlarged hepatocytes have pale eosinophilic or amphophilic intracytoplasmic, PAS-positive, diastase-resistant inclusions (Figs. 14.3–14.5, e-Fig. 14.5), often surrounded by a clear zone (6,74). Resembling Lafora bodies (17,74,75,94,99) or

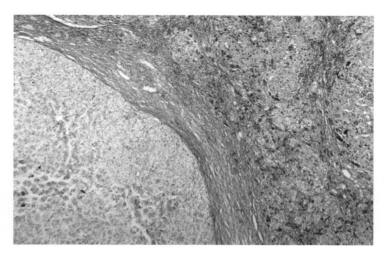

FIGURE 14.4   Glycogenosis IV. Note macroregenerative nodule developing in the background of cirrhotic liver (PAS original magnification ×100).

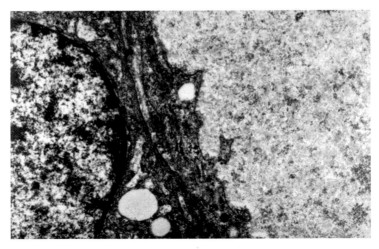

FIGURE 14.5 Glycogenosis IV. Ultrastructure showing glycogen particles dispersed in cytoplasm.

ground-glass cells, they are present throughout the parenchyma. Fibrosis and cirrhosis develop early. Liver cell adenoma has been described (3).

Galactosemia

Galactosemia is a result of deficiency of galactose-1-phosphate uridyl-transferase (76). When milk is introduced in the diet, neonates present with failure to thrive, vomiting, hepatosplenomegaly, jaundice, and ascites. If diagnosed early, the disease is reversible with diet correction (4). Untreated patients develop cirrhosis, cataracts, mental retardation, and HCC (133).

PATHOLOGY. Hepatic changes can be indistinguishable from acute tyrosinemia, with diffuse steatosis, subsequent marked cholestasis, bile ductular proliferation, and striking pseudoacinar transformation of liver cells. Extramedullary hematopoiesis and mild hemosiderosis may also be seen. Steatosis diminishes with time. Pericellular fibrosis and cirrhosis develop, often in months (e-Figs. 14.6, 14.7).

Hereditary Fructose Intolerance

Two hereditary forms affect the liver. Fructose-1-phosphate aldolase (aldolase B) deficiency is most common (12,53), and deficiency of fructose-1, 6-biphosphatase (22) also occurs. Children present, after introduction of fructose-containing formula, with abdominal pain, nausea and vomiting, and failure to thrive. They have fructosemia, fructosuria, hypophos-phatemia, and metabolic acidosis. Diagnosis may be delayed in some children who develop a natural aversion to fructose-containing foods (102).

PATHOLOGY. Liver changes are nonspecific until perivenular steatosis and cholestasis develop. Many hepatocytes contain amylopectin (Fig. 14.3). Mildly fibrotic portal tracts show ductular reaction. Giant cell hepatitis develops in neonates, with progression to fibrosis and cirrhosis. Electron microscopy is virtually diagnostic (Fig. 14.5) (109).

DISORDERS OF GLYCOPROTEIN AND PROTEIN METABOLISM

Mucopolysaccharidoses

These rare lysosomal storage diseases are a result of deficiency of enzymes that degrade connective tissue mucopolysaccharides (74). There are at least ten subtypes.

PATHOLOGY. Histologic changes are subtle and nonspecific (38,67,92). Pale slightly basophilic cytoplasm of hepatocytes, Kupffer cells, and biliary epithelial cells reflect the presence of enlarged lysosomes filled with the deposited mucopolysaccharides (64). Alcian blue and colloidal iron are helpful. Kupffer cells show diffuse staining, whereas hepatocytes are more granular patterned (64,74,109). Pericellular fibrosis and cirrhosis develop (105).

Mucolipidoses

Lysosomes are affected because of variable mucopolysaccharide, glycoprotein, and lipid metabolic defects (74), with at least four mucolipidosis types (mucolipidosis I, sialidosis, gargoylism, Hurler disease).

Neuraminidase (sialidase) deficiency is demonstrable in peripheral leukocytes and cultured fibroblasts. Affected children usually present with developmental retardation, gargoyle-like facial features, and dysostosis. They develop peripheral neuropathy, muscular weakness, corneal opacities, and impaired hearing.

PATHOLOGY. Liver macrophages are enlarged with foamy cytoplasm and prominent Kupffer cells. Ultrastructurally, hepatocytes, Kupffer cells, and biliary epithelium have vacuolar lysosomes containing granular and flocculent material (74,109).

ENDOPLASMIC RETICULUM STORAGE DISEASES

α1-Antitrypsin Deficiency

α1-Antitrypsin (α1-AT), a glycoprotein, is a protease inhibitor that is primarily synthesized in hepatocytes. The gene is on chromosome 14, with as many as 70 allelic forms. Normal phenotype is Pi (protease inhibitor) MM (74). The two major forms are the homozygous, phenotype PiZZ, and heterozygous, PiMZ and PiSZ. PiZZ has a single amino acid, lysine, substitution for glutamine at position 342, causing the secretion of a defective

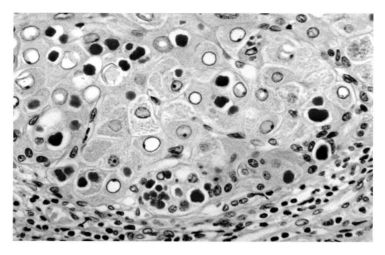

FIGURE 14.6 α1-Antitrypsin deficiency. Note numerous α1-antitrypsin globules in the periseptal hepatocytes (periodic acid–Schiff after diastase original magnification ×200).

enzyme and the accumulation of α1-AT in endoplasmic reticulum. Liver disease occurs mostly in homozygous patients (8,30,31,32).

Both heterozygous (PiMZ) and homozygous (PiZZ) forms have the characteristic and diagnostic PAS-positive, diastase-resistant hepatocyte globules, mostly in zone 1 (Fig. 14.6). The globules range from 1 to 40 mm, and when abundant and large enough, are seen in hematoxylin-eosin–stained slides as round, eosinophilic globules. Smaller globules require PAS/D for visualization (15,24,54,55). Distribution, however, may be uneven and can be highlighted immunohistochemically with specific monoclonal α1-AT antibody (24,103). Similar globules have been described with congestion, usually in zone 3, in PiMM individuals (15,114).

Homozygous α1-AT deficiency can manifest in neonates with hepatomegaly, cholestasis, jaundice, neonatal hepatitis, paucity of bile ducts, or bile ductular proliferation, mimicking many other conditions (59). As many as 30% of children with neonatal hepatitis of unknown cause have abnormal Pi phenotypes. Disease progresses in 20% to 30%, with fibrosis and cirrhosis developing as early as 4 months of age (137). Early changes can even be seen in the fetal liver (90).

Homozygous adults are mostly men older than age 50 years presenting with advanced chronic liver disease or cirrhosis (116). Panlobular emphysema occurs in 80% to 90%. Other associations include membranoproliferative glomerulonephritis, hematuria, Wegener granulomatosis, and systemic vasculitis (5,52). Liver injury results from the direct effect of accumulated α1-AT material in hepatocytes (54,90,107,137). In homozygotes as well as in transgenic mouse models, α1-AT can be in various tissues in addition to the liver (26,42). HCC occurs with or without cirrhosis

(30,44,46,116). α1-AT deficiency can occur with other liver diseases, including alcoholic liver disease, hepatitis B and C, and autoimmune hepatitis (44,45,68,110,113,119).

PATHOLOGY. Liver biopsy may be diagnostic in neonates in whom the clinical diagnosis is unclear, with characteristic globules demonstrable histochemically and immunohistochemically (24,26,57,63,114) (e-Figs. 14.8–14.13). Nonspecific liver changes include mild chronic hepatitis, fibrosis, and cirrhosis, sometimes interpreted as cryptogenic cirrhosis if the characteristic globules are not seen. HCC can develop (46,54) (e-Figs. 14.14, 14.15). Electron microscopy demonstrates granular electron-dense material in dilated, rough endoplasmic reticulum (50).

α1-Antichymotrypsin Deficiency

Low serum levels of both α1-AT and α1-antichymotrypsin can be demonstrated. Inheritance is autosomal dominant, and the liver can show signs of chronic hepatitis and cirrhosis (47).

PATHOLOGY. Granular or globular eosinophilic intracytoplasmic material, similar to that seen in α1-AT deficiency can be seen, and electron microscopy confirms the presence of the material in dilated endoplasmic reticulum (86).

Afibrinogenemia and Hypofibrinogenemia

The relatively rare autosomal recessive disorders afibrinogenemia and hypofibrinogenemia are characterized by intracytoplasmic fibrinogen inclusions (Fig. 14.7), confirmed with specific antibody (23). Ultrastructurally,

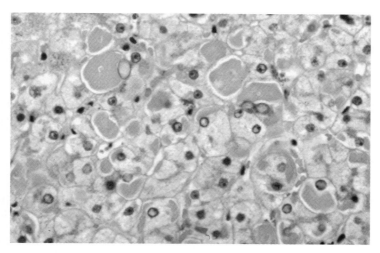

FIGURE 14.7   Fibrinogen globules in the liver of a patient with hypofibrinogenemia (hematoxylin-eosin, original magnification ×400).

fibrinogen is deposited in the cisterns of the rough endoplasmic reticulum in a finger-like pattern.

DISORDERS OF LIPOPROTEIN AND LIPID METABOLISM

β-Lipoprotein Deficiency

This autosomal codominant disorder results from deficiency of apoprotein B100, a lipoprotein primarily synthesized in the liver, and a component of both low-density lipoprotein (LDL) and very-low-density lipoprotein (VLDL) (5,11). Patients lack LDL and VLDL. Patients have steatorrhea and fat malabsorption, acanthocytosis, retinitis pigmentosa, and ataxic neuropathic disease, all developing during infancy. Liver transplantation has been used (10).

PATHOLOGY. There is variable hepatic steatosis, and some patients develop fibrosis and cirrhosis (5).

Familial High-Density Lipoprotein Deficiency (Tangier Disease)

This deficiency of α-lipoprotein and high-density lipoprotein, with low cholesterol levels and esterified cholesterol accumulation in macrophages, is an autosomal recessive disorder (16). Tonsillar enlargement, generalized lymphadenopathy, hepatosplenomegaly, and peripheral neuropathy are seen, with xanthomas and thrombocytopenia (69).

PATHOLOGY. Cholesterol crystal deposits impart a striking orange coloration to tissues. Microvesicular steatosis and foamy cellular changes, as well as birefringent, needle-shaped crystals, are typical (35,51).

Familial Hypercholesterolemia

This autosomal dominant inherited disorder has a high concentration of LDL (20), with cholesterol accumulating in tendons, skin, and arteries. Xanthomas and atheromas usually develop.

PATHOLOGY. Neutral lipids and cholesterol are present in the hepatocytes and Kupffer cells, sometimes seen as microvesicular steatosis (21).

Familial Hyperlipoproteinemia

Familial hyperlipoproteinemia patients have high blood levels of various lipoproteins, with lipoproteins in macrophages of various organs, including bone marrow, spleen, and liver (20).

PATHOLOGY. Hepatocytes and Kupffer cells contain variable numbers of fat droplets, with foamy portal histiocytes. Ultrastructurally, nonspecific mitochondria and endoplasmic reticulum changes are seen (21).

LYSOSOMAL STORAGE DISEASES

Gaucher Disease

Gaucher disease (cerebroside lipidosis) is one of the most common lysosomal storage diseases, with three clinical types. Mutations of β-glucosidase structural gene localize to chromosome 1. Enzyme replacement treatment, as well as bone marrow transplantation and liver transplantation, has been successful (7,142).

Type I (chronic nonneuronopathic), particularly prevalent in Ashkenazi Jews, affects children and adolescents. Hepatosplenomegaly and pancytopenia are complicated by skeletal manifestations, including spontaneous fractures, degenerative hip disease, and aseptic necrosis.

Type II (neonatal) usually leads to death before age 2. Neurologic symptoms are seen early, with later hepatosplenomegaly, lymphadenopathy, spasticity, and cranial nerve involvement.

Type III (adults) typically has hepatosplenomegaly with eventual progressive mental deterioration. Death occurs in the second to fourth decades.

PATHOLOGY. The principal hepatic change is in zone 3 Kupffer cells and portal histiocytes (Fig. 14.8, e-Figs. 14.16–14.19). Cytoplasm is distended by linear amphophilic material highlighted with antibody for KP-1, a histiocytic marker. Hepatocytes become compressed and atrophic, with secondary pericellular fibrosis progressing to cirrhosis, often manifesting as portal hypertension (74). Elongated lysosomes with accumulated deposits of glucocerebroside are seen ultrastructurally. Mild iron deposition seen consists of individual ferritin micelles (109).

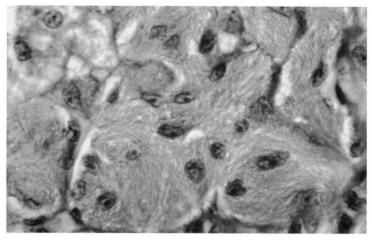

FIGURE 14.8 Gaucher disease. Note numerous histiocytes with striated cytoplasm (hematoxylin-eosin, original magnification ×200).

Sphingomyelin Lipidosis (Niemann-Pick Disease)

Niemann-Pick disease results from impaired sphingomyelinase activity with subsequent tissue accumulation of sphingomyelin. Of several variants, the first four are autosomally inherited (84,85). The sphingomyelinoses differ at least partly because the enzyme is deficient in types A and B, but enzymatic activity is within normal range in types C, D, and E (88). Liver transplantation has been used (41,132).

Type A (acute neuronopathic) is most common, manifesting in infancy with vomiting, failure to thrive, hepatosplenomegaly, bronchopneumonia, osteoporosis, anemia, thrombocytopenia, and olive discoloration of the skin. One third of patients have macular degeneration with a characteristic cherry-red spot. Progressive neurologic degeneration leads to death by the age of 4. Type B (chronic form without central nervous system involvement) lacks neurologic symptoms but has hepatosplenomegaly. Type C (subacute form with central nervous system involvement) has a later onset, usually by age 2 years, and a progressive course. Patients die in childhood or adolescence (140). Type D (Nova Scotia form) has intellectual deterioration starting at school age, with transient jaundice during infancy. The course is progressive with development of spasticity, mental retardation, and seizures. Death is usually before age 15 years. Type E (indeterminate adult form) affects adults, who have hepatosplenomegaly but no neurologic symptoms.

PATHOLOGY. Reticuloendothelial cells throughout the body are enlarged. Enlarged Kupffer cells contain sphingomyelin seen as tiny cytoplasmic vacuoles. Cells also contain lipofuscin and ceroid, giving them a brown tinge on routine sections. Intrahepatic cholestasis may be seen (Fig. 14.9, e-Figs. 14.20–14.23). Niemann-Pick also presents as neonatal

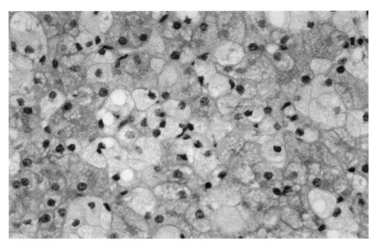

FIGURE 14.9   Niemann-Pick disease. Note Kupffer cells and foamy histiocytes containing deposits of sphingomyelin (hematoxylin-eosin, original magnification ×200).

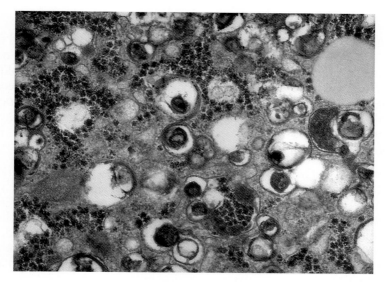

FIGURE 14.10   Niemann-Pick. Ultrastructure showing lipid vacuoles, including many myelin-like figures.

hepatitis. Fibrosis is seen, but true cirrhosis is uncommon (138,140). Foam cells are autofluorescent and birefringent under polarized light and stain with fat stains in frozen material. Ultrastructural findings are characteristic, but not pathognomonic, with dense 1- to 5-mm lipid inclusions forming concentric laminated myelin-like figures with a periodicity of approximately 5 nm (Fig. 14.10) (109).

GANGLIOSIDOSES

Three gangliosidosis types are recognized: GM1, GM2, and GM3 (100, 144).

GM1 Gangliosidosis

GM1 gangliosidosis has two forms: infantile (type I) and juvenile (type II), both a result of absence or deficient activity of lysosomal isoenzyme GM1 galactosidase (100,108). Type I affects infants who have hepatomegaly, progressive psychomotor retardation, seizures, failure to thrive, and characteristic facial abnormalities. Half have macroglossia and a macular cherry-red spot. Death is by age 2 years in type I and between 3 and 8 years in type II.

PATHOLOGY. Epithelial cells, including hepatocytes and renal glomerular cells, show fine vacuolation (74,109). Bone marrow foam cells and lymphocyte vacuolation are seen. Histiocytes throughout the body show lipid accumulation. Ultrastructurally, Kupffer cells contain distinctive granulofibrillar material, and both hepatocytes and Kupffer cells have membrane-bound inclusions.

GM2 Gangliosidosis, Including Tay-Sachs Disease

GM2 gangliosidosis has accumulation of GM2 ganglioside in neural tissue (109). Type I, infantile or Tay-Sachs disease, the most severe type, results from the absence of hexosaminidase A and is most common in Ashkenazi Jews. Newborns present with apathy, weakness, and difficulty feeding. Spasticity with subsequent quadriplegia, excessive drooling, and focal or generalized convulsions can follow. Visual abnormalities develop with a characteristic cherry-red spot, disorderly eye movements, optic nerve degeneration, and blindness.

PATHOLOGY. On light microscopy, hepatocytes are unremarkable. Ultrastructurally, they show membrane-bound inclusions (109).

Type II, Sandhoff disease, is caused by hexosaminidase A and B deficiency, and GM2 accumulation in neural tissue and other organs. There is no ethnic predilection. In neonates, motor development is delayed, with mild hepatomegaly and cardiovascular symptoms. Psychomotor retardation is progressive; optic atrophy and cherry-red spots develop early. Affected children often die from aspiration before age 3.

Pathology. On routine light microscopy, changes are subtle and nondiagnostic. Ultrastructurally, lysosomal lipid accumulates in hepatocytes and lymphocytes (109).

Type III, the juvenile form, has partial deficiency of hexosaminidase A. Children present between age 2 and 6 years with locomotor ataxia, impaired speech, and reduced or lost intellectual abilities. Extrapyramidal rigidity, grand mal seizures, decerebrate rigidity, and somnolence develop, typical of late stage disease.

Pathology. Histologic findings are minimal and entirely nonspecific.

Glycosphingolipid Lipidosis (Fabry Disease)

An X-linked disorder, glycosphingolipid lipidosis (Fabry disease) is caused by deficiency of the lysosomal hydrolase α-galactosidase, with subsequent accumulation of ceramide trihexoside in various tissues (74,121). Signs and symptoms first occur in childhood or adolescence, with paresthesias, hypohidrosis, and cutaneous angiokeratomas. Kidney and cardiovascular system involvement lead to death.

PATHOLOGY. Kupffer cells, portal macrophages, and sinusoidal endothelial cells are light tan and filled with a mixture of PAS-positive cholesterol and ceramide. Ultrastructurally, concentric laminated inclusions can be seen in Kupffer cells, portal macrophages, and hepatocytes (74,109).

Sulfatide Lipidosis (Metachromatic Leukodystrophy) (117)

PATHOLOGY. Foamy histiocytes are present with metachromatic granules mostly in portal histiocytes, but also in Kupffer cells and hepatocytes. The gallbladder has the most striking changes, however, with numerous foamy histiocytes in the lamina propria (129).

FATTY ACID OXIDATION DISORDERS

Systemic Carnitine Deficiency (78)

PATHOLOGY. The liver shows diffuse panacinar microvesicular and macrovesicular Steatosis with portal and septal fibrosis. Sometimes there is only minimal change or mild portal inflammation. Electron microscopy is not contributory.

WOLMAN AND CHOLESTEROL ESTER STORAGE DISEASES

Wolman Disease

Failure to thrive, abdominal distention, vomiting, severe diarrhea, and steatorrhea are seen in the first year of life with hepatosplenomegaly, ascites, and malnutrition (96). Enlarged adrenal glands with calcifications can be seen with imaging studies. Internal organs, including liver, are yellow.

PATHOLOGY. Kupffer cells and histiocytes contain abundant cholesterol and cholesterol ester. Liver cells show predominantly microvesicular steatosis, caused by neutral lipid accumulation demonstrable in frozen sections with fat stains (83); with polarized light, the cholesterol has striking birefringence.

Cholesterol Ester Storage Disease

Cholesterol ester storage disease is milder than Wolman disease. Patients have hepatomegaly and occasionally splenomegaly (33,39).

PATHOLOGY. Liver histology is similar to that of Wolman disease. Kupffer cells and portal histiocytes are foamy appearing, highlighted by PAS reaction. Mild fibrosis may be present, but cirrhosis is rare.

Ceramide Deficiency (Farber Lipogranulomatosis) (97,139)

PATHOLOGY. Granulomatous infiltrates are present in multiple organs, including the liver. They contain foamy lymphocytes, foamy histiocytes, and histiocytes with faintly granular PAS-positive material. Fibrosis may develop (139). Ultrastructurally, histiocytes contain filamentous or tubular structures called Farber bodies. The presence of so-called banana bodies has been documented in Schwann cells, not in the liver.

PEROXISOMAL DISORDERS

Primary Hyperoxaluria

Type I is a result of deficiency of alanine-glyoxylate aminotransferase, which occurs almost exclusively in liver peroxisomes. Type II is exceedingly rare and caused by d-glycerate dehydrogenase deficiency (73). Urinary calcium oxalate stones form, and calcium oxalate accumulates in heart, bones, arteries, retina, and bone marrow. Cardiac arrhythmias, vascular disease, bone fractures, and hepatosplenomegaly, from extramedullary hematopoiesis, are seen (72). Liver transplantation corrects the defect (115,145).

PATHOLOGY. The liver changes are nonspecific, with increased lipofuscin and hemosiderin, especially after renal hemodialysis (73). Oxalate crystals are not seen.

Zellweger Syndrome, Neonatal Adrenoleukodystrophy, and Infantile Refsum Disease

Zellweger syndrome, neonatal adrenoleukodystrophy, and infantile Refsum disease all involve impaired assembly of peroxisomes (125,131). Zellweger syndrome is characterized by a striking lack of peroxisomes in the liver (19,93). Patients present with facial dysmorphism, atrophy, seizures, and neurologic impairment. Neonatal adrenoleukodystrophy and Refsum disease are milder variants of Zellweger syndrome, and patients have less striking dysmorphic changes (73,111).

PATHOLOGY. The liver findings are nonspecific and variable, with mild steatosis, prominent Kupffer cells, focal liver cell necrosis, cholestasis, hemosiderosis, and sometimes, portal and periportal fibrosis (59,111,126) (e-Figs. 14.24, 14.25). Peroxisome absence and the presence of lamellated lysosomes are the principal ultrastructural findings (e-Fig. 14.26).

Pseudo-Zellweger Syndrome

Pseudo-Zellweger syndrome has been described in a child with an isolated enzyme defect involving 3-oxacyl coenzyme A thiolase. The liver showed steatosis with portal fibrosis. Ultrastructurally, both hepatocytes and Kupffer cells contained numerous enlarged peroxisomes with associated lamellar intracytoplasmic and intralysosomal inclusions (58).

Zellweger-Like Syndrome

Zellweger-like syndrome has been described in a child who died of liver failure. Ultrastructural examination revealed the presence of normal-sized peroxisomes and enlarged mitochondria (111).

METABOLIC DISORDERS AFFECTING AMINO ACID METABOLISM

Tyrosinemia

Tyrosinemia is an autosomal recessive disease caused by a defect of fumarylacetoacetase. It can be acute or chronic (82). The serum tyrosine level is elevated in both forms. Patients have hypoglycemia, hypophosphatemia, glucosuria, and radiologic manifestations of rickets. The serum α-fetoprotein level may also be elevated. Neonates present with fulminant liver failure, including bleeding, hypoglycemia, and renal tubular dysfunction. Death often occurs during the first year, even if the diet has been corrected. Chronic tyrosinemia is characterized by growth retardation, gastrointestinal symptoms, cirrhosis and hepatic failure, and multiple renal tubular defects. Patients surviving longer than 2 years have a significant risk for HCC. Death usually occurs in the first decade. The acute, fulminant form of tyrosinosis resembles submassive and massive hepatic necrosis. Liver transplantation is the treatment of choice (91,95).

PATHOLOGY. Histopathologic features are nonspecific. There is marked cholestasis with significant pseudoacinar transformation (Fig. 14.11) and pericellular fibrosis. Focal or extensive microvesicular steatosis can be seen; with progression, cirrhosis develops. Liver cell dysplasia, macroregenerative nodules, and multifocal HCC occur (34,36). Electron microscopy confirms fat droplets, cholestasis, enlarged and pleomorphic mitochondria, and pericellular collagen.

Cystinosis

Cystinosis, a rare autosomal recessive condition, results from a defect of the carrier-mediated transport system for cystine, with accumulation of l-cystine in lysosomes (74). Three forms of cystinosis have been identified: nephrogenic (infantile) cystinosis, intermediate or adolescent cystinosis with late onset, and benign cystinosis. The nephrogenic (infantile) form usually develops 6 to 12 months after birth, with renal tubular dysfunction of Fanconi type, leading to progressive renal failure. Cystine crystals deposit in the kidney, cornea, and conjunctiva. Ocular deposits cause photophobia. Hepatosplenomegaly and variceal bleeding occur in older children. The intermediate or adolescent form of cystinosis usually presents after age

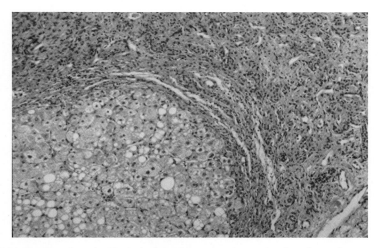

FIGURE 14.11 Tyrosinemia. Cholestasis and occasional pseudoacinar formation are present (hematoxylin-eosin, original magnification ×100).

5 years. These patients have longer survival despite several clinical manifestations, including retinal depigmentation, mild renal failure, and deposits of cystine crystals in the conjunctiva and bone marrow. Benign cystinosis is asymptomatic, and patients have normal life expectancy.

PATHOLOGY. Crystals of cystine are best seen in unstained frozen sections of liver or, because they are water soluble, in alcohol-fixed tissue. The crystals are in Kupffer cell lysosomes, particularly in zone 3 (Fig. 14.12A, e-Fig. 14.27). The crystals are birefringent (Fig. 14.12B), and in some cases electron microscopy may be useful (74).

Cystathionine β-Synthase Deficiency (Homocystinuria)

Homocystinuria is an autosomal recessive metabolic disorder resulting from cystathionine β-synthase deficiency. Patients have varied signs and

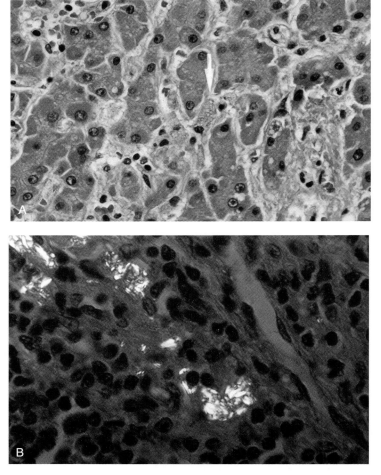

FIGURE 14.12 Cystinosis. Note numerous crystals of cystine in Kupffer cells (hematoxylin-eosin, original magnification ×200).

symptoms, including ocular abnormalities, skeletal abnormalities, mental retardation, and propensity for arterial thrombosis. Hepatomegaly may be present, but liver test values are not significantly altered.

PATHOLOGY. Steatosis is present, particularly in zone 3. Portal fibrosis and fibrotic thickening of portal arterioles is seen (74).

MISCELLANEOUS METABOLIC DISORDERS

Cystic Fibrosis

Cystic fibrosis (CF) is a relatively common, autosomal recessive disorder, characterized by impaired secretions from exocrine glands, including pancreas, salivary glands, and secretory glands in the gastrointestinal tract and lungs. Liver manifestations are not particularly common, and liver biopsy is not often performed. Secondary changes and complications involve the gastrointestinal tract, the biliary system, with gallstone formation, and the liver (2,98,106,135,141). The primary condition is generally known before liver biopsy is performed.

PATHOLOGY. Neonates can present with giant cell hepatitis. Later on, fatty change is prominent and is particularly severe in malnourished children. Most common, however, is irregular biliary fibrosis with multifocal fibrous scarring and proliferation of bile ductules, sometimes with dilated lumen filled with granular eosinophilic, inspissated material (101,113) (e-Figs. 14.28, 14.29). Inflammation is not typical. Biliary-type cirrhosis develops in 5% to 10% of patients. Complications include bile duct stenosis, resembling primary sclerosing cholangitis, as well as adenocarcinoma of the extrahepatic bile duct and amyloidosis (2,113).

Several relatively uncommon syndromes affecting the liver are summarized in Table 14.2.

DISORDERS OF PORPHYRIN METABOLISM

Disorders of porphyrin metabolism result from impaired synthesis of porphyrins and heme, traditionally classified as hepatic and erythropoietic forms, depending on the site of the metabolic defect (74). Histopathologic changes in the liver can be seen in acute intermittent porphyria (AIP), porphyria cutanea tarda (PCT), and erythropoietic protoporphyria (EPP) (9,130). Most porphyrias are inherited in an autosomal dominant fashion. An acquired form of PCT has also been documented. The hepatic porphyrias have a spectrum of clinical manifestations, including neurologic lesions with abdominal colicky pain, constipation, peripheral neuropathy, and neuropsychiatric episodes. Photosensitivity is common. Porphyrias are triggered by many drugs, including barbiturates, estrogens, oral contraceptives, and alcohol (29). A strong association exits between PCT and either hepatitis B virus or hepatitis C virus infection, with the implication

TABLE 14.2 Miscellaneous Metabolic Disorders

	Systemic Findings	Liver Findings
Shwachman syndrome (18,128)	Pancreatic insufficiency Failure to thrive Neutropenia, anemia Thrombocytopenia	Steatosis Fibrosis Cirrhosis
Alpers disease (74)	Progressive brain atrophy	Hepatomegaly Steatosis (micro) Submassive/ massive necrosis Fibrosis
Aarskog syndrome (1)		Hemosiderin Cirrhosis
Congenital total lipodystrophy (63,80,127)	Absence of adipose tissue Insulin-resistant diabetes mellitus Hyperlipidemia Muscular hypertrophy Acanthosis nigricans	Hepatosplenomegaly Steatosis Fibrosis Cirrhosis
Familial hepatosteatosis (104,123,136)	High levels of total lipids and fatty acids Immotile cilia syndrome	Kernicterus Jaundice Steatosis (macro)
Leprechaunism (Donohue syndrome) (37,40,43,77)	Insulin receptor gene mutation Typical facial features Mental/motor retardation Failure to thrive	Increased glycogen Steatosis Hemosiderin Cholestasis
Albinism (2 forms)		
1. Hermansky-Pudlak syndrome (65,74,124)	Autosomal recessive Bleeding diathesis Pulmonary fibrosis Renal failure Cardiomyopathy	Clusters of macrophages/ Kupffer cells Ceroid pigment Yellow autofluores-cence under UV light
2. Chediak-Higashi syndrome (143)	Autosomal recessive Albinism Recurrent infections Peripheral neuropathies Hemorrhage	Hepatosplenomegaly Cytoplasmic granules/giant lysosomes

TABLE 14.3	Diagnostic Histologic and Ultrastructural Findings in Porphyrias Affecting the Liver	
Type	Histologic Findings	Ultrastructure
Porphyria cutanea tarda (PCT)	Hepatocytes: Needle-shaped inclusions	Needle-shaped inclusions
Erythropoietic porphyria (EPP)	Hepatocytes, Kupffer cells, bile ducts: Dark brown pigment Autofluorescence with UV light (Maltese cross pattern)	Non-membrane-bound crystals (starburst pattern)

that these viruses may play a role in both pathogenesis and progression (13,49,66,120).

Human immunodeficiency virus (HIV) may also have a role in pathogenesis of PCT (87). The key histopathologic features of the porphyrias are summarized in Table 14.3.

PATHOLOGY. The PCT liver shows variable steatosis, with zone 1 iron deposition (Fig. 14.13, e-Figs. 14.30, 14.31). Mild portal inflammation and occasional liver cell necrosis may also be seen (25,29,83). Characteristic needle-shaped intracytoplasmic crystals, a mixture of porphyrinogens, porphyrins, and uroporphyrins, can sometimes be shown by ferric ferricyanide reduction test but are best seen in unstained paraffin sections (48). The crystals are birefringent and ultrastructurally show variable electron

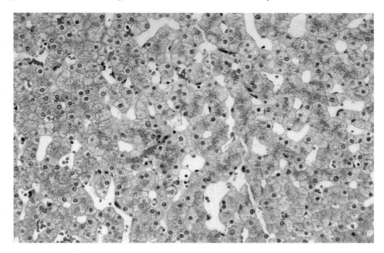

FIGURE 14.13 Porphyria cutanea tarda. Note clusters of histiocytes with hemosiderin (hematoxylin-eosin, original magnification ×200).

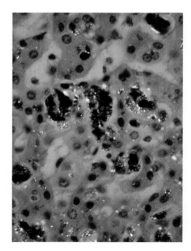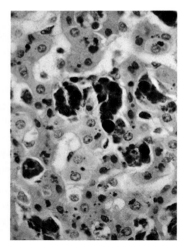

FIGURE 14.14 Erythropoietic porphyria. Dark brown pigment, showing autofluorescent Maltese cross pattern with ultraviolet light (UV light, original magnification ×40).

density. Fibrosis and cirrhosis can develop, especially in cases associated with chronic viral hepatitis B or C (84). Excess alcohol ingestion as a triggering factor in PCT has also been documented (13,66). Patients with longstanding PCT and fibrosis or cirrhosis have an increased risk of developing HCC (122,130).

Similar, but milder, changes are seen in AIP. Ultrastructurally, mitochondrial changes are prominent, with large electron-dense granules. Lipofuscin is also abundant and admixed with ferritin. Myelin-like figures may also be present (74). HCC has been documented with AIP (79).

The liver in EPP is grossly black. Histologically, there are striking deposits of dark brown pigment in liver cells, bile ducts, bile canaliculi, and Kupffer cells. The pigment has characteristic red birefringence (Maltese cross pattern) (Fig. 14.14) and, in unstained frozen sections, red autofluorescence (81). Fibrosis and cirrhosis develop. An association between EPP and histiocytosis X has been documented (60). Electron microscopy shows that crystals are non-membrane bound, with a so-called starburst pattern.

REFERENCES

1. Aarskog D. A familial syndrome of short stature associated with facial dysplasia and genital anomalies. J Pediatr 1970;77:856–861.
2. Abdul-Karim FW, King TA, Dahms BB, et al. Carcinoma of the extrahepatic biliary system in an adult with cystic fibrosis. Am J Clin Pathol 1983;80:752–754.
3. Alshak NS, Cocjin J, Podesta L, et al. Hepatocellular adenoma in glycogen storage disease type IV. Arch Pathol Lab Med 1994;118:88–91.
4. Appelbaum NM, Thaler MM. Reversibility of extensive liver damage in galactosemia. Gastroenterology 1975;69:496–502.

5. Avigan MI, Ishak KG, Gregg RE, et al. Morphologic features of the liver in abetalipoproteinemia. Hepatology 1984;4:1223–1226.

6. Bannayan GA, Dean WJ, Howell RR. Type IV glycogen storage disease. Light-microscopic, electron microscopic, and enzymatic study. Am J Clin Pathol 1976;66:702–709.

7. Barton NW, Brady RO, Dumbrosia JM, et al. Replacement therapy for inherited enzyme deficiency-macrophage-targeted glucocerebrosidase for Gaucher's disease. N Engl J Med 1991;324:1464–1470.

8. Bell H, Schrumpf E, Fagerhol MK. Heterozygous alpha-1-antitrypsin deficiency in adults with chronic liver disease. Scand J Gastroenterol 1990;25:788–792.

9. Biempica L, Kosower N, Ma HH, et al. Hepatic porphyrias. Cytochemical and ultrastructural studies of liver in acute intermittent porphyria and porphyria cutanea tarda. Arch Pathol 1974;98:336–343.

10. Bieri JG, Hoeg JM, Schafer J, et al. Vitamin A and vitamin E replacement in abetalipoproteinemia. Ann Intern Med 1984;100:238–239.

11. Black DD, Hay RV, Rohwer-Nutter PL, et al. Intestinal and hepatic apolipoprotein 13 gene expression in abetalipoproteinemia. Gastroenterology 1991;101:749–755.

12. Black JA, Simpson K. Fructose intolerance. Br J Med 1967;2:138–141.

13. Bloomer JR. The liver in protoporphyria. Hepatology 1988;8:402–407.

14. Borowitz SM, Green HL. Cornstarch therapy in patients with type III glycogen storage disease. J Pediatr Gastroenterol Nutr 1987;6:631–634.

15. Bradfield JWB, Blenkinsopp WK. Alpha-1-antitrypsin globules in liver and PiM phenotype. J Clin Pathol 1977;30:579–584.

16. Brook JG, Lees RS, Yules JH, et al. Tangier disease (alpha-lipoprotein deficiency). JAMA 1977;238:332–334.

17. Bruguera M, Lamar C, Bernet M, et al. Hepatic disease associated with ground-glass inclusions in hepatocytes after cyanamide therapy. Arch Pathol Lab Med 1986;110: 906–910.

18. Brueton MJ, Mavromichalis J, Goodchild MC, et al. Hepatic dysfunction in association with pancreatic insufficiency and cyclical neutropenia. Shwachman-Diamond syndrome. Arch Dis Child 1977;52:76–78.

19. Brul S, Westerveld A, Strijland A, et al. Genetic heterogeneity in the cerebrohepatorenal (Zellweger) syndrome and other inherited disorders with a generalized impairment of peroxisomal functions. J Clin Invest 1988;81:1710–1715.

20. Bruton OC, Kanter AJ. Idiopathic familial hyperlipidemia. Am J Dis Child 1951;82: 153–159.

21. Buja M, Kovanen PT, Bilheimer DW. Cellular pathology of homozygous familial hypercholesterolemia. Am J Pathol 1979;327–345.

22. Burmeister LA, Valdivia T, Nuttal FQ. Adult hereditary fructose intolerance. Arch Intern Med 1991;151:773–776.

23. Callea F, De Vos R, Tagni R, et al. Fibrinogen inclusions in liver cells: a new type of ground-glass hepatocyte. Immune light and electron microscopic characterization. Histopathology 1986;10:65–73.

24. Callea F, Fevery J, Massi G, et al. Storage of alpha-1-antitrypsin in intrahepatic bile duct cells in alpha-1-antitrypsin deficiency (PiZ phenotype). Histopathology 1985;9:99–108.

25. Campo E, Bruguera M, Rodes J. Are there diagnostic histologic features of porphyria cutanea tarda in liver biopsy specimens? Liver 1990;10:185–190.

26. Carlson JA, Rogers BB, Sifers RN, et al. Accumulation of PiZ alpha 1-antitrypsin causes damage in transgenic mice. J Clin Invest 1989;83:1409–1412.

27. Coire CF, Qizilbash AH, Castelli MF. Hepatic adenomata in type Ia glycogen storage disease. Arch Pathol Lab Med 1987;111:166–169.

28. Conti JA, Kemeny N. Type Ia glycogenosis associated with hepatocellular carcinoma. Cancer 1992;69:1320–1322.

29. Cortes JM, Oliva H, Paradinas FJ, et al. The pathology of the liver in porphyria cutanea tarda. Histopathology 1980;4:471–485.

30. Cox DW, Smyth S. Risk for liver disease in adults with alpha 1-antitrypsin deficiency. Am J Med 1983;74:221–227.

31. Crowley JJ, Sharp HL, Freier EF, et al. Fatal liver disease associated with alpha 1-antitrypsin deficiency PiM1/PiMduarte. Gastroenterology 1987;93:242–244.

32. Crystal RG. Alpha 1-antitrypsin deficiency, emphysema, and liver disease. J Clin Invest 1990;85:1343–1352.

33. D'Agostino D, Bay L, Gallo G, et al. Cholesterol ester storage disease: clinical, biochemical, and pathological studies of four new cases. J Pediatr Gastroenterol Nutr 1985;7:446–450.

34. Day DL, Letouneau JG, Allan BT, et al. Hepatic regenerating nodules in hereditary tyrosinemia. AJR Am J Roentgenol 1987;149:391–393.

35. Dechelotte P, Kantelip B, de Laguillamie BV. Tangier disease. A histological and ultra-structural study. Pathol Res Pract 1985;180:424–430.

36. Dehner LP, Snover DC, Sharp HL, et al. Hereditary tyrosinemia type I (chronic form): pathologic findings in the liver. Hum Pathol 1989;20:149–159.

37. Dekaban A. Metabolic and chromosomal studies in leprechaunism. Arch Dis Child 1965;40:632–636.

38. Dekaban AS, Constantopoulos G, Herman MM, et al. Mucopolysaccharidosis type V (Scheie syndrome). Arch Pathol Lab Med 1976;100:237–245.

39. DiBisceglie AM, Ishak KG, Rabin L, et al. Cholesteryl ester storage disease: hepatopathology and effects of therapy with lovastatin. Hepatology 1990;11:764–772.

40. Donohue WL, Uchida I. Leprechaunism: a euphemism for a rare familial disorder. J Pediatr 1954;45:505–519.

41. Duloze P, Delvin EE, Glorieaax FH, et al. Replacement therapy for inherited enzyme deficiency. Liver orthotopic transplantation in Niemann–Pick disease type A. Am J Med Genet 1977;1:229–239.

42. Dycaico MJ, Grant SGN, Felts K, et al. Neonatal hepatitis induced by alpha-1-antitrypsin: a transgenic mouse model. Science 1988;242:1409–1412.

43. Elsas LJ. Leprechaunism: an inherited defect in high-affinity insulin receptor. Am J Hum Genet 1985;37:73–88.

44. Elzouki A-NY, Eriksson S. Risks of hepatobiliary diseases in adults with severe a1-antitrypsin deficiency (PiZZ). Is chronic viral hepatitis B and C an additional risk factor for cirrhosis and hepatocellular carcinoma? J Hepatol 1996;8:989–994.

45. Elzouki A-NY, Segelmark M, Wieslander G, et al. Strong link between alpha1-antitrypsin PiZ allele and Wegener's granulomatosis. J Intern Med 1994;236:543–548.

46. Eriksson S, Carlson J, Velez R. Risk of cirrhosis and primary liver cancer in alpha 1-antitrypsin deficiency. N Engl J Med 1992;314:736–739.

47. Eriksson S, Lindmark B, Lilja H. Familial alpha 1-antichymotrypsin deficiency. Acta Med Scand 1986;220:447–453.

48. Everback L, Lunvall O. Properties and distribution of liver fluorescence in porphyria cutanea tarda (PCT). Virchows Arch A Pathol Anat Histopathol 1970;350:293–302.

49. Fargion S, Piperno A, Capellini MD, et al. Hepatitis C virus and porphyria cutanea tarda: evidence of a strong association. Hepatology 1992;16:1322–1326.

50. Feldmann G, Bignon J, Chahinian P, et al. Hepatocyte ultrastructural changes in alpha 1-antitrypsin deficiency. Gastroenterology 1974;67:1214–1224.

51. Ferrans VJ, Fredrickson DS. Pathology of Tangier disease. Am J Pathol 1975;78:101–136.

52. Fortin PR, Fraser RS, Watts CS, et al. Alpha-1 antitrypsin deficiency and systemic necro-tizing vasculitis. J Rheumatol 1991;18:1613–1616.

53. Froesch ER, Wolf HP, Baitsch H. Hereditary fructose intolerance. An inborn defect of hepatic fructose-1-phosphate splitting aldolase. Am J Med 1963;34:151–167.

54. Geller SA, Nichols WS, Dycaico MJ, et al. Histopathology of alpha 1-antitrypsin liver disease in a transgenic mouse model. Hepatology 1990;12:40–47.

55. Geller SA, Nichols WS, Kim S, et al. Hepatocarcinogenesis is the sequel to hepatitis in Z2 alpha 1-antitryspin transgenic mice: histopathological and DNA ploidy studies. Hepatology 1994;19:389–397.

56. Gerson B, Hemphill JM, Rock RC. Creatine kinase and lactate dehydrogenase in type II glycogenosis (Pompe disease). Arch Pathol Lab Med 1977;101:213–215.

57. Ghishan FK, Greene HL. Liver disease in children with PiZZ alpha 1-antitrypsin deficiency. Hepatology 1988;8:307–310.

58. Goldfischer S, Collins H, Rapin I, et al. Pseudo-Zellweger syndromes: deficiencies in several peroxisomal oxidative activities. J Pediatr 1986;108:25–32.

59. Goldfischer S, Moore CL, Johnson AB, et al. Peroxisomal and mitochondrial defects in the cerebro-hepatorenal syndrome. Science 1973;182:62–64.

60. Graham-Brown RAC, Scheuer PJ, Sarkany I. Histiocytosis X and erythropoietic protoporphyria. J R Soc Med 1984;77:238–240.

61. Greene HL. Glycogen storage disease. Semin Liver Dis 1982;2:291–301.

62. Greene HL, Brown BI, McClenathan DT, et al. A new variant of type IV glycogenosis: deficiency of branching enzyme activity without apparent progressive liver disease. Hepatology 1988;8:302–306.

63. Harbour JR, Rosenthal P, Smuckler EA. Ultrastructural abnormalities of the liver in total lipodystrophy. Hum Pathol 1981;12:856–862.

64. Haust MD. Crystalloid structure of hepatic mitochondria in children with heparin sulfate mucopolysaccharidosis (Sanfilippo type). Exp Mol Biol 1968;8:123–134.

65. Hermansky F, Pudlak P. Albinism associated with hemorrhagic diathesis and unusual pigmented reticular cells in the bone marrow: report of two cases with histochemical studies. Blood 1959;14:162–169.

66. Herrero C, Vicente A, Bruguera M, et al. Is hepatitis C virus infection a trigger of porphyria cutanea tarda? Lancet 1993;341:288–289.

67. Hobbs JR, Hugh-Jones K, Barrett AJ, et al. Reversal of clinical features of Hurler's disease and biochemical improvement after treatment by bone marrow transplantation. Lancet 1981;2:709–712.

68. Hodges JR, Millward-Sadler GH, Barbatis C, et al. Heterozygous MZ alpha 1-antitrypsin deficiency in adults with chronic hepatitis and cirrhosis. N Engl J Med 1981;304:557–560.

69. Hoffman HN, Fredrickson DS. Tangier disease (familial high destiny lipoprotein deficiency). Clinical and genetic features in two adults. Am J Med 1965;39:582–593.

70. Howell RR, Kaback MM, Brown BI. Type IV glycogen storage disease. Branching enzyme deficiency in skin fibroblasts and possible heterozygote detection. J Pediatr 1971;78:638–642.

71. Howell RR, Stevenson RE, Ben-Menachem Y. Hepatic adenomata with type I glycogen storage disease. JAMA 1976;236:1481–1484.

72. Hricick DE, Hussain R. Pancytopenia and hepatomegaly in oxalosis. Arch Intern Med 1984;144:167–168.

73. Hughes JL, Poulos A, Robertson E, et al. Pathology of hepatic peroxisomes and mitochondria in patients with peroxisomal disorders. Virchows Arch A Pathol Anat Histopathol 1990;416: 255–264.

74. Ishak KG, Sharp HL. Metabolic errors and liver disease. In: MacSween RNM, Anthony A, Scheuer PJ, et al., eds. Pathology of the Liver. 3rd Ed. Edinburgh: Churchill Livingstone, 1994:123–219.

75. Ishihara T, Yokota T, Yamashita Y, et al. Comparative study of the intracytoplasmic inclusions in Lafora disease and type IV glycogenosis by electron microscopy. Acta Pathol Jpn 1987;37:1591–1601.

76. Isselbacher KJ, Anderson ER, Kurakoski K, et al. Congenital galactosemia, a single enzymatic block in galactose metabolism. Science 1956;123:635.

77. Kallo IL, Lakatos I, Szijart L. Leprechaunism (Donohue's syndrome). J Pediatr 1965;66: 372–379.

78. Karpati G, Carpenter S, Engel AG, et al. The syndrome of systemic carnitine deficiency. Clinical, morphologic, biochemical and pathophysiologic features. Neurology 1975;25:16–24.

79. Kauppinen R, Mustajoki P. Acute hepatic porphyria and hepatocellular carcinoma. Br J Cancer 1988;57:117–120.

80. Klar A, Livni N, Gross-Kieselstein E, et al. ultrastructural abnormalities of the liver in total lipodystrophy. Arch Pathol Lab Med 1987;111:197–199.

81. Klatskin G, Bloomer JR. Birefringence of hepatic pigment deposits in erythropoietic protoporphyria. Gastroenterology 1974;67:294–302.

82. Kvittingen EA. Tyrosinemia type I: an update. J Inher Metab Dis 1991;14:554–562.

83. Lefkowitch JH, Grossman ME. Hepatic pathology in porphyria cutanea tarda. Liver 1983; 3:19–29.

84. Levran O, Desnick RJ, Schuchman EH. Niemann-Pick disease: a frequent massive mutation in the acid sphingomyelinase gene of Ashkenazi type A and B patients. Proc Natl Acad Sci USA 1991;88:3748–3752.

85. Levran O, Desnick RJ, Schuchman EH. Niemann-Pick type B disease. Identification of a single codon deletion in the acid sphingomyelinase gene and genotypic/phenotypic correlations in type A and B patients. J Clin Invest 1991;88:806–810.

86. Lindmark B, Millward-Saddler H, Callea F, et al. Hepatocyte inclusions of a1-antichymotrypsin in a patient with partial deficiency of a1-antichymotrypsin and chronic liver disease. Histopathology 1990;16:211–225.

87. Lobato MN, Berger TG. Porphyria cutanea tarda associated with the acquired immunodeficiency syndrome. Arch Dermatol 1988;124:1009–1010.

88. Long RG, Lake RD, Pettit JE, et al. Adult Niemann-Pick disease. Its relationship to the syndrome of the sea-blue histiocyte. Am J Med 1977;62:627–635.

89. Malatack JJ, Iwatsuki S, Gartner C, et al. Liver transplantation for type I glycogen storage disease. Lancet 1983;1:1073–1075.

90. Malone M, Mieli-Vergani G, Mowat AP, et al. The fetal liver in PiZZ alpha-1-antitrypsin phenotype: a report of five cases. Pediatr Pathol 1989;9:623–631.

91. Manowski Z, Silver MM, Roberts EA, et al. Liver cell dysplasia and early liver transplantation in hereditary tyrosinemia. Mod Pathol 1990;3:694–701.

92. Martin JJ, Ceuterick C. Prenatal pathology in mucopolysaccharidoses: a comparison with postnatal cases. Clin Neuropathol 1983;2:122–127.

93. Martinez RD, Martin-Jimenez R, Matalon R. Zellweger syndrome. Paediatrics 1991; 6:91–93.

94. McAdams AJ, Hug G, Bove KE. Glycogen storage disease, types I to X. Criteria for morphologic diagnosis. Hum Pathol 1974;5:463–487.

95. Mieles LA, Esquivel CO, Van Thiel DH, et al. Liver transplantation in tyrosinemia. A review of 10 cases from the University of Pittsburgh. Dig Dis Sci 1990;35:153–157.

96. Miller R, Bialer MG, Rogers JF, et al. Wolman's disease. Report of a case, with multiple studies. Arch Pathol Lab Med 1982;106:41–45.

97. Moser HW, Moser AB, Chen WW, et al. Ceramidase deficiency: Farber lipogranulomatosis. In: Scriver CR, Beaudet AL, Sly WS, et al., eds. The metabolic basis of inherited disease. 6th Ed. New York: McGraw-Hill, 1980:1645–1654.

98. Nagel RA, Javaid A, Meire HB, et al. Liver disease and bile duct abnormalities in adults with cystic fibrosis. Lancet 1989;2:1422–1425.

99. Nishimura RN, Ishak KG, Reddick R, et al. Lafora disease: diagnosis by liver biopsy. Ann Neurol 1979;8:409–415.

100. O'Brien JS. Ganglioside-storage disease. N Engl J Med 1971;284:893–896.

101. O'Brien S, Keogan M, Casey M, et al. Biliary complications of cystic fibrosis. Gut 1992;33:387–391.

102. Odievre M, Gertil C, Gautier M, et al. Hereditary fructose intolerance in childhood: diagnosis, management and course in 55 patients. Am J Dis Child 1978;132:605–608.

103. Palmer PE, Wolfe HJ, Dayal Y, et al. Immunocytochemical diagnosis of a1-antitrypsin deficiency. Am J Surg Pathol 1978;2:275–281.

104. Paolucci F, Cinti S, Cangiotti A, et al. Steatosis associated with immotile cilia syndrome: an unrecognized relationship. J Hepatol 1992;14:317–324.

105. Parfrey NA, Hutchins GM. Hepatic fibrosis in the mucopolysaccharidoses. Am J Med 1986;81:825–829.

106. Park RW, Grand RJ. Gastrointestinal manifestations of cystic fibrosis. A review. Gastroenterology 1981;81:1143–1161.

107. Perlmutter DH. Cellular basis for liver injury in alpha-1-antitrypsin deficiency. Hepatology 1991;13:172–1185.

108. Petrelli M, Blair JD. The liver in GM1 gangliosidosis types 1 and 2. A light and electron microscopic study. Arch Pathol 1975;99:111–116.

109. Phillips MJ, Poucell S, Patterson J, et al. The liver. An atlas and text of ultrastructural pathology. New York: Raven Press, 1987.

110. Pittschieler K. Liver disease and heterozygous alpha-1-antitrypsin deficiency. Acta Pediatr Scand 1991;80:323–327.

111. Poll-The BT, Saudubray JM, Ogier HA, et al. Infantile Refsum disease: an inherited peroxisomal disorder. Comparison with Zellweger syndrome and neonatal adrenoleukodystrophy. Eur J Pediatr 1987;146:477–483.

112. Propst T, Propst A, Dietze O, et al. High prevalence of viral infection in adults with homozygous and heterozygous alpha 1-antitrypsin deficiency and chronic liver disease. Ann Intern Med 1992;117:641–645.

113. Psacharopoulos HT, Howard ER, Portmann B, et al. Hepatic complications of cystic fibrosis. Lancet 1981;2:78–80.

114. Qizilbash A, Young-Pong O. Alpha 1 antitrypsin liver disease and differential diagnosis of PAS-positive, diastase-resistant globules in liver cells. Am J Clin Pathol 1983;79: 697–702.

115. Raby RA, Tyszka TS, Williams JW. Reversal of cardiac dysfunction secondary to type I primary hyperoxaluria after combined liver–kidney transplantation. Am J Med 1991;90: 498–504.

116. Rakela J, Goldschmiedt M, Ludwig J. Late manifestation of chronic liver disease in adults with alpha-1-antitrypsin deficiency. Dig Dis Sci 1987;32:1358–1362.

117. Rattazi MC, Davidson RG. Prenatal diagnosis of metachromatic leukodystrophy by electrophoretic and immunologic techniques. Pediatr Res 1977;11:1030–1035.

118. Reed GB, Dixon JEP, Nestein HB, et al. Type IV glycogenosis. Lab Invest 1968;19:546–557.

119. Roberts EA, Cox DW, Medline A, et al. Occurrence of alpha-1-antitrypsin deficiency in 155 patients with alcoholic liver disease. Am J Clin Pathol 1984;82:424–427.

120. Rochi E, Gibertini P, Cassanelli M, et al. Hepatitis B virus infection in porphyria cutanea tarda. Liver 1986;6:153–157.

121. Rodriqez FH, Hoffman EO, Ordinario AT, et al. Fabry's disease in a heterozygous woman. Arch Pathol Lab Med 1985;109:89–91.

122. Salata H, Cortes JM, de Salamnca RE, et al. Porphyria cutanea tarda and hepatocellular carcinoma. Frequency of occurrence and related factors. J Hepatol 1985;1:477–487.

123. Satran L, Sharp HL, Sehenken JR, et al. Fatal neonatal hepatic steatosis. A new familial disorder. J Pediatr 1969;75:39–46.

124. Schinella RA, Greco MA, Garay SM, et al. Hermansky-Pudlak syndrome. A clinicopathologic study. Hum Pathol 1985;16:366–376.

125. Schutgens RBH, Hegmans HSA, Wanders RJA, et al. Peroxisomal disorders: a newly recognized group of genetic diseases. Eur J Pediatr 1986;144:430–440.

126. Scotto JM, Hadchouel M, Odievre M, et al. Infantile phytanic acid storage disease, a possible variant of Refsum's disease: three cases, including ultrastructural studies of the liver. J Inherited Metab Dis 1982;5:83–90.

127. Senior B, Gellis SS. The syndromes of total lipodystrophy and partial lipodystrophy. Pediatrics 1964;33:593–612.

128. Shwachman H, Diamond LK, Oski FA, et al. The syndrome of pancreatic insufficiency and bone marrow insufficiency. J Pediatr 1964;65:645–663.

129. Siegel EG, Lucke H, Schauer W, et al. Repeated upper gastrointestinal hemorrhage caused by metachromatic leukodystrophy of the gall bladder. Digestion 1992;51:121–124.

130. Siersema PD, Kate FJW, Mulder PGH, et al. Hepatocellular carcinoma in porphyria cutanea tarda: frequency and factors related to its occurrence. Liver 1992;12:56–61.

131. Singh I, Johnson GH, Brown FR III. Peroxisomal disorders: biochemical and clinical diagnostic considerations. Am J Dis Child 1988;142:1297–1301.

132. Smanik EJ, Tavill AS, Jacobs GH, et al. Orthotopic liver transplantation in two adults with Niemann-Pick and Gaucher's diseases. Hepatology 1993;17:42–49.

133. Smetana HF, Olen E. Hereditary galactose disease. Am J Clin Pathol 1962;38:3–25.

134. Smit GPA, Fernandes J, Leonard JV, et al. The long-term outcome of patients with glycogen storage diseases. J Inher Dis 1990;13:411–418.

135. Strandvik B, Hjelte L, Gabrielsson N, et al. Sclerosing cholangitis in cystic fibrosis. Scand J Gastroenterol 1988;23:121–124.

136. Suprun H, Freundlich E. Fatal familial steatosis of myocardium, liver and kidneys in three siblings. Acta Pediatr Scand 1981;70:247–252.

137. Sveger T. Prospective study of children with a1-antitrypsin deficiency: eight-year-old follow-up. J Pediatr 1989;104:91–94.

138. Tamaru J, Iwasaki I, Horie H, et al. Niemann-Pick disease associated with liver disorders. Acta Pathol Jpn 1985;35:1267–1272.

139. Tanaka T, Takahashi K, Hakozaki H, et al. Farber's disease (disseminated lipogranulomatosis): a pathological histochemical and ultrastructural study. Acta Pathol Jpn 1979;29:135–155.

140. Tassoni JP, Fawaz KA, Johnston DE. Cirrhosis and portal hypertension in a patient with adult Niemann-Pick disease. Gastroenterology 1991;100:567–569.

141. Travis WD, Castile R, Vawter G, et al. Secondary (AA) amyloidosis in cystic fibrosis. Am J Clin Pathol 1986;85:419–424.

142. Tsai P, Lipton JM, Sahdev I, et al. Allogeneic bone marrow transplantation in severe Gaucher disease. Pediatr Res 1992;31:503–507.

143. Valenzuela R, Aikawa M, O'Regan S, et al. Chediak–Higashi syndrome in a black infant. A light and electron microscopic study with special emphasis on erythrophagocytosis. Am J Clin Pathol 1976;65:483–494.

144. Volk BW, Adachi M, Schneck L. The gangliosidoses. Hum Pathol 1975;6:555–569.

145. Watts RWS, Morgan SH, Dampure CJ, et al. Combined hepatic and renal transplantation in primary hyperoxaluria type I: clinical report of nine cases. Am J Med 1991;90: 179–188.

15

HEMOCHROMATOSIS AND OTHER IRON-RELATED DISORDERS

Hereditary hemochromatosis (HH), a condition of abnormal iron absorption, is among the most common hereditary disorders in humans. Its incidence is higher than the combined incidences of cystic fibrosis, phenylketonuria, and muscular dystrophy (7,13,39). HH is the most common hereditary disorder in Caucasians, and approximately 1 million Americans are homozygous for this condition. HH remains significantly underdiagnosed because of the persisting misconception that it is rare. The pathologist may be the first to detect HH, helping to prevent cirrhosis (Table 15.1).

Iron is not demonstrable in the normal liver using standard histochemical methods such as the Perls reaction. Stainable iron is abnormal. Iron is most often secondary from the breakdown of red blood cells, as in chronic hemolytic anemias or after repeated transfusions, characteristically in Kupffer cells and portal tract macrophages (19,30) (Fig. 15.1).

Predominantly hepatocytic iron deposition may signify HH and, if untreated, will progress to cirrhosis and possibly to hepatocellular carcinoma (HCC) (18,25,33). HH can often be histologically differentiated from other causes of iron accumulation (19,47). Alcoholic liver disease, however, often mimics the pattern of iron deposition in HH. Differentiation requires supplemental studies, such as serum ferritin and iron-binding capacity determinations, or, most reliably, chemical assay of the liver biopsy for iron content and subsequent calculation of the hepatic iron index (HII) (46).

TERMINOLOGY

Primary hemochromatosis, hemochromatosis, and hereditary hemochromatosis (HH) are synonyms for the inherited condition in which hepatocyte iron deposition predominates with deposition of excess iron in other organs, such as the pancreas, other endocrine organs, and the heart. Excess iron absorption is not related to the level of iron stores in the body.

In contrast, hemosiderosis, siderosis, and secondary hemosiderosis refer to acquired excess iron deposition with varying amounts of

TABLE 15.1	Key Features of Hereditary Hemochromatosis

1. Hereditary hemochromatosis is a common disorder!
2. It is uncommon in normally menstruating women
3. Early detection can prevent cirrhosis and hepatocellular carcinoma
4. Transferrin saturation determination has high sensitivity for disease detection, but is not specific
5. Hepatic iron content is proportional to body stores; hepatic iron assay is not specific, however
6. Granular iron deposits are abnormal in a liver biopsy
7. Hematoxylin-eosin staining does not adequately display deposited iron
8. In hereditary hemochromatosis, iron deposits are primarily in hepatocytes
9. In early hereditary hemochromatosis, iron deposits are in zone 1 (periportal) hepatocytes, with progressive involvement of zones 2 and 3 as the disease progresses
10. In secondary hemosiderosis, iron deposits are primarily in Kupffer cells
11. Alcoholics may demonstrate the pattern of iron deposition usually seen in hereditary hemochromatosis
12. Hepatic iron index, based on hepatic iron assay, is highly useful
13. Hepatic iron index can be determined using formalin-fixed, paraffin-embedded liver

hemosiderin in macrophages and without associated tissue damage until the amount of iron is excessive.

HH and secondary hemosiderosis are usually separable, because of both the pattern of distribution and the amount of iron present. Sometimes the findings in secondary hemosiderosis and HH may be indistinguishable, with varying hepatocyte iron deposition. Examples include alcoholism

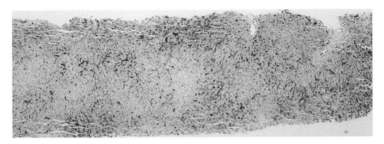

FIGURE 15.1   Secondary hemochromatosis in a 24-year-old man with sickle cell disease, with iron granules mostly in Kupffer cells and portal tract macrophages (Perls reaction, original magnification ×200).

(8,9,42), chronic hemolytic anemia, generally with many red blood cell transfusions over many years (4,5,19,38), and porphyria cutanea tarda (15,20,28,37,41), as well as some cases of chronic hepatitis.

BASIC ASPECTS OF IRON METABOLISM

A healthy adult man has approximately 5 g (90 mmol) of total body iron, almost all in hemoglobin, myoglobin, or various enzymes, with approximately 20% as ferritin or hemosiderin in the reticuloendothelial system. The liver has one third of total body iron, almost all in hepatocytes, with approximately 2% in Kupffer cells. Kupffer cell iron derives from red cell breakdown, whereas hepatocyte iron originates from free hemoglobin, from hemoglobin bound to haptoglobin, and from transferrin. Hepatocyte iron occurs in several biochemical forms, including ferritin, hemosiderin, heme, and in the intracellular transit pool as elemental iron. Iron is also stored in bone marrow and striated muscle.

The mechanism of normal iron absorption, primarily in proximal small intestine mucosa, is not completely understood (8,13,23,43). When iron stores are depleted, absorption increases. Conversely, absorption falls when iron stores are increased. Iron absorption is modulated by the rate of cell uptake and intracellular transfer, the degree of cellular retention, and the rate of release to the portal circulation. The daily diet has 15 to 20 mg of iron, yet only approximately 1 mg is absorbed each day by males and only approximately 2 mg by females of reproductive age. Iron is absorbed both as heme iron and nonheme iron. Normal iron loss occurs principally via the intestinal tract. In females, menstruation and pregnancy also cause iron loss. Hepatocytes have specific receptor-mediated mechanisms for iron uptake.

Ten to fifteen percent of white Americans are heterozygous for hemochromatosis (13,23,43), and as many as 0.25% are homozygous. Heterozygotes can have the histopathologic and clinical features of hereditary hemochromatosis, particularly when iron or alcohol intake is increased, or when alleles for hereditary anemias or porphyria cutanea tarda, which also increase iron absorption, are inherited independently (1b).

MORPHOLOGIC DETERMINATION
OF HEPATIC IRON CONTENT

Iron is not easily seen with hematoxylin-eosin until there is relatively heavy deposition (e-Fig. 15.1). Even with markedly increased iron stores, the amount will almost always be significantly underestimated with hematoxylin-eosin. For this reason, and because HH is a relatively common disorder, iron staining should be performed on almost all liver biopsy samples, allowed for potential family studies and, presumably, the prevention of chronic liver disease.

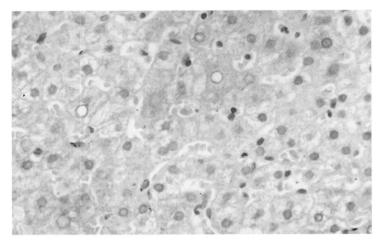

FIGURE 15.2   Ferritin appearing as a delicate blue discoloration of hepatocyte (Perls reaction, original magnification ×200).

Perls histochemical method is widely used because of its high sensitivity and specificity, and relative ease of performance. Hepatocytes without increased iron stores can demonstrate a diffuse, pale blue discoloration with Perls and other iron stains; this is intracellular ferritin, and, in the absence of granules, should not be interpreted as abnormal iron accumulation (Fig. 15.2). Both ferritin and hemosiderin are ferric compounds. Ferritin is barely discernible with low magnification objectives. The presence of distinct iron granules is abnormal, and the cause should be determined. Artifactually precipitated pigment is sometimes misinterpreted as mild iron deposition (Fig. 15.3). Clues include seeing the pigment on cell or nuclear membranes, within nuclei or in sinusoidal space. Iron deposition is evaluated in terms of (a) the grade, or amount, of stainable iron present; (b) its distribution in the liver, in terms of acinar zones and portal structures; and (c) the presence or absence of associated fibrosis, and, if present, the degree. The commonly used grading schemes use a scale of 0 to 4+. In recent years, image analysis has been used to morphometrically separate HH from other causes of iron overload (46).

CHEMICAL DETERMINATION OF HEPATIC IRON CONTENT: THE HEPATIC IRON INDEX (HII)

Special handling is not needed to ensure accurate determination of iron concentration. Formalin-fixed, paraffin-embedded tissue can be reliably studied (40). The raw value of iron concentration is not particularly useful, however, in distinguishing HH from other conditions, such as chronic alcoholism. Determination of the HII allows for differentiating HH homozygotes from heterozygotes and from alcoholics (6,24,46).

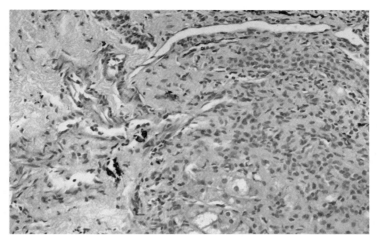

FIGURE 15.3   Artifact mimicking iron deposition. Note that the granules are not confined to cytoplasm and can even be seen overlapping nuclear membranes (Perls reaction, original magnification ×400).

The HII is defined as μmol/g dry weight liver divided by patient age (in years) (6).

In individuals homozygous for hereditary hemochromatosis, the HII is greater than 2, whereas heterozygotes and individuals with iron deposition associated with alcoholic liver disease have an HII less than 2. Normal individuals generally have a calculated HII less than 1.0.

HEREDITARY HEMOCHROMATOSIS

Hereditary hemochromatosis is an autosomal recessive disorder principally determined by a gene abnormality on chromosome 6, near the A locus for the HLA system (3,4,7,8,16,21–23,31,32,43). Virtually all HH patients and their relatives have a single mutation in the hemochromatosis gene. Patients with HH have increased frequency of HLA-A3, HLA-B14, HLA-A3, and HLA-B77. As many as 85% of HH patients are homozygous for the C282Y mutation in HFE, the hemochromatosis gene (11,23,43). HH has a gene frequency of 1:20, a heterozygosity frequency of 1:10, and a homozygosity frequency of 1:400.

Iron absorption increases inappropriately because of increased iron transfer across intestinal epithelial cells, possibly due to a primary defect of the epithelial cell itself. A similar mechanism is obtained with prolonged or repeated alcohol-induced gastritis and enteritis. The accumulated iron is hepatotoxic and likely causes peroxidative injury to organelle membrane phospholipids, particularly lysosomes. Iron may also affect other organelles, such as mitochondria and microsomes. Excess iron stimulates

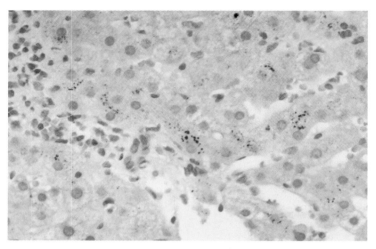

FIGURE 15.4   Hereditary hemochromatosis, early, with iron deposition in zone 1 (periportal) hepatocytes (Perls reaction, original magnification ×100).

collagen synthesis increase, and fibrosis can develop without histologically significant cell injury.

HH generally becomes clinically manifest in the fifth and sixth decades of life, typically affecting men of Mediterranean descent. There may be involvement of various endocrine organs (e-Fig. 15.2), the skin, the heart, and the skeletal system.

Histopathology

Portal tracts show variable inflammatory cell infiltration, particularly seen with concurrent disease such as hepatitis C, porphyria cutanea tarda or α1-antitrypsin deficiency (e-Figs. 15.3–15.5). In advanced hemochromatosis, iron is demonstrable in bile duct epithelial cells.

Iron deposition occurs first in zone 1 (periportal) hepatocytes (e-Figs. 15.6–15.13), with little or no involvement of Kupffer or endothelial cells (Fig. 15.4). Stainable iron can be seen as early as adolescence, particularly in males. Early, the granules tend to border the canaliculi (canalicular shadowing) (Fig. 15.5, e-Fig. 15.14). This becomes less prominent with increasing iron (e-Fig. 15.15). This pattern is highly suggestive of HH but not pathognomonic and is also seen, for example, in alcohol-associated iron deposition, along with significant Kupffer cell deposition. With a history or morphologic evidence of excess alcohol ingestion and liver cell iron deposition. HII should be determined (44,46).

With long-standing HH, iron deposits progressively increase and eventually are in Kupffer cells and macrophages, as well as biliary epithelial cells (Figs. 15.6 and 15.7). Liver architecture is undisturbed early. With involvement of zones 2 and 3, fibrosis begins, with periportal septa

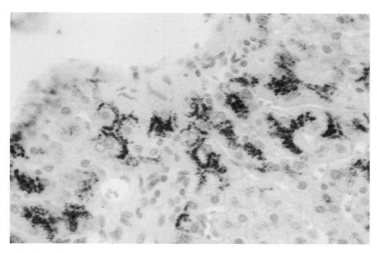

FIGURE 15.5 Hereditary hemochromatosis, showing iron granules outlining canaliculi (Perls reaction, original magnification ×400).

(Fig. 15.6) and then fine septa irregularly dissecting the liver. The classic cirrhosis of HH is micronodular, but macronodular, or irregular, cirrhosis is seen often. Ductular reaction (proliferation) is generally not prominent.

In cirrhosis, areas of nodules appear may be iron-free. These iron-free zones may be the foci from which HCC develops (17). Iron-free zones may also contribute to variation in HII determinations (2), and histologic correlation should always be made. HCC generally develops in HH cirrhosis but can also develop before cirrhosis develops (25,33,35).

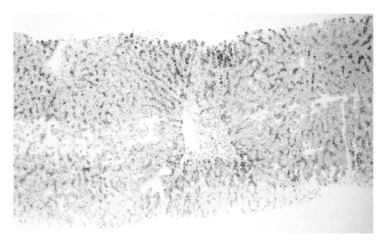

FIGURE 15.6 Hereditary hemochromatosis, advanced, with iron deposition throughout the lobule as well as in bile duct epithelial cells (Perls reaction, original magnification ×100).

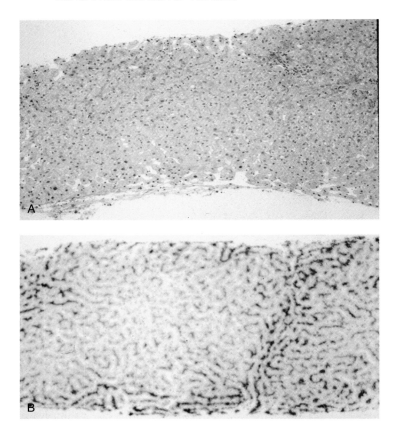

FIGURE 15.7 Hereditary hemochromatosis, with marked iron deposition demonstrating how iron granules can be relatively inapparent with hematoxylin-eosin (**A**. hematoxylin-eosin, original magnification ×200; **B**. Perls reaction, original magnification ×40).

In the heterozygote, the liver biopsy may be indistinguishable from early-stage homozygote HH, with heavy iron deposition in zone 1 hepatocytes but not in Kupffer cells, portal macrophages, or bile duct epithelial cells, and without fibrosis.

NEONATAL HEMOCHROMATOSIS

This rare perinatal syndrome is thought to be a result of antenatal liver disease that causes abnormal intrauterine iron metabolism, as well as subsequent iron overload of the liver and other tissues in the body. This condition may be seen in stillborns or in liveborns, and is not related to HH (12,26,36,48). Presentation includes hemorrhagic diathesis, edema, hypoalbuminemia, and hypoglycemia, and mortality is high. The liver generally shows significant parenchymal loss with irregular patchy or confluent collapse. Acinar transformation, giant cell formation, and regenerative nodules are seen (30,39).

SECONDARY HEMOSIDEROSIS

Iron overload is seen after long-term transfusion, with excess dietary iron, and in various forms of cirrhosis. Iron is principally in Kupffer cells and portal tract macrophages (e-Fig. 15.16). Eventually, in prolonged iron overload, as after many years of transfusions, iron is also in hepatocytes, and the biopsy may be indistinguishable from HH, although generally Kupffer cell iron deposition is more marked than in HH (Fig. 15.1). Fibrosis can develop.

Mild hepatic iron deposition is often seen in cirrhosis, in the absence of clinical history of an iron overload disorder. In some cirrhotic livers, iron overload may be accentuated after portacaval shunt, but this is not a universal phenomenon (14,34).

REFERENCES

1. Adams PC, Powell LW. Porphyria cutanea tarda and HLA-linked hemochromatosis—all in the family? Gastroenterology 1987;92:2033–2035.
2. Argani P, Furth EE. Intrahepatic iron variation may greatly affect the hepatic iron index. Int J Surg Pathol 1996;3:263–266.
3. Bacon BR, Schilsky ML, New knowledge of hereditary pathogenesis of hemochromatosis and Wilson Disease. Adv Intern Med 1999;44:91–116.
4. Bannerman RM, Keusch G, Kreimer-Birnbaum M, et al. Thalassemia intermedia, with iron overload, cardiac failure, diabetes mellitus, hypopituitarism and porphyrinuria. Am J Med 1967;42:476–486.
5. Barry M, Scheuer PJ, Sherlock S, et al. Hereditary spherocytosis with secondary haemochromatosis. Lancet 1968;2:481–485.
6. Bassett ML, Halliday JW, Powell LW. Value of hepatic iron measurements in early hemochromatosis and determination of the critical iron level associated with fibrosis. Hepatology 1986;6:24–29.
7. Bassett ML, Halliday JW, Powell LW. Genetic haemochromatosis. Semin Liver Dis 1984;4:217–227.
8. Batts K. Iron overload syndromes and the liver. Mod Pathol 2007;20(Suppl 1):S31–39.
9. Beutler E, Gelbart R, West C, et al. Mutation analysis in hereditary hemochromatosis. Blood Cell Mol Dis 1996;22:187–194.
10. Beutler E. The significance of the 187G (H63D) mutation in hemochromatosis. Am J Hum Genet 1997;61:762–764.
11. Beutler E, Felitti V, Koziol J, et al. Penetrance of the 845G to A (C282Y) HFE hereditary hemochromatosis mutation. Lancet 2002;359:211–218.
12. Blisard KS, Bartow SA. Neonatal hemochromatosis. Hum Pathol 1986;17:376–383.
13. Conrad ME, Umbreit JN, Moore EG, et al. Hereditary hemochromatosis: a prevalent disorder of iron metabolism with elusive etiology. Am J Hematol 1994;47:218–224.
14. Conn HO. Postcaval anastomosis and hepatic hemosiderin deposition: a prospective, controlled investigation. Gastroenterology 1972;62:61–72.

15. Cortes JM, Oliva H, Paradinas FL, et al. The pathology of the liver in porphyria cutanea tarda. Histopathology 1980;4:471–485.

16. Cullen LM, Anderson GJ, Ramm GA, et al. Genetics of hemochromatosis. Annu Rev Med 1999;50:87–98.

17. Deugnier YM, Charalambous P, Le Quilleuc D, et al. Preneoplastic significance of hepatic iron-free foci in hereditary hemochromatosis: a study of 185 patients. Hepatology 1993;18:1363–1369.

18. Deugnier YM, Guyader D, Crantock L, et al. Primary liver cancer in hereditary hemochromatosis: a clinical, pathological, and pathohereditary study of 54 cases. Gastroenterology 1993;104:228–234.

19. Deugnier Y, Turlin B. Pathology of hepatic iron overload. World J Gastroenterol 2007;13:4755–4760.

20. Fargion S, Piperno A, Cappellini MD, et al. Hepatitis C virus and porphyria cutanea tarda: evidence of a strong association. Hepatology 1992;16:1322–1326.

21. Feder JN, Gnirke A, Thomas W, et al. A novel MHC class-I like gene is mutated in patients with hereditary haemochromatosis. Nat Genet 1996;13:399–408.

22. Feder JN, Isuchihasi Z, Irrinki A, et al. The hemochromatosis founder mutation in HLA-H disrupts 6-2 microglobulin interaction and cell surface expression. J Biol Chem 1997;272:14025–14028.

23. Fleming RE, Britton RS, Waheed A, et al. Pathogenesis of hereditary hemochromatosis. Clin Liv Dis 2004;8:755–773.

24. George PM, Conaghan C, Angus HB, et al. Comparison of histological and biochemical hepatic iron indexes in the diagnosis of hereditary haemochromatosis. J Clin Pathol 1996;49:159–163.

25. Goh J, Gallagy G, McEntee G, et al. Hepatocellular carcinoma arising in the absence of cirrhosis in hereditary hemochromatosis. Eur J Gastroenterol Hepatol 1999;11:915–919.

26. Goldfischer S, Grotsky HW, Chang CH, et al. Idiopathic neonatal iron storage involving the liver, pancreas, heart and endocrine and exocrine glands. Hepatology 1981;1:58–64.

27. Hsing AW, McLaughlin JK, Olsen JH, et al. Cancer risk following primary hemochromatosis: a population-based cohort study in Denmark. Int J Cancer 1995;60:160–162.

28. James KR, Cortes JM, Paradinas FJ. Demonstration of intracytoplasmic needle-like inclusions in hepatocytes with porphyria cutanea tarda. J Clin Pathol 1980;33:899–900.

29. Jazwinska EC, Cullen LM, Busfield F, et al. Haemochromatosis and HLA-H. Nat Genet 1996;14:249–251.

30. Johnson BF. Hemochromatosis resulting from prolonged oral iron therapy. N Engl J Med 1968;278:1100.

31. Jouanelle AM, Gandon G, Jezequel P, et al. Haemochromatosis and HLA-H. Nat Genet 1996;14:251–252.

32. Jouanelle AM, Fergelot P, Gandon G, et al. A candidate gene for hemochromatosis: frequency of the C28Y and H63D mutations. Hum Genet 1997;100:544–547.

33. Ko C, Dissalah N, Berger J, et al. Prevalence of hepatic iron overload association with hepatocellular cancer in end-stage liver disease: results from the National Hemochromatosis Transplant Registry. Liver Int 2007;27:1394–1401.

34. Koff RS, Go TB, Oliai A. Hepatic hemosiderosis after portacaval shunt surgery in alcoholic cirrhosis: a sometime thing. Gastroenterology 1972;63:834–836.

35. Kohler HH, Kohter T, Kusel V, et al. Hepatocellular carcinoma in a patient with hereditary hemochromatosis and noncirrhotic liver. A case report. Pathol Res Pract 1999; 195:509–513.

36. Knisely AS. Neonatal hemochromatosis. Adv Pediatr 1992;39:383–403.

37. Lefkowitch JH, Grossman ME. Hepatic pathology in porphyria cutanea tarda. Liver 1983;3:19–29.

38. MacDonald RA, Mallory GK. Hemochromatosis and hemosiderosis: study of 211 autopsied cases. Arch Intern Med 1960;105:686–700.

39. Nichols GM, Bacon BR. Hereditary hemochromatosis: pathogenesis and clinical features of a common disease. Am J Gastroenterol 1989;84:851–862.

40. Olynyk JK, O'Neill R, Britton RS, et al. Determination of hepatic iron concentration in fresh and paraffin-embedded tissue: diagnostic implications. Gastroenterology 1994;106:674–677.

41. Piperno A, D'Alba R, Roffi L, et al. Hepatitis C virus infection in patients with idiopathic hemochromatosis (IH) and porphyria cutanea tarda (PCT). Arch Virol 1992;4(Suppl): 215–216.

42. Powell LW. The role of alcoholism in hepatic iron storage disease. Ann NY Acad Sci 1975;252:124–134.

43. Roetto A, Camaschella C. New insights into iron homeostasis through the study of non-HFE hereditary haemochromatosis. Best Practice Res Clin Haematol 2005;18:235–250.

44. Sallie RW, Reed WD, Shilkin KB. Confirmation of the efficacy of hepatic tissue iron index in differentiating hereditary haemochromatosis from alcoholic liver disease complicated by alcoholic haemosiderosis. Gut 1991;32:207–210.

45. Simon M, Le Mignon L, Fauchet R, et al. A study of 609 HLA haplotypes marking for the hemochromatosis gene: (1) mapping of the gene near the HLA-A locus and characters required to define a heterozygous population and (2) hypothesis concerning the underlying cause of hemochromatosis-HLA association. Am J Hum Genet 1987;41:89–105.

46. Summers KM, Halliday JW, Powell LW. Identification of homozygous hemochromatosis subjects by measurement of hepatic iron index. Hepatology 1990;12:20–25.

47. Turlin B, Devgnier Y. Evaluation and interpretation of iron in the liver. Semin Diagn Pathol 1998;15:237–245.

48. Whitington PF. Neonatal hemochromatosis: a congenital alloimmune hepatitis. Semin Liver Dis 2007;27:243–250.

49. Yaouang J, el Kahloun A, Chorney M, et al. Familial screening for hereditary haemochromatosis by means of DNA markers. J Med Genet 1992;29:320–322.

16

COPPER STORAGE DISORDERS (WILSON DISEASE, INDIAN CHILDHOOD CIRRHOSIS, AND MENKES DISEASE)

WILSON DISEASE

Wilson disease (WD), or hepatolenticular degeneration, is the principal disorder of copper metabolism affecting the liver (12,25,30,40,42). A high index of suspicion for this disorder is needed since both the clinical manifestations and biopsy findings may vary. This neurologically debilitating and ultimately fatal disease should be considered in the evaluation of every young patient with unexplained liver disease. Most patients present between the ages of 5 and 30 years, but the disease occurs as late as the seventh decade (17,40). The usual clinical laboratory tests are not specific (Table 16.1), and the liver biopsy may be the only way to establish the diagnosis (25).

WD follows tissue injury caused by copper overload in liver and other organs because of decreased excretion of copper in the biliary tract (7,27). Increasing amounts of copper are excreted in the urine, but a positive copper balance remains and copper is deposited in the liver and brain, as well as in other tissues, including the cornea (Kayser-Fleischer rings), kidneys, striated muscle, bones, and joints. The liver is universally affected, although clinical manifestations are not always prominent.

Clinical features vary greatly, with hepatic, neurologic, hematologic, and psychiatric manifestations (4,5,10,12,17,28,30,38,40,46,49) (Table 16.2). Most patients present with hepatic disease, often in a manageable stage (25,30,46). Neuropsychiatric presentations indicate advanced disease, with some patients not having had signs or symptoms of liver disease despite considerable evidence of liver injury, including cirrhosis (17,42).

Copper accumulates in liver cell lysosomes beginning in early childhood and is then released into the blood stream. This is a gradual process,

TABLE 16.1	Clinical Laboratory Tests in Wilson Disease
Test	Result
Serum ceruloplasmin	Decreased, may be normal (ceruloplasmin can be an acute-phase reactant)
Serum copper (nonceruloplasmin)	Increased (total serum copper is decreased; however, the ceruloplasmin-free fraction is increased)
Urine copper	Increased (not specific for Wilson disease)
Incorporation of radiocopper into ceruloplasmin	Decreased (specific)

and signs and symptoms can begin in middle adolescence, with increasing fatigue, jaundice, and elevated serum transaminase values. This chronic hepatitis picture is clinically indistinguishable from other forms of chronic hepatitis. As many as 50% of patients are cirrhotic at presentation (25,26,40,44). Hepatocellular carcinoma may develop (8,24,36).

Approximately 25% of patients present with an acute hepatitis picture. This can be severe and accompanied by acute hemolytic anemia, most likely caused by the rapid release of copper into the circulation. Fulminant hepatitis, with severe hemolytic anemia, coagulopathy, renal insufficiency, and often death, is occasionally seen in teenagers without prior evidence of liver disease (4,13,18,38,43,46,49). This form can go unrecognized because of the acuteness and severity of presentation; in fatal cases autopsy may not be performed or the histologic features, which are nonspecific, may not suggest WD.

TABLE 16.2	Patterns of Presentation in Wilson Disease	
Fulminant hepatitis	Hemolytic anemia
	Coagulopathy
	Renal insufficiency
	Death
Acute hepatitis	Fatigue
	Variable degrees of jaundice
	Transaminase value elevation
Chronic hepatitis	Fatigue
	Jaundice usual
	Transaminase value elevation
Cirrhosis	Indistinguishable from other cirrhoses

Genetics

This autosomal recessive disorder occurs in 1 in 30,000 births, with a carrier frequency of 1 in 400. The gene is localized to chromosome 13, where it is in linkage disequilibrium with a red blood cell enzyme esterase D, as well as with the gene for retinoblastoma. The specific locus is thought to be at the ATP7B site (7,9,12,23,34,37). Mutations, frequently found in affected individuals, are thought to be quite heterogeneous (12,21). The gene encodes a putative copper-transporting protein that is almost exclusively expressed in the liver (9). Gene mutations lead to copper accumulation as a result of production of defective liver-specific copper transporter (4,7,12,48) that cannot adequately deliver copper into the bile, leading to its accumulation in tissues (16,39). There is no evidence of a genetically derived deficiency of ceruloplasmin production (11). Various phenotypic presentations are associated with specific mutations (37). WD has been associated with other genetically determined conditions, such as Gilbert disease and thalassemia minor, both of which can contribute to masking of the more serious diagnosis.

The earliest, but nonspecific, laboratory finding is the elevation of serum transaminase values, often before signs or symptoms are manifest (40). Low serum ceruloplasmin levels suggest the diagnosis, but ceruloplasmin is an acute-phase reactant and values can be normal, even in well-established WD. Serum copper values are almost always decreased, although the ceruloplasmin-free fraction is increased. Urine copper determination can screen for WD, but increased values are nonspecific. Most specific is measurement of incorporation of orally administered radiocopper into ceruloplasmin. In WD this incorporation is decreased, but the test is not widely available.

The diagnosis is often established by the presence of Kayser-Fleischer corneal rings when seen with reduced serum ceruloplasmin levels. Neither is specific or universal, and determination of hepatic copper concentration may be required (3,22). In WD, copper levels of 250 to 3,000 μg/g dry weight can be demonstrated, although heterozygotes have values near reference range. Copper levels can be reliably quantified from formalin-fixed paraffin-embedded tissue (19). There may be considerable variation in copper content in the cirrhotic liver, particularly in fibrous tissue-rich, hepatocyte-poor samples that are submitted for assay (15,20,33), and values less than 250 μg/g dry weight should not exclude the diagnosis (16). Copper increases in the liver in other conditions (Table 16.3).

Pathology

Histologic alterations may be seen in biopsies obtained at all stages of the disease but vary considerably from patient to patient (1,2,25,26,40,41,44). The most constant feature is the variability of the findings.

Although the hallmark of WD is the accumulation of copper in hepatocytes, both copper and copper-associated protein (26,39) may not be histochemically demonstrable in many cases, and either copper assay or

TABLE 16.3	Conditions Associated with Elevated Hepatic Copper Levels

Primary biliary cirrhosis
Primary sclerosing cholangitis
Chronic large-duct obstruction
Biliary atresia
Intrahepatic cholestasis of childhood
Indian childhood cirrhosis
Cirrhosis and chronic active hepatitis (less common)

ultrastructural studies of the liver biopsy may be required to confirm the diagnosis, particularly in precirrhotic stages (16).

EARLY STAGE. There may be only mild hepatocellular damage, with slight variation in cell and nuclear size, including increased numbers of binucleate hepatocytes, which can resemble mild acute viral hepatitis. Individual swollen hepatocytes as well as isolated acidophilic bodies are sometimes seen, most prominent in zone 1 but observed throughout the lobule. Portal inflammation may be slight or absent. Slight macrovesicular steatosis with no particular distribution pattern is often, but not invariably, associated with increased numbers of glycogenated nuclei (e-Figs. 16.1–16.3). This latter feature is seen mostly in zone 1 (Fig. 16.1). In less than 25% of case, minimal copper is present in zone 1 hepatocytes (Fig. 16.2). Rarely, the picture of submassive necrosis is seen.

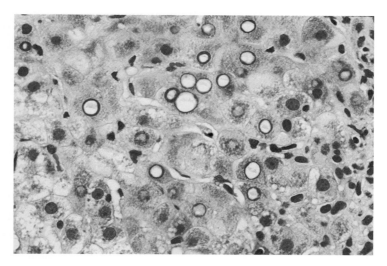

FIGURE 16.1   Photomicrograph of Wilson disease showing prominence of glycogenated nuclei in zone 1 (periportal) hepatocytes (hematoxylin-eosin, original magnification ×400).

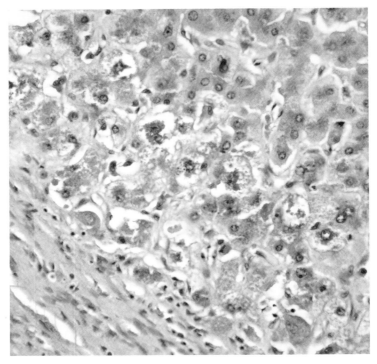

FIGURE 16.2   Photomicrograph of Wilson disease showing copper deposition in zone 1 hepatocytes (rubeanic acid, original magnification ×400).

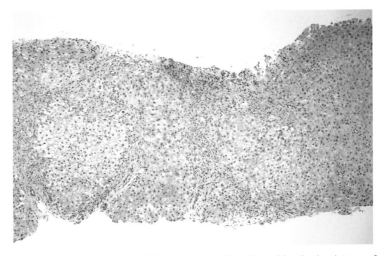

FIGURE 16.3   Photomicrograph of Wilson disease showing a histologic picture of chronic hepatitis with interface hepatitis (piecemeal necrosis) (hematoxylin-eosin, original magnification ×100).

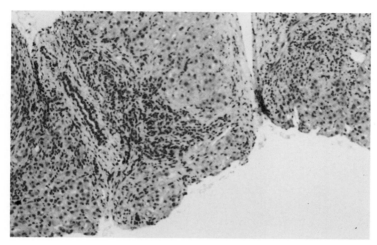

FIGURE 16.4 Photomicrograph of Wilson disease showing macronodular cirrhosis (hematoxylin-eosin, original magnification ×100).

PRECIRRHOTIC STAGE. Inflammation and hepatocyte necrosis can increase with progression (1,2,23,40,41,44). Portal inflammation, with prominent interface hepatitis and necrosis, particularly in zone 1, occurs. Lymphocytes are prominent, and polymorphonuclear leukocytes may be seen. There is increased portal collagen and fibrosis extending into the lobule. The biopsy can resemble chronic viral or autoimmune hepatitis (Fig. 16.3, e-Fig. 16.4). Early-stage changes can persist. Steatosis, microvesicular as well as macrovesicular, is seen. Multinucleate giant hepatocytes can form. Uncommonly, there are lipofuscin-like coarse copper granules, but in zone 1 rather than 3 (1,2, 26,40,41).

CIRRHOTIC STAGE. Micronodular cirrhosis progressively transforms to mixed or predominantly macronodular pattern with broad bands of parenchymal collapse (Fig. 16.4, e-Figs. 16.5–16.9). Early and precirrhotic stage changes are admixed. Hepatocytes are variable with anisonucleosis and necrosis, and many polymorphonuclear leukocytes, may be seen. Mallory hyalin is common (Fig. 16.5, e-Fig. 16.10), most often in paraseptal hepatocytes but also elsewhere in the nodule, often with ballooned cells. Ductular reaction is quite prominent, and cholestasis is common (Fig. 16.6, e-Figs. 16.7, 16.8, 16.11). Copper-associated protein and/or copper can be histochemically demonstrated in many cases, typically irregularly distributed (e-Fig. 16.12) (15,19,20,25,32, 33,45).

FULMINANT STAGE. In the absence of clinical or morphologic evidence of some other cause for fulminant hepatic failure, WD should always be considered. The biopsy is indistinguishable from that of other forms of fulminant hepatic failure (4,13,28,38). Parenchymal collapse and regenerative nodules are seen. Many cirrhotic WD patients have fulminant failure (42). With massive necrosis and few viable liver cells, copper assay may not be useful.

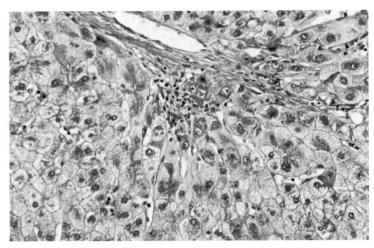

FIGURE 16.5   Photomicrograph of Wilson disease showing Mallory hyalin in zone 1 hepato-cytes (hematoxylin-eosin, original magnification ×400).

Histochemistry

Copper-associated protein can be demonstrated with Victoria blue, orcein (Shikata), or Gomori aldehyde–fuchsin. Copper can be seen after staining with rhodanine, rubeanic acid, or Timm silver sulfide. A recently developed method for demonstrating copper is a modification of the rhodanine stain, but is technically easier to perform and can be completed in 2 hours rather than overnight (e-Figs. 16.12, 16.13) (14). Fetal liver is useful as control tissue for copper stains. Absence of copper or copper-associated protein, demon-strated by histochemical methods, does not exclude the diagnosis of WD (16,25,35) (Table 16.4). The key features of WD are summarized in Table 16.5.

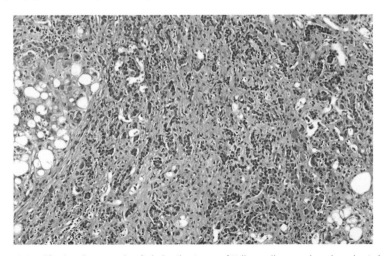

FIGURE 16.6   Photomicrograph of cirrhotic stage of Wilson disease showing ductular reac-tion and cholestasis (hematoxylin-eosin, original magnification ×100).

TABLE 16.4 Histochemical Techniques Used to Identify Copper and Copper-Binding Protein

Name	Product Stained	Appearance
Emanuele/Goodman	Copper	Orange-red
Rhodanine	Copper	Orange-red
Rubeanic acid	Copper	Green-black
Timm silver sulfide	Copper, zinc, and iron[a]	Brown–black
Orcein	Copper-binding protein	Black
Victoria blue	Copper-binding protein	Blue-purple

[a]This stain is not specific for copper, but it is more sensitive than rhodanine and rubeanic acid.

INDIAN CHILDHOOD CIRRHOSIS

Indian Childhood Cirrhosis, a disease of young children with high mortality, occurs almost exclusively in India (6,47). Genetic factors likely play a role, although increased copper ingestion from household water supplies may also contribute. Hepatocellular swelling may be prominent early. Mallory hyalin is usually found, with scattered foci of necrosis and focal accumulation of neutrophils. Pericellular fibrosis, similar to that of alcoholic liver disease, is seen, but steatosis is not prominent. Hepatocytes generally contain large amounts of copper and copper-associated protein. Cirrhosis ultimately ensues.

MENKES DISEASE (KINKY HAIR DISEASE)

Menkes disease is caused by a defective gene that regulates copper metabolism. Copper accumulates at higher than normal levels in the kidney and intestinal lining, but at abnormally low levels in the brain and liver, and,

TABLE 16.5 Key Features of Wilson Disease

1. Consider Wilson disease with unexplained liver disease in a young person
2. Histology highly variable
3. Distribution of copper and copper-associated protein highly variable; may not be demonstrable in all cases
4. Steatosis and glycogenated nuclei commonly seen
5. May mimic acute hepatitis and chronic hepatitis
6. Cirrhosis
7. Hepatocellular carcinoma

consequently, the liver is not affected (12,29,30). The responsible gene is closely related to that of WD (12,48).

REFERENCES

1　Aaseth J, Flaten TP, Andersen O. Hereditary iron and copper deposition: diagnostics, pathogenesis and therapeutics. Scand J Gastroenterol 2007;42:673–681.

2.　Anderson PJ, Popper H. Changes in hepatic structure in Wilson's disease. Am J Pathol 1960;36:483–497.

3.　Bacon BR, Schilsky ML. New knowledge of genetic pathogenesis of hemochromatosis and Wilson disease. Adv Intern Med 1999;44:91–116.

4.　Berman DH, Leventhal RI, Gavaler JS, et al. Clinical differentiation of fulminant Wilson's disease from other causes of hepatic failure. Gastroenterology 1991;100:1129–1134.

5.　Brewer GJ. Recognition, diagnosis, and management of Wilson disease. Proc Soc Exp Biol Med 2000;223:39–46.

6.　Bhusnurmath SR, Walia BNS, Singh S, et al. Sequential histopathologic alterations in Indian childhood cirrhosis treated with d-penicillamine. Hum Pathol 1991;22:653–658.

7.　Bowcock AM, Farrer LA, Herbert JM, et al. Eight closely linked loci place the Wilson disease locus within 13q14-q21. Am J Hum Genet 1988;43:664–674.

8.　Cheng WSC, Govindarajan S, Redeker AG. Hepatocellular carcinoma in a case of Wilson's disease. Liver 1992;12:42–45.

9.　Cuthbert JA. Wilson's disease: a new gene and an animal model for an old disease. J Investig Med 1995;43:323–336.

10.　Cuthbert JA. Wilson disease. Update of a systemic disorder with protean manifestations. Gastroenterol Clin North Am 1998;27:655–681.

11.　Czaja MJ, Weiner FR, Schwarzenberg SJ, et al. Molecular studies of ceruloplasmin deficiency in Wilson's disease. J Clin Invest 1987;80:1200–1204.

12.　Daniel KG, Harbach RH, Guida WC, et al. Copper storage diseases: Menkes, Wilson's, and cancer. Front Biosc 2004;9:2652–2662.

13.　Davies SE, Williams R, Portmann B. Hepatic morphology and histochemistry of Wilson disease presenting as fulminant hepatic failure: a study of 11 cases. Histopathology 1989; 15:385–394.

14.　Emanuele P, Goodman ZD. A simple and rapid stain for copper in liver tissue. Ann Diagn Pathol 1998;2:125–126.

15.　Faa G, Nurchi V, Demelia L, et al. Uneven hepatic copper distribution in Wilson's disease. J Hepatol 1995;22:303–308.

16.　Ferenci P, Steindl-Munda P, Vogel W, et al. Diagnostic value of quantitative copper determination in patients with Wilson's disease. Clin Gastroenterol Hepatol 2005;3:811–818.

17.　Ferenci P, Czlonkowska A, Merle U, et al. Late-onset Wilson's disease. Gastroenterology 2007;132:1294–1298.

18.　Ferlan-Marolt V, Stepee S. Fulminant Wilsonian hepatitis unmasked by disease progression: report of a case and review of the literature. Dig Dis Sci 1999;44:1054–1058.

19.　Goldfischer S, Sternlieb I. Changes in the distribution of hepatic copper in relation to the progression of Wilson's disease (hepatolenticular degeneration). Am J Pathol 1968;53: 883–901.

20.　Goldfischer S, Popper H, Sternlieb I. The significance of variations in the distribution of copper in liver disease. Am J Pathol 1980;99:715–730.

21.　Haas, R, Gutierraz-Rivero B, Knoche J, et al. Mutation analysis in patients with Wilson disease: identification of 4 novel mutations. Mutation in brief no. 250. Online. Hum Mutat 1999;14:88.

22.　Hall P de la M, Dilena B, Padbury R. Hepatic copper studies in "native" livers. Hepatology 1996;24:423A.

23. Houwen RH, Schaeffer H, Te-Meerman GJ, et al. Close linkage of the Wilson's disease 6WS to D13S12 in the chromosomal region 13q 21 and not to EDD in 13q 14. Hum Genet 1990;85:560–562.

24. Iwadate H, Ohira H, Suzuki T, et al. Hepatocellular carcinoma associated with Wilson's disease. Intern Med 2004;43:1042–1045.

25. Langner C, Denk H. Wilson disease. Virchows Arch 2004;445:111–118.

26. Ludwig J, Moyer TP, Rakela J. The liver biopsy diagnosis of Wilson disease. Am J Clin Pathol 1994;102:443–446.

27. McCardle HJ, Bingham MJ, Summer K, et al. Cu metabolism in the liver. Adv Exp Med Biol 1999;448:29–37.

28. McCullough AJ, Fleming CR, Thistle JL, et al. Diagnosis of Wilson's disease presenting as fulminant hepatic failure. Gastroenterology 1983;84:161–167.

29. Menkes JH. Menkes disease and Wilson disease: two sides of the same copper coin. II: Wilson disease. Eur J Paediatric Neurol 1999;3:245–253.

30. Merle U, Schaefer M, Ferenci P, et al. Clinical presentation, diagnosis and long-term outcome of Wilson's disease: a cohort study. Gut 2007;56:115–120.

31. Monaco AP, Chelly J. Menkes and Wilson diseases. Adv Genet 1995;33:233–253.

32. Mulder TPJ, Janssens AR, Verspaget HW, et al. Metallothionein concentration in the liver of patients with Wilson's disease, primary biliary cirrhosis, and liver metastases of colorectal cancer. J Hepatol 1992;16:346–350.

33. Nartey NO, Frei JV, Cherian MG. Hepatic copper and metallothionein distribution in Wilson's disease (hepatolenticular degeneration). Lab Invest 1987;57:397–401.

34. Petrokhin K, Fischer SG, Pirastu M, et al. Mapping, cloning and genetic characterization of the region containing the Wilson disease gene. Nat Genet 1993;5:338–343.

35. Pillon L, Lecca S, Van Eyken P, et al. Value of histochemical stains for copper in the diagnosis of Wilson disease. Histopathology 1998;33:28–33.

36. Polio J, Enriquez RE, Chow A, et al. Hepatocellular carcinoma in Wilson's disease. J Clin Gastroenterol 1989;11:220–224.

37. Pyeritz RE. Genetic heterogeneity in Wilson disease: lessons from rare alleles. Ann Intern Med 1997;127:21–26.

38. Sallie R, Katsiyiannakesh L, Baldwin D, et al. Failure of simple biochemical studies to reliably differentiate fulminant Wilson disease from other causes of fulminant hepatic failure. Hepatology 1992;16:1206–1211.

39. Schaefer M, Gitlin JD. Genetic disorders of membrane transport. IV. Wilson disease and Menkes disease. Am J Physiol 1999;276(2 Pt 1):G311–G314.

40. Scheinberg IH, Sternlieb I. Wilson's Disease. Philadelphia: WB Saunders, 1984.

41. Sternlieb I. Evolution of the hepatic lesion in Wilson's disease (hepatolenticular degeneration). Progr Liver Dis 1972;4:511–525.

42. Sternlieb I. Perspectives on Wilson's disease. Hepatology 1990;12:1234–1239.

43. Sternlieb I. Hepatic copper toxicosis. J Gastroenterol Hepatol 1989;4:175–181.

44. Stromeyer FW, Ishak KG. Histology of the liver in Wilson's disease. Am J Clin Pathol 1980;73:12–24.

45. Sumithran E, Looi LM. Copper-binding protein in liver cells. Hum Pathol 1985;16:677–682.

46. Taly AB, Meenakshi-Sunderam S, Sinha S, et al. Wilson disease: description of 282 patients evaluated over 3 decades. Medicine (Baltimore) 2007;86:112–121.

47. Tanner MS, Portmann B, Mowat AP, et al. Increased hepatic copper concentration in Indian childhood cirrhosis. Lancet 1979;1:1203–1205.

48. Tanzl RE, Petrokhim K, Chernov I, et al. The Wilson's disease gene is a copper transporting ATPase with homology to the Menkes disease gene. Nat Genet 1993;5:344–350.

49. Walshe JM. Wilson's disease presenting with features of hepatic dysfunction: a clinical analysis of eighty-seven patients. Q J Med 1989;70:253–263.

17

SMALL BILE DUCT DISORDERS

The principal disorders affecting intrahepatic bile ducts are primary biliary cirrhosis (PBC) and primary sclerosing cholangitis (PSC). They show similar histologic changes and reflect, to some extent, immune-mediated bile duct injury and, eventually, bile duct destruction and loss. They are also alike as progressive, chronic liver diseases leading to liver failure in either the precirrhotic or the cirrhotic stage. Clinically, they can also behave similarly as chronic, relentless, cholestatic disorders, with similar patterns of biochemical abnormalities. Medical treatment is generally not effective, and liver transplantation is often the only life-saving measure. However, the conditions differ in terms of the patients affected.

PRIMARY BILIARY CIRRHOSIS

Primary biliary cirrhosis (PBC) is a progressive nonsuppurative destructive cholangitis affecting mostly middle-aged women, with peak incidence between 40 and 60 years (30). The onset is usually insidious, with patients asymptomatic for years. In contrast with PSC, with its strong association with inflammatory bowel disease, there are no known predecessor disorders. Patients frequently present with cholestatic itching, which can be disabling. Jaundice is usually not seen early; cholestasis in the biopsy is a poor prognostic sign (22,24,25). PBC can be associated with various autoimmune conditions, including sicca syndrome, CREST (calcinosis, Raynaud phenomenon, esophageal motility disorders, sclerodactyly, and telangiectasia) syndrome, celiac sprue, membranous glomerulonephritis, and interstitial lung disease (3,5,10,21,23,27,29). Hepatocellular carcinoma is uncommon (7,9,26). Elevated serum alkaline phosphatase value and high titers of antimitochondrial antibody (AMA) are virtually diagnostic.

Antimitochondrial antibodies are a family of immunoglobulins, including anti-M2, anti-M4, anti-M8, and anti-M9, all of which are directed against different epitopes and all of which may be associated with primary biliary cirrhosis. Anti-M2, the antibody against the multienzyme complexes at the inner mitochondrial membrane, is present in all PBC patients; its presence is considered highly specific and virtually diagnostic (24).

Despite the presence of AMA, the etiopathogenesis of PBC is unclear. Autoimmune mechanisms may have a role in its development. Impairment of cell-mediated immunity, particularly involving the T-lymphocyte population, circulating immune complexes, and complement activation, has been implicated (13,14). There is up-regulation of human leukocyte antigen (HLA) class I antigens as well as aberrant expression of HLA class II antigens on bile duct epithelium in PBC. This is not specific and is seen in other immunologically mediated bile duct conditions, including acute allograft rejection and graft versus host disease (GVHD).

The possibility that PBC is an atypical manifestation of different infectious diseases, such as tuberculosis or sarcoidosis, has been considered. A possible association with *Escherichia coli*, which is antigenically similar to biliary epithelium, has been suggested (molecular mimicry) (12). *Chlamydia pneumoniae* has also been implicated in the pathogenesis of PBC (1,19).

The diagnosis is usually established clinically. Liver biopsy confirms the diagnosis but is particularly useful for determining the stage of the disease and in monitoring progression.

Pathology

Four distinct stages are generally recognized although there is a significant overlap among them, and as the disease progresses those overlapping features can be found in any given biopsy. Several staging classifications have been proposed (Table 17.1) (18,24). The Scheuer staging method emphasizes an early, florid bile duct injury stage with subsequent bile ductular proliferation (reaction) as particularly important in the development of the histopathologic changes (23,25). The Ludwig approach, in contrast, emphasizes the inflammatory cell component (18).

Despite the commonly accepted name, cirrhosis is only the last stage in the development of the disease, and PBC encompasses a wide spectrum

TABLE 17.1 **Staging of Primary Biliary Cirrhosis**
Scheuer staging:
Stage 1. The florid duct lesion (portal inflammation)
Stage 2. Ductular proliferation (periportal expansion and inflammation)
Stage 3. Scarring with bridging, septal fibrosis
Stage 4. Cirrhosis
Ludwig staging:
Stage 1. Portal hepatitis
Stage 2. Periportal hepatitis
Stage 3. Bridging necrosis/fibrosis
Stage 4. Cirrhosis

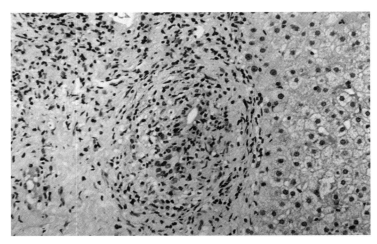

FIGURE 17.1   Early (stage 1) primary biliary cirrhosis. Florid bile duct injury and associated predominantly mononuclear inflammatory infiltrate in the portal tract (hematoxylin-eosin, original magnification ×400).

of relentlessly progressive changes. Stage 1 (early primary biliary cirrhosis) is characterized by florid duct lesion and portal inflammation (e-Figs. 17.1–17.4). Bile duct injury is segmental, affecting small and medium-sized interlobular bile ducts. Bile duct epithelium is irregularly involved. Hyperplasia of the epithelium occurs early in association with infiltration by mature lymphocytes. The basement membrane is disrupted, and bile duct rupture takes place. The injured bile duct is usually surrounded by inflammatory infiltrate predominantly composed of lymphocytes, plasma cells, some histiocytes, and a variable number of eosinophils (23,24). Lymphoid aggregates may form, sometimes including true lymphoid follicles with germinal centers, resembling those seen in chronic hepatitis C infection (see Chapter 9) (Fig. 17.1).

In as many as 40% of stage 2 early-stage biopsies (e-Figs. 17.5–17.11) characteristic, but not pathognomonic, epithelioid and histiocytic noncaseating granulomas can be seen immediately adjacent to a damaged bile duct (Figs. 17.2, 17.3, e-Figs. 17.5–17.9, 17.11) (17). Granulomas can also be seen in later stages but are uncommon with advanced fibrosis. The absence of granulomatous bile duct damage does not exclude the diagnosis (23,24). Because the bile duct injury in PBC is segmental, any biopsy may fail to show diagnostic changes, and step sections, and occasionally a subsequent biopsy, may be required (Fig 17.4).

The stage of bile duct injury and portal inflammation is followed by extension of the inflammatory infiltrate beyond the limiting plate into the lobule, strongly resembling the lymphocytic interface hepatitis (lymphocytic piecemeal necrosis) of various forms of chronic hepatitis, particularly chronic hepatitis C. Kupffer cells are frequently prominent, and varying

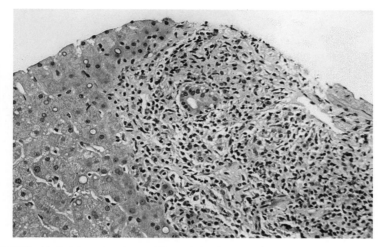

FIGURE 17.2   Early (stage 1) primary biliary cirrhosis. Granulomatous inflammation and bile duct injury (hematoxylin-eosin, original magnification ×200).

degrees of parenchymal inflammation, with sinusoidal inflammation, are invariably present. Lobular foci of necrosis can be seen, with accumulations of lymphocytes and even scattered small granulomas or clusters of histiocytes (Fig. 17.5, e-Figs. 17.5–17.11). Cholestasis is usually not prominent in early PBC. Once significant fibrosis or frank cirrhosis has developed, parenchymal inflammatory activity is usually minimal.

Early PBC can sometimes be associated with portal hypertension, perhaps because of narrowing of intrahepatic portal vein branches by the

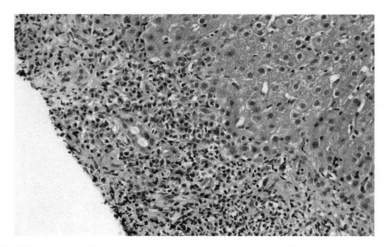

FIGURE 17.3   Primary biliary cirrhosis. Extensive interface hepatitis is present (lymphocytic piecemeal necrosis) (hematoxylin-eosin, original magnification ×200).

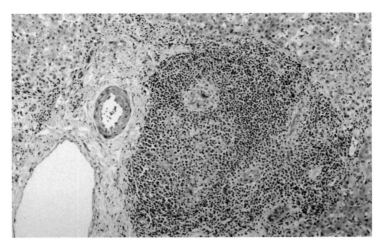

FIGURE 17.4 Primary biliary cirrhosis. Smaller bile ducts are affected, and some of them have already disappeared (hematoxylin-eosin, original magnification ×200).

inflammatory process. In some patients, nodular hyperplasia may contribute to portal hypertension (Fig. 17.6) (4).

Late primary biliary cirrhosis (periportal or progressive stage) is manifested not only by more extensive bile duct injury but also by expansion of the portal tracts with associated lymphocytic piecemeal necrosis, as well as marked bile ductular reaction (proliferation), giving rise to so-called biliary interface hepatitis. Superimposed on this is increasing fibrosis, sometimes

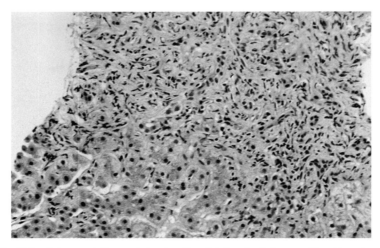

FIGURE 17.5 Primary biliary cirrhosis. Focal bile ductular proliferation is present (hematoxylin-eosin, original magnification ×200).

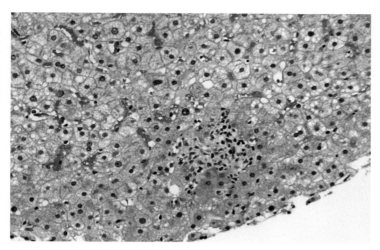

FIGURE 17.6   Primary biliary cirrhosis. Mild lobular inflammation and microgranulomas are present (hematoxylin-eosin, original magnification ×200).

referred to as "fibrotic interface hepatitis" (24,25). These three changes interrupt the limiting plate and are generally easily seen.

Prolonged cholate stasis gives a characteristic appearance to the periportal/paraseptal hepatocytes (e-Figs. 17.12–17.14). They are slightly enlarged and pale, with rarefied cytoplasm, sometimes containing abundant copper-associated protein (e-Fig. 17.15), demonstrable with Victoria blue or orcein stain. Mallory hyalin may also be present. In fully developed stage 3 and 4 PBC, intracanalicular cholestasis can be prominent and most of the original interlobular bile ducts are no longer seen. Granulomatous inflammatory injury may affect the remaining bile ducts. Clusters of xanthomatous and pseudoxanthomatous cells are also seen.

However, the most significant and characteristic feature of late-stage PBC is progressive bile duct loss (Fig. 17.7). The normal portal tract generally has at least one interlobular bile duct with one to two accompanying hepatic artery branches (see Chapter 4). The site of the original bile ducts is sometimes marked by collections of histiocytes or lymphoid aggregates, adjacent to undamaged arteries. The fibrous scarring typical of PSC is not seen in PBC. Eventually fibrous septa extend from portal tracts and intersect parenchymal architecture, with development of irregular (jigsaw puzzle-shaped) regenerative nodules (Fig. 17.8, e-Figs. 17.6–17.18).

PBC can recur after liver transplantation (e-Figs. 17.19–17.22).

Differential Diagnosis

Several conditions affecting the liver show variable degrees of bile duct injury. In addition to PBC and PSC, other conditions, such as suppurative cholangitis, sarcoidosis, graft versus host disease (GVHD), and acute cellular and

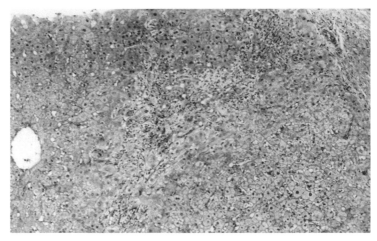

FIGURE 17.7   Primary biliary cirrhosis. Slender fibrous septa (late stage 3, 4), and periseptal cholestasis and cholate stasis (hematoxylin-eosin, original magnification ×100).

chronic ductopenic rejection have bile duct injury as a significant feature. In each of these, the injury may be destructive and progressive, leading to bile duct loss.

In contrast, some degree of bile duct damage, without loss, may be seen in viral hepatitis, particularly hepatitis C and autoimmune hepatitis, some drugs/toxins, HIV-associated cholangiopathy (with or without

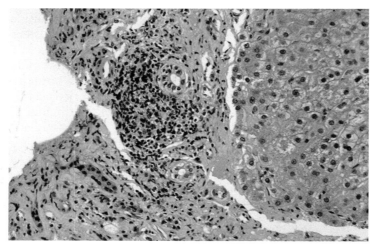

FIGURE 17.8   Primary sclerosing cholangitis (PSC). Bile duct injury in the early (stage I) of PSC. Bile duct epithelium is irregular and atrophic (hematoxylin-eosin, original magnification ×200).

cryptosporidiosis), sepsis and septicemia, toxic shock syndrome, parasitic infestation, and Hodgkin disease.

The progressive periportal stage of PBC can be difficult to differentiate from chronic hepatitis with periportal activity. In most forms of chronic hepatitis, there is only mild bile duct epithelial injury and no recognizable bile duct loss. Lobular activity with focal necrosis, acidophilic body formation, and inflammation is usually more pronounced in chronic viral hepatitis than in PBC. Differentiating between PBC and autoimmune hepatitis can also be difficult. Clinical information is invaluable in these cases.

PRIMARY SCLEROSING CHOLANGITIS

Primary sclerosing cholangitis (PSC) is characterized by the presence of inflammation and fibrosis with segmental stricturing along the biliary tree. In many patients there is little or no intrahepatic bile duct change until late in the disease, and in part for this reason, the biopsy is not a standard for diagnosis. Small duct PSC is a variant that affects only intrahepatic bile ducts (20). In small duct PSC, liver biopsy is the principal means of establishing the diagnosis.

Approximately 70% of patients with PSC also have inflammatory bowel disease (IBD), mostly ulcerative colitis (UC). Conversely, fewer than 10% of patients with UC have associated PSC. PSC can sometimes precede the onset of PSC. PSC occurs at any age, with peak incidence in the fourth decade, with an incidence in males twice that of in females (25). The onset may be insidious, with malaise associated with increased serum alkaline phosphatase values. In contrast with PBC, there are no specific associated serum antibodies. In approximately 65% of patients, however, high titers of perinuclear antineutrophil cytoplasmic antibody (p-ANCA) are demonstrable and anti–smooth muscle antibody (SMA) titer may be increased (8). Approximately 10% of chronic PSC patients develop cholangiocarcinoma.

The etiopathogenesis of PSC is not well understood. Both nonimmune and autoimmune mechanisms are thought to contribute (15). Although PSC and IBD often occur concurrently, they can also occur independently of each other, suggesting that different factors influence their occurrence. Familial cases indicate some genetic predisposition with associated HLA-B8 and DR2 and DR3 haplotypes. In a few cases, PSC and autoimmune hepatitis occur simultaneously, so-called overlap syndrome (28).

Although the diagnosis of PSC can sometimes be established on liver biopsy, definitive diagnosis is most often based on characteristic cholangiographic findings. The biliary tree is distorted with alternating segments of extrahepatic bile duct stenosis and dilatation, imparting a typical and virtually diagnostic "beaded" appearance. Other possible causes of secondary sclerosing cholangitis must be excluded including previous biliary tract surgery or prior instances of cholecystitis and cholelithiasis. They may have similar histopathologic and cholangiographic findings.

Pathology

Early (stage 1) changes (e-Figs. 17.23–17.27) may be inconspicuous and, even when present, not seen in all portions of the liver, with resultant unremarkable biopsies (20). Interlobular bile ducts may show only mild epithelial irregularity with focal atrophy. The hyperplastic epithelial changes seen in PBC are not seen in PSC. Instead, partial lumen obliteration and focal branching of bile ducts occur (Fig. 17.9). Portal tracts have a mild chronic inflammatory cell infiltrate, mostly lymphocytes, confined to the portal tract. Interface hepatitis is unusual. Lymphoid aggregates are seen but without germinal centers. Granulomas are only rarely seen.

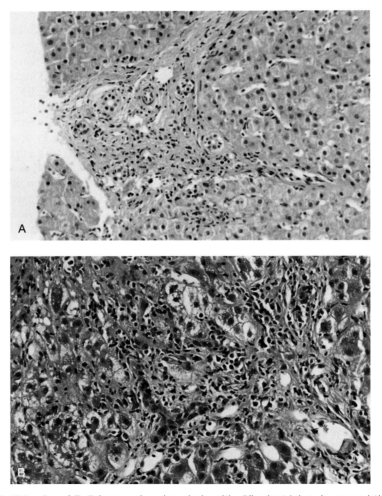

FIGURE 17.9 **A** and **B.** Primary sclerosing cholangitis. Bile duct injury is very subtle, with epithelial atrophy, pleomorphic epithelial nuclei, and early branching of the intrahepatic ducts (hematoxylin-osin, original magnification ×200).

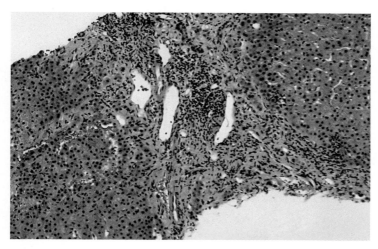

FIGURE 17.10   Primary sclerosing cholangitis. The inflammatory infiltrate in the portal tract is predominantly mononuclear, and only focal interface hepatitis is present (hematoxylin-eosin, original magnification ×200).

Stage 2 PSC (e-Fig. 17.28) is characterized by more extensive inflammatory interface hepatitis, sometimes mimicking chronic hepatitis C or autoimmune hepatitis. Bile ductular proliferation is usual but may be minimal and only focal. Mild fibrosis of the portal tracts may be evident (Fig. 17.10, e-Figs. 17.29–17.33). Parenchymal changes are prognostically more important than bile duct alterations (19) (Fig. 17.11).

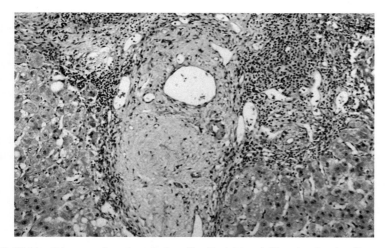

FIGURE 17.11   Primary sclerosing cholangitis. Portal tract fibrosis, slender fibrous septa and "smudgy" fibrous scar, the site of the original interlobular bile duct (hematoxylin-eosin, original magnification ×200).

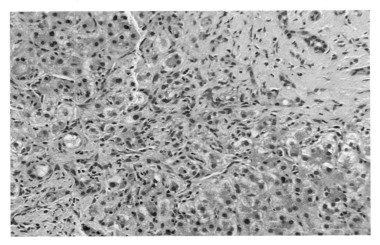

FIGURE 17.12 Primary sclerosing cholangitis (PSC). Focal bile ductular proliferation and periseptal cholestasis and cholate stasis are present, usually in the late stages (stage 3, 4) of PSC (hematoxylin-eosin, original magnification ×200).

Stage 3 PSC has a characteristic, but not pathognomonic, pattern of periductal fibrosis (e-Figs. 17.28–17.31). The "onion skinning" pattern of fibrosis becomes more obvious in later stages but can be present earlier (e-Fig. 17.28). Ultimately, there is bile duct loss and complete replacement of the bile duct with a characteristic fibrous scar, described as "smudgy" (Fig. 17.12 e-Figs. 17.32–17.35). Unfortunately, this is not uniformly distributed and often is not seen in biopsy samples.

At this stage progressive, biliary-type fibrosis is more extensive and portal-to-portal bridging usual (e-Figs. 17.33–17.35). The inflammatory infiltrate is less prominent. With loss of many interlobular bile ducts, portal tracts contain only arteries and portal tributaries. Periportal/periseptal hepatocytes show cholate stasis, similar to that of PBC, with accumulation of copper and copper-binding protein (e-Fig. 17.36) and occasionally Mallory hyalin (e-Fig. 17.37). Despite extensive loss of interlobular bile ducts, there is little bile ductule proliferation. Centrolobular cholestasis is only seen when large bile ducts are affected.

Stage 4 PSC has extensive biliary-type fibrosis imparting the typical picture of biliary-type cirrhosis (e-Fig. 17.38) (11). The advanced stages of PBC and PSC may be indistinguishable, and the correct diagnosis requires clinical information.

PSC can recur after liver transplantation (e-Figs. 17.39, 17.40)

Differential Diagnosis

Secondary (acquired) sclerosing cholangitis can be indistinguishable from PSC. Secondary sclerosing cholangitis was seen in most patients who were treated with intra-arterial infusions of fluorodeoxyuridine for metastatic adenocarcinoma (6). Patients with AIDS can have various bile duct changes, including true cholangiopathy (AIDS cholangiopathy), as well as acalculous cholecystitis and sclerosing cholangitis, sometimes with papillary stenosis. These occur with or without either cryptosporidiosis or cytomegalovirus infection.

In immune deficiency syndromes in children, such as familial combined immunodeficiency and immunodeficiency with hyperimmunoglobulin M, the features of sclerosing cholangitis may be present. Superimposed bacterial/opportunistic infection in these conditions can also cause changes that resemble PSC. GVHD, autoimmune cholangitis, portal vein thrombosis, and Langerhans cell histiocytosis (histiocytosis X) can all cause changes that resemble PSC.

REFERENCES

1. Abdulkarim A, Petrovic L, Kim WR, et al. Primary biliary cirrhosis: an infectious disease caused by *Chlamydia pneumoniae*? J Hepatol 2004;40(3):380–384.
2. Baggenstoss AH, Foulk WT, Butt HR, et al. The pathology of primary biliary cirrhosis with emphasis on histogenesis. Am J Clin Pathol 1964;42:259–276.
3. Ballardini G, Mirakian R, Bianchi FB, et al. Aberrant expression of HLA-DR antigens on bile duct epithelium in primary biliary cirrhosis: relevance to pathogenesis. Lancet 1984; 2:1009–1013.
4. Colina F, Pinedo F, Solis JA, et al. Nodular regenerative hyperplasia of the liver in early histological stages of primary biliary cirrhosis. Gastroenterology 1992;102:1319–1324.
5. Culp KS, Fleming CR, Duffy J, et al. Autoimmune association in primary biliary cirrhosis. Mayo Clin Proc 1982;57:365–370.
6. Demetris AJ, Markus BH, Esquivel C, et al. Pathologic analysis of liver transplantation for primary biliary cirrhosis. Hepatology 1988;8:939–947.
7. Farinati F, Floreans A, DeMaria N, et al. Hepatocellular carcinoma in primary biliary cirrhosis. J Hepatol 1994;21:315–316.
8. Farrant JM, Hayllar KM, Wilkinson ML, et al. Natural history and prognostic variables in primary sclerosing cholangitis. Gastroenterology 1991;100:1710–1717.
9. Gores GJ. Yes, hepatocellular cancer does occur in primary biliary cirrhosis. Liver Transpl 2002;8:570–571.
10. Gores GJ, Moore SB, Fisher LD, et al. Primary biliary cirrhosis: associations with class II major histocompatibility complex antigens. Hepatology 1987;7:889–892.
11. Jeffrey GP, Reed DW, Carrello S, et al. Histological and immunohistochemical study of the gall bladder lesion in primary sclerosing cholangitis. Gut 1991;32:424–429.
12. Jones DE, Palmer JM, Burt AD, et al. Bacterial motif DNA as an adjuvant for the breakdown of immune self-tolerance to pyruvate dehydrogenase complex. Hepatology 2002; 36:679–686.
13. Kaplan MM. Primary biliary cirrhosis: past, present, and future. Gastroenterology 2002; 123:1392–1394.
14. Keefe NA, Gershwin ME. Immunopathogenesis of primary biliary cirrhosis. Semin Liver Dis 2002;22:291–302.
15. Lee TJ, Wanless IR, Tsui FW, et al. Apoptosis of biliary epithelial cells in primary biliary cirrhosis and primary sclerosing cholangitis. Liver 2002;22:228–234.
16. Ludwig J, Dickson ER, McDonald GS. Staging of chronic non-suppurative destructive cholangitis (syndrome of primary biliary cirrhosis). Virchows Arch A Pathol Anat 1978; 379:103–112.

17. Ludwig J. New concepts in biliary cirrhosis. Semin Liver Dis 1987;7:293–301.

18. Mackay IR, Gershwin ME. Primary biliary cirrhosis: considerations on pathogenesis based on identification of the M2 autoantigens. Springer Semin Immunopathol 1990; 12:101–119.

19. Marangoni A, Donati M, Cavrini F, et al. *Chlamydia pneumoniae* replicates in Kupffer cells in mouse model of liver infection. World J Gastroenterol 2006;28:12(40):6453–6457.

20. Markus BH, Dickson ER, Grambsch PM, et al. Efficacy of liver transplantation in patients with primary biliary cirrhosis. N Engl J Med 1989;320:1709–1713.

21. McMahon RF, Babbs C, Warnes TW. Nodular regenerative hyperplasia of the liver, CREST syndrome and primary biliary cirrhosis: an overlap syndrome? Gut 1989;30:1430–1433.

22. Michieletti P, Wanless IR, Katz A, et al. Are patients with antimitochondrial antibody negative primary biliary cirrhosis a distinct syndrome of autoimmune cholangitis? Gut 1994;35:260–265.

23. Portmann B, Popper H, Neuberger J, et al. Sequential and diagnostic features in primary biliary cirrhosis based on serial histologic study in 209 patients. Gastroenterology 1985; 88:1777–1790.

24. Sherlock S, Scheuer PJ. The presentation and diagnosis of 100 patients with primary biliary cirrhosis. Lancet 1987;2:493–496.

25. Shimizu M, Yuh K, Aoyama S, et al. Immunohistochemical characterization of inflammatory infiltrates at the site of bile duct injury in primary biliary cirrhosis. Liver 1986;6:1–6.

26. Singson RC, Fraiman M, Geller SA. Hepatocellular carcinoma with fibrolamellar pattern in a patient with autoimmune cholangitis. Mt Sinai J Med 1999;66:109–112.

27. Wee A, Ludwig J, Coffey RJJ, et al. Hepatobiliary carcinoma associated with primary sclerosing cholangitis and chronic ulcerative colitis. Hum Pathol 1985;16:719–726.

28. Wiesner RH, Grambsch PM, Dickson ER, et al. Primary sclerosing cholangitis: natural history, prognostic factors and survival analysis. Hepatology 1989;10:430–436.

29. Wiesner RH, LaRusso NF, Ludwig J, et al. Comparison of the clinicopathologic features of primary sclerosing cholangitis and primary biliary cirrhosis. Gastroenterology 1985;88: 108–114.

30. Yamada S, Howe S, Scheuer PJ. Three-dimensional reconstruction of biliary pathways in primary biliary cirrhosis: a computer-assisted study. J Pathol 1987;152:317–323.

18

LARGE BILE DUCT DISORDERS

Disorders affecting the large extrahepatic bile ducts are common. Modern biochemical tests and sophisticated imaging techniques often make liver biopsy unnecessary in contrast with past years when large duct obstruction (LDO) was one of the most important indications for liver biopsy.

LARGE DUCT OBSTRUCTION

Acute Large Bile Duct Obstruction

Acute large bile duct obstruction (LDO) often has a dramatic clinical presentation with sudden onset of jaundice and right upper quadrant abdominal pain, generally due to obstruction of the common hepatic duct or the ampulla of Vater.

Histopathologic changes are characteristic but not pathognomonic. They can be seen with obstruction of the right or left hepatic ducts as well as the smaller intrahepatic ducts into which portal tract interlobular ducts drain. When either intrahepatic duct obstruction or obstruction above the point of juncture of the right and left hepatic ducts is suspected, biopsy of tissue from both liver lobes may be useful. Changes will be bilateral with obstructions below the juncture of the right and left hepatic ducts, but will be one-sided when only one is involved or when the obstructed duct is intrahepatic.

Acute LDO is most commonly associated with gallstones and can persist after passage of the gallstone. Any process causing obstruction or stenosis of the bile ducts can lead to similar changes, including neoplasms (13), strictures following surgical procedures (8), and congenital biliary atresia (see Chapter 6), for example. Rare causes include inflammatory bile duct polyps, choledochal cyst or diverticulum, parasites such as *Clonorchis sinensis*, annular pancreas compressing the common duct, and pancreatitis and its complications (7,10,11,16,21,23).

PATHOLOGY. The earliest change, seen as early as 2 or 3 days after onset, is canalicular cholestasis, predominantly in zone 3 of the acinus (Fig. 18.1). The bile is visible as green or brown-green pigment in the form of bile plugs or bile thrombi. In addition, the perivenular (zone 3) area has

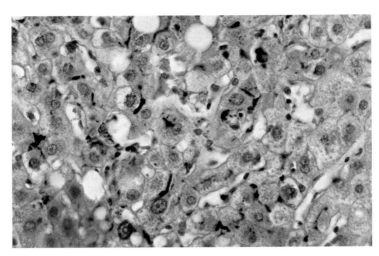

FIGURE 18.1 Acute large bile duct obstruction (early, first couple of days). Centrolobular canalicular cholestasis and mild reactive changes in the hepatocytes (hematoxylin-eosin, original magnification ×200).

prominent, bile-laden Kupffer cells. In resolving acute LDO, the bile plugs disappear first, but pigment-rich Kupffer cells may persist for weeks. Periodic acid–Schiff–positive Kupffer cells may be the only remaining evidence of cholestasis after resolution of the obstruction (23).

In acute LDO, hepatocytes are not primarily damaged. If obstruction and cholestasis persist, however, secondary reactive changes become prominent (4). Cholestasis up-regulates class I human leukocyte antigen expression in hepatocytes leading to focal liver cell injury and necrosis (6). Zone 3 hepatocytes have distended, swollen cytoplasm, and liver cell nuclei vary in size with nuclear hyperchromasia. The cytoplasm of some hepatocytes becomes rarified with fine, weblike reticulation, traditionally recognized, and described as "feathery degeneration" (Fig. 18.2). Individual liver cells may be necrotic (acidophilic bodies). Mitoses are common. Ultrastructurally there is hypertrophy of endoplasmic reticulum.

In the first week after onset of LDO, portal tracts are edematous, with pale, loose connective tissue and early fibroblast proliferation (Fig. 18.3, e-Figs. 18.1–18.4). Interlobular or septal bile ducts can show reactive epithelial changes including irregularity of epithelium, variation in size and nuclear hyperchromasia, and, occasionally, true necrosis. Bile duct epithelium may later become atrophic, particularly once periductal fibrosis is well developed. In spite of this, interlobular bile duct loss is exceedingly rare (Fig. 18.4).

The portal tract inflammatory infiltrate varies. Early, there is little or no inflammatory cell accumulation. When present, lymphoid and histiocytic cells predominate (Fig. 18.4). As LDO persists, the number of polymorphonuclear leukocytes (PMNs) increases in number, usually accompanying

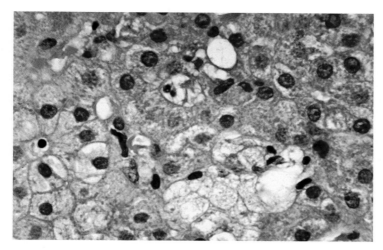

FIGURE 18.2   Large bile duct obstruction (first week). Centrolobular cholestasis and feath-ery degeneration of some hepatocytes (hematoxylin-eosin, original magnification ×200).

so-called marginal bile ductular proliferation. Proliferating bile ductules are themselves chemotactic and nonspecifically stimulate a PMN response in many conditions associated with ductular proliferation.

Marginal bile ductular reaction (proliferation) is a reliable, but not pathognomonic, feature of LDO, seen in more than 80% of portal tracts (e-Fig. 18.4). Although proliferated bile ductules may have a dilated lumen, there is usually no visible bile. When dilated ductules are prominent, sepsis

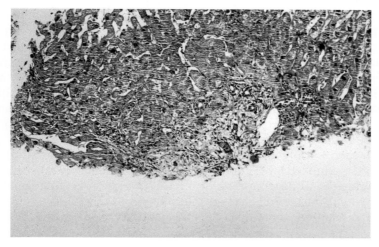

FIGURE 18.3   Acute large bile duct obstruction (early, first 2 to 3 days). Portal tract is edematous and contains only mild predominantly mononuclear inflammatory infiltrate (hematoxylin-eosin, original magnification ×100).

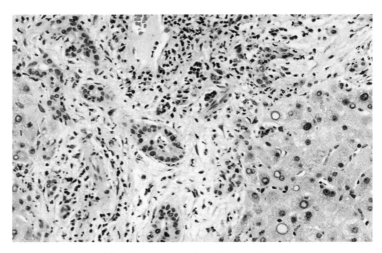

FIGURE 18.4   Acute large bile duct obstruction (first week). Edematous portal tract with inflammatory infiltrate composed of lymphocytes, histiocytes, and polymorphonuclear leukocytes and with associated marginal bile ductular proliferation (hematoxylin-eosin, original magnification ×200).

and septicemia should also be considered (17). Superimposed acute cholangitis with intraluminal PMNs and chronic inflammatory cells focally infiltrating the bile duct epithelium can be seen. Proliferated ductules, especially before a luminal space is apparent, can be highlighted with keratin immunohistochemistry, using CK19 or keratin AE 1,3.

The origin of ductules is controversial. Possibilities include (a) multiplication of pre-existing bile ductules, (b) proliferation from a putative progenitor (stem) cell, and (c) metaplasia of periportal hepatocytes. It may be that they are all active at different stages (9,24,27,29–31). Multiplication of the pre-existing bile ductules seems more important in acute cholestasis, whereas ductular periportal metaplasia is more often associated with chronic cholangiopathies, including primary biliary cirrhosis and primary sclerosing cholangitis. Hepatocytes undergo phenotypic changes with expression of biliary-type cytokeratin, integrins, blood group antigens, and tissue peptide antigen (20,29–31). Cholestatic rosette formation is commonly seen (Fig. 18.5).

Periportal bile lakes or bile infarcts are the hallmark of LDO, although seen in only a small percentage of patients. Bile within the bile lake is often admixed with fibrin. Hepatocytes immediately adjacent show variable degrees of degeneration and lytic-type necrosis. Bile can escape from bile ducts into portal tracts as bile extravasation with local histiocytic phagocytic reaction, sometimes causing giant cell reaction (Fig. 18.6).

Long-Standing Large Duct Obstruction

The clinical diagnosis of long-standing LDO obstruction is rarely problematic.

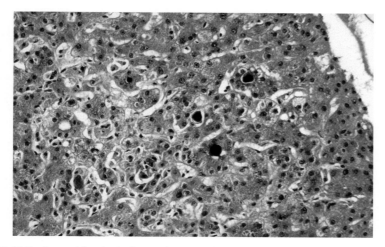

FIGURE 18.5   Large bile duct obstruction. In addition to reactive changes and feathery degeneration, occasional cholestatic rosettes are formed (hematoxylin-eosin, original magnification ×400).

PATHOLOGY. In long-standing LDO, lasting weeks to months, fibrosis gradually replaces the portal inflammatory infiltrate. A characteristic pattern of periductal, concentric fibrosis, similar to that of primary sclerosing cholangitis, develops (Figs. 18.7, 18.8). Portal-to-portal fibrous bridging ensues, and secondary biliary cirrhosis eventually develops. Liver cell injury is not prominent, and fibrous septa are highly irregular. The nodules that

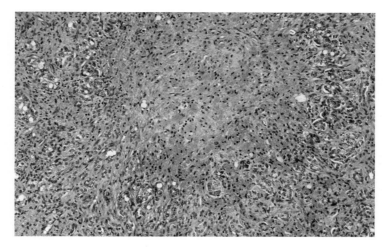

FIGURE 18.6   Large bile duct obstruction. Bile infarct formation is pathognomonic of bile duct obstruction (hematoxylin-eosin, original magnification ×200).

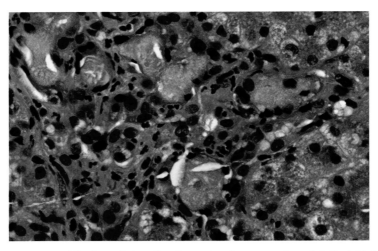

FIGURE 18.7 Large bile duct obstruction (long-standing, several weeks). Portal inflammation and fibrosis and bile ductular proliferation (hematoxylin-eosin, original magnification ×400).

form are not circular as are typical regenerative nodules of cirrhosis following hepatitis and have a geographic or jigsaw-puzzle appearance (e-Figs. 18.5, 18.6) (5,7,8). In the absence of portal-to-central shunting and true regenerative nodules, secondary biliary cirrhosis is not a true cirrhosis and initially manifests as portal hypertension without hepatocellular dysfunction (see Chapter 20). Cholestasis has an inhibitory effect on liver cell regeneration by

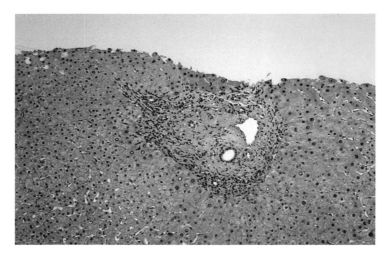

FIGURE 18.8 Large bile duct obstruction (long-standing, at least several weeks). Periductal concentric fibrosis. Only reactive epithelial changes are present in the bile duct (hematoxylin-eosin, original magnification ×200).

interfering with expression of growth-promoting genes (4,28). The term *biliary fibrosis* is more appropriate than biliary cirrhosis in these cases.

Other parenchymal changes can be seen with long-standing cholestasis secondary to LDO. Feathery degeneration (Fig. 18.2), and cholestatic rosettes (Fig. 18.5), representing a circular arrangement of hepatocytes around a central bile plug, may be seen. Antibody directed against cytokeratin CAM 5.2 will highlight these tubule-like structures. Clusters of foamy (xanthomatous) cells are seen. Perpiportal or paraseptal hepatocytes are pale and rarified (cholate stasis). These hepatocytes often have increased copper-associated protein, demonstrated with Victoria blue or orcein (Shikata) stain (14,25,26). Mallory hyalin can be present (Fig. 18.9), but, unlike in alcoholic liver disease, the intracytoplasmic hyalin is almost invariably periportal or paraseptal and not distributed throughout the lobule (see Chapter 13). Portal and periportal fibrosis develops (e-Figs. 18.7–18.9). Fibrous septa are usually regular, broad, and paucicellular, with loosely arranged collagen fibers.

The changes of acute LDO are entirely reversible. When LDO is eliminated, the inflammatory and reactive changes and the cholestasis resolve within a few weeks. However, the reversibility of established fibrosis is somewhat controversial (1,5). Extensive fibrosis of established secondary biliary cirrhosis is probably irreversible, but there have been reports of resolution of biliary cirrhosis in children (32).

Cholangitis Associated with Bile Duct Obstruction

PMNs accompany bile ductular proliferation following prolonged LDO in the connective tissue (acute pericholangitis). True acute ascending

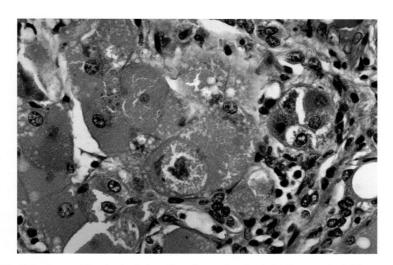

FIGURE 18.9 Large bile duct obstruction (long-standing). Mallory material is present in some periportal hepatocytes with swollen cytoplasm (hematoxylin-eosin, original magnification ×400).

cholangitis, rare with modern antibiotic therapy, should be diagnosed only when numerous PMNs fill the bile duct lumen. In ascending cholangitis there may also be suppurative necrosis of the bile duct epithelium and eventual abscess formation.

Differential Diagnosis of Intrahepatic Cholestasis

Cholestasis is the presence of visible bile in liver tissue and can be canalicular (intracanalicular), intracellular (intrahepatocytic) or can involve ducts and/or ductules.

Canalicular (intracanalicular) cholestasis is the most frequently observed form of acute cholestasis. In LDO, canalicular cholestasis is seen within a few days of onset. Green or green-yellow bile plugs are in dilated canaliculi, particularly in zone 3. Histochemical stains can be used to demonstrate bile, but canalicular cholestasis is generally easily recognized with hematoxylin-eosin. In prolonged cholestasis, the cytoplasm of liver cells also contains bile pigment (intracytoplasmic cholestasis). With excessive accumulation of bile, liver cells form tubular, glandlike structures (cholestatic liver cell rosettes) (19).

Canalicular cholestasis is not pathognomonic for LDO and can be seen in other conditions, including acute hepatitis, whether viral or drug-induced, preservation (harvesting) injury in liver transplantation patients, and "pure" cholestatic syndromes associated with oral contraceptives, benign recurrent cholestasis, pregnancy, sepsis, and some malignancies including Hodgkin disease and other lymphoproliferative disorders. Several drugs can also cause a pure cholestatic jaundice in the absence of other morphologic changes (15).

Chronic cholestasis is often associated with long-standing chronic biliary diseases. Even in the absence of bile in the canaliculi and hepatocytes, cytoplasmic changes develop secondary to compromised bile flow, so-called cholate stasis (22). The term and the concept of cholate stasis are not universally accepted, despite the constellation of changes that are easily recognized, including swelling and rarefaction of the hepatocytes in periportal or paraseptal areas. These swollen cells contain a variable amount of finely granular copper-associated protein within autophagic vacuoles, demonstrated with Victoria blue or orcein stains (14,25,26). There may also be excessive metallic copper, stainable with rubeanic acid or rhodamine methods. Hepatocytes can contain Mallory hyaline–like material (12).

Cholate stasis is seen as a pale rim of hepatocytes at the periphery of the nodule. There is usually associated ductular proliferation.

Ductal and, when present, ductular cholestasis are commonly seen in sepsis, as well as in acute pancreatitis, and can follow ischemic cholangitis in the early posttransplantation period. In congenital hepatic fibrosis and bile duct hamartomas, larger bile duct–like structures can contain bile in their lumen in the absence of obstructive changes, hepatitis, or other causes of cholestasis.

Intrahepatic Cholestasis

The list of conditions contributing to intrahepatic cholestasis is extensive and includes congenital and inherited syndromes as well as various acquired disorders (see Chapter 26) (8,18).

REFERENCES

1. Abdel-Aziz G, Lebeau G, Rescan PY, et al. Reversibility of hepatic fibrosis in experimentally induced cholestasis in rat. Am J Pathol 1990;137:1333–1342.
2. Afroudakis A, Kaplowitz N. Liver histopathology in chronic common bile duct stenosis due to chronic alcoholic pancreatitis. Hepatology 1981;1:65–72.
3. Bouche H, Housset C, Dumont J-L, et al. AIDS-related cholangitis. Diagnostic features and course in 15 patients. J Hepatol 1993;17:34–39.
4. Bucher NLR, Robinson GS, Farmer SR. Effects of extracellular matrix on hepatocyte growth and gene expression: implication for hepatic regeneration and repair of liver injury. Semin Liver Dis 1990;10:11–19.
5. Bunton GL, Cameron R. Regeneration of liver after biliary cirrhosis. Ann N Y Acad Sci 1963;111:412–421.
6. Calmus Y, Arvieux C, Gane P, et al. Cholestasis induces major histocompatibility class I expression in hepatocytes. Gastroenterology 1992;102:1371–1377.
7. Desmet VJ. Cholestasis: extrahepatic obstruction and secondary biliary cirrhosis. In: MacSween RNM, Anthony PP, Scheuer PJ, et al., eds. Pathology of the Liver. 3rd Ed. Edinburgh: Churchill Livingstone, 1994:425–477.
8. Desmet VJ, Callea F. Cholestatic syndromes of infancy and childhood. In: Zakim D, Boyer TD, eds. Hepatology. A Textbook of Liver Disease, vol 2, 2nd Ed. Philadelphia: WB Saunders, 1990:1355–1395.
9. De Vos R, Desmet V. Ultrastructural characteristics of novel epithelial cell types identified in human pathologic liver specimens with chronic ductular reaction. Am J Pathol 1992;6:1441–1450.
10. Ecktein RP, Bambach CP, Stiel D, et al. Fibrolamellar carcinoma as a cause of bile duct obstruction. Pathology 1988;20:326–331.
11. Flinn WR, Olson DF, Oyasu R, et al. Biliary bacteria and hepatic histopathologic changes in gallstone disease. Ann Surg 1977;185:593–597.
12. Gerber MA, Orr W, Denk H, et al. Hepatocellular hyaline in cholestasis and cirrhosis: its diagnostic significance. Gastroenterology 1973;64:89–98.
13. Gerber MA, Thung SN, Bodenheimer HC Jr, et al. Characteristic histologic triad in liver adjacent to metastatic neoplasm. Liver 1986;6:85–88.
14. Gurasciao P, Yentis F, Cevikbas U, et al. Value of copper-associated protein in diagnostic assessment of liver biopsy. J Clin Pathol 1983;36:18–23.
15. Herrmann G, Lorenz M, Kirkowa-Reimann, et al. Morphological changes after intra-arterial chemotherapy of the liver. Hepatogastroenterology 1987;34:5–9.
16. Lee KC, Sakai K, Kinoshita H, et al. Resection of hepatocellular carcinoma with obstructive jaundice caused by compression of the common hepatic duct. J Surg Oncol 1988;39:201–205.
17. Lefkowitch JH. Bile ductular cholestasis: an ominous histopathologic sign related to sepsis and "cholangitis lenta". Hum Pathol 1982;13:19–24.
18. Ludwig J, Kim CH, Wiesner RH, et al. Floxuridine-induced sclerosing cholangitis: an ischemic cholangiopathy? Hepatology 1989;9:215–218.
19. Nagore N, Howe S, Scheuer PJ. Liver cell rosettes: structural differences in cholestasis and hepatitis. Liver 1989;9:43–51.

20. Nakanuma Y, Sasaki M. Expression of blood group-related antigens in the intrahepatic biliary tree and hepatocytes in normal livers and various hepatobiliary diseases. Hepatology 1989;10:174–178.

21. Pol S, Romana CA, Richard S, et al. Microsporidia infection in patients with the human immunodeficiency virus and unexplained cholangitis. N Engl J Med 1993;328:95–99.

22. Popper H. Morphological and immunological studies on chronic aggressive hepatitis and primary biliary cirrhosis. In: Smith M, Williams R, eds. Immunology of the Liver. London: Heinemann, 1971:17–27.

23. Scheuer PJ, Lefkowitch J. Biliary Disease. In: Liver Biopsy Interpretation. 5th Ed. London: WB Saunders, 1994.

24. Sell S. Is there a liver stem cell? Cancer Res 1990;50:3811–3815.

25. Sipponen P. Orcein positive hepatocellular material in long-standing biliary diseases. 1. Histochemical characteristics. Scand J Gastroenterol 1976;11:545–552.

26. Sipponen P. Orcein positive hepatocellular material in long-standing biliary diseases. II. Ultrastructural studies. Scand J Gastroenterol 1976;11:553–557.

27. Slott PA, Liu MH, Tavoloni N. Origin, pattern and mechanism of bile duct proliferation following biliary obstruction in the rat. Gastroenterology 1990;99:466–477.

28. Tracy TF Jr, Bailey PV, Goerke ME, et al. Cholestasis without cirrhosis alters regulatory liver gene expression and inhibits hepatic regeneration. Surgery 1991;34:280–289.

29. Van Eyken P, Desmet VJ. Development of intrahepatic bile ducts, ductular metaplasia of hepatocytes, and cytokeratin patterns in various types of human hepatic neoplasms. In: Sirica AE, ed. The Role of Cell Types in Hepatocarcinogenesis. Boca Raton: CRC Press, 1992:227–263.

30. Van Eyken P, Sciot R, Desmet VJ. A cytokeratin immunohistochemical study of cholestatic liver disease: evidence that hepatocytes can express 'bile duct-type' cytokeratins. Histopathology 1989;15:125–135.

31. Volpes R, Van den Oord JJ, Desmet VJ. Distribution of the VLA family of integrins in normal and pathological human liver tissue. Gastroenterology 1991;101:200–206.

32. Yeong ML, Nicholson GI, Lee SP. Regression of biliary cirrhosis following choledochal cyst drainage. Gastroenterology 1988;10:332–335.

19

VASCULAR DISORDERS

Some conditions affecting the hepatic vasculature are extrahepatic, such as congestive heart failure and systemic hypotension. Abnormalities of the vascular system can also be seen in the liver biopsy; examples are Budd-Chiari syndrome and venoocclusive disease (VOD), as well as peliosis hepatis and endothelialitis of liver allograft rejection (Table 19.1).

HEPATIC ARTERY

The hepatic artery rarely is a cause of clinical or morphologic liver disease, since the major blood flow to the liver is via the portal vein. Ischemic liver disease based on the hepatic artery is often a function of decreased hepatic artery blood flow rather than reduction of lumen size, as in heart failure.

Atherosclerosis

Atherosclerosis affects the hepatic artery just as it does the rest of the arterial system, and atherosclerotic changes of the hepatic artery branches can sometimes be observed in portal tracts in liver biopsies (e-Fig. 19.1); atherosclerotic liver disease, however, in and of itself, does not occur. The liver is remarkably resistant to anoxia. Significant hepatic artery atherosclerosis will not affect the liver unless the portal or hepatic vein system is compromised.

Hepatic Ischemia

With hepatic ischemia, biochemical changes suggest hepatitis, with significant and rapid elevations in the serum aminotransferase values (20). Ischemic hepatitis occurs with myocardial infarction, cardiac arrhythmias, or hypotension. The morphologic features are characteristic and virtually diagnostic, consisting of zone 3 (centrolobular) hepatocytic coagulative necrosis (5,54). A relatively sharp demarcation can be seen (Fig. 19.1, e-Fig. 19.2). Nuclear pyknosis, karyorrhexis, and eosinophilic necrosis occurs, usually with sparing of sinusoidal cells. With severe and prolonged ischemia, zone 2 can also be involved (14). However, it should be remembered that both zone 2 and zone 3 arc from the portal tracts (see Chapter 2). Necrosis in the midportion of the limiting plate, at the interface between the portal

TABLE 19.1	Vascular Disorders of the Liver in Terms of Their Localization in the Liver Biopsy

Hepatic artery
  Atherosclerosis
  Ischemic hepatitis
  Hepatic artery thrombosis or ligation
  Hepatic infarction
  Vasculitis
  Amyloidosis
  Hepatic allograft rejection
Portal vein
  Portal vein thrombosis
    Prehepatic
    Intrahepatic
  Pyelophlebitis
  Hepatoportal sclerosis
  Hepatic allograft rejection
  Zahn infarct
  Nodular hyperplasia and cirrhosis
  Hereditary hemorrhagic telangiectasia (Osler-Weber-Rendu syndrome)
Sinusoids
  Sinusoidal dilatation
    Pregnancy/contraceptive pill related
    Hodgkin disease
    Space-occupying lesion
    AIDS
  Peliosis hepatis
  Sinusoidal thrombosis
  Amyloidosis and light chain disease
  Terminal hepatic venules (central veins)
  Right heart failure (congestive heart failure)
  Systemic hypotension (shock liver)
  Ischemic hepatitis
  Hepatic venous outflow obstruction
    Budd–Chiari syndrome
    Venoocclusive disease

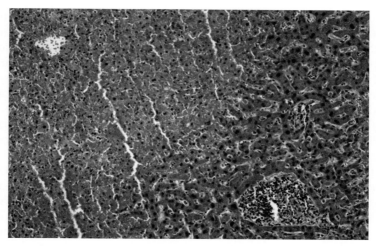

FIGURE 19.1   Zone 3 (centrolobular) ischemic necrosis in a chronically ill patient with intermittent hypotension in whom biopsy was performed to exclude the possibility of concurrent viral hepatitis. There is a relatively sharp line of demarcation between the ischemic zone and the viable zone 2 (hematoxylin-eosin, original magnification ×200).

tract and the hepatocytes, is common as a reflection of predominantly zone 3 necrosis and is not necessarily representative of diffuse hepatic necrosis (Fig. 19.2).

Phagocytosed cell material in Kupffer cells can be demonstrated after a few days with diastase–periodic acid–Schiff (dPAS) reaction. Other changes

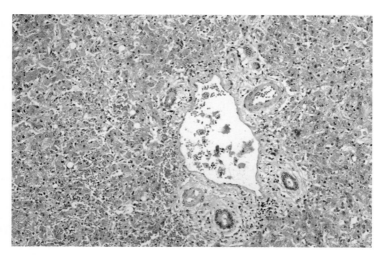

FIGURE 19.2   Ischemic necrosis in a patient with cardiogenic shock showing involvement of the central, zone 3 portion of the limiting plate (hematoxylin-eosin, original magnification ×200).

include canalicular cholestasis adjacent to the necrosis, and eosinophilic hyaline globules, resembling those of α1-antitrypsin deficiency (32) as well as mild steatosis and early regenerative changes. With right-sided heart failure, sinusoids are dilated and congested. Uncommonly, a picture similar to that of hepatic vein obstruction (Budd–Chiari), with red blood cells filling the liver cord in place of the removed hepatocytes, is seen and the biopsy-derived diagnosis may be misleading. In patients who recover, the histologic structure is restored. Sometimes perivenular fibrosis remains, particularly with recurrent or prolonged heart failure, and there may be associated calcification.

Hepatic artery thrombosis, involving the extrahepatic portion of the hepatic artery, can occur after trauma, including that related to surgery and catheterization. Rarely, arteritis, embolization or tumor invasion occurs. Trauma can also lead to hepatic artery aneurysm. Infusion of chemotherapeutic agents can also cause hepatic artery thrombosis. Oral contraceptives have also been implicated as causal, with intrahepatic arterial branch intimal hyperplasia (43).

Intrahepatic thrombi can be seen in association with disseminated intravascular coagulopathy (DIC) or thrombotic thrombocytopenic purpura (TTP). Patients with these conditions, and indeed most thrombotic disorders, however, are rarely, if ever, subject to liver biopsy.

Hepatic Infarction

Hepatic infarction is uncommon and exceedingly rare in liver biopsy samples (23,52). Extensive coagulative necrosis affects one or more lobules (e-Fig. 19.2).

Vasculitis

The systemic arteritides, including periarteritis nodosa (e-Fig. 19.3), systemic lupus erythematosus (53), rheumatoid arthritis, and others, as well as drug-induced vasculitis, can potentially, but rarely, affect the liver (19,65). Liver biopsy helps identify concurrent or complicating conditions. A form of vasculitis affecting the portal vein and its tributaries is characteristic of acute allograft rejection and is discussed in Chapter 25.

Amyloidosis

Amyloidosis is discussed in Chapter 21.

PORTAL VEIN

Luminal obstruction is the basis of most portal vein disorders, occurring at any level of the portal vein system. Consequences depend on site and extent. With an intact hepatic artery system, portal vein obstruction may not have significant clinical or morphologic manifestations. Instead, prehepatic portal vein obstruction with portal hypertension may ensue.

Prehepatic Portal Vein Obstruction

The effects on the liver are variable and often minor (12). There are no consistent liver biopsy patterns (25). Indeed, the liver may not show any changes with portal vein compromise. In elderly patients, however, with advanced atherosclerosis, hepatic ischemia, particularly affecting zone 3, will be seen after portal vein thrombosis. Similarly, associated heart failure or mechanical hepatic vein obstruction causes zone 3 necrosis. Prehepatic portal vein obstruction can be (a) congenital; (b) caused by intra-abdominal inflammatory disorders causing pylephlebitis (27); (c) seen with hypercoagulable states; (d) hormone related, including pregnancy and oral contraceptive pill usage; (e) associated with myeloproliferative disorders (50,62); (f) after trauma, including surgery; (g) with cirrhosis; (h) with neoplasm, particularly hepatocellular carcinoma; (i) from mass compression effect, generally from tumors; and (j) as a sequel to hepatic vein outflow obstruction (7).

Intrahepatic Portal Vein Obstruction

Intrahepatic portal vein obstruction may be associated with the same long list of conditions as prehepatic portal vein obstruction. In addition, intrahepatic portal vein obstruction can follow intrahepatic abscess formation, sarcoidosis, schistosomiasis, and other less common conditions. Often, the cause cannot be established. The clinical diagnosis may be quite difficult to establish, and venous flow studies may be required (6).

Thrombi are seen in portal vein tributaries. Because of the irregular distribution of changes, biopsy is often not helpful. Septic thrombi occur with acute pylephlebitis. Nodular hyperplasia can follow occlusion of intrahepatic portal vein branches and may be seen in the liver biopsy without evidence of the causative thrombus (41,53,54,61) (see Chapter 4). Inflammatory change of the intrahepatic portal vein, as seen in acute allograft rejection and graft versus host disease, is generally not associated with thrombosis (38).

Hepatoportal Sclerosis

Hepatoportal sclerosis is a rare and distinct clinicopathologic entity characterized by sclerosis of the intrahepatic portal veins that causes noncirrhotic portal hypertension (23,33,37) (see Chapter 20).

The intrahepatic portal venous system can have degrees of fibrosis and occlusion, leading to presinusoidal obstruction. The fibrosis can also affect the prehepatic portal vein, which generally does not become completely occluded (43). The changes are irregularly distributed and vary from mild intimal thickening to complete occlusion, with or without thrombus formation. Some portal vein sclerosis is seen with aging.

Zahn Infarcts

Zahn infarcts are best recognized macroscopically and typically in autopsy material, as a sequel to a space-occupying lesion, most often metastatic carcinoma. Mild to moderate liver cell plate atrophy with associated sinu-soidal dilatation is seen, without necrosis (22). This is only rarely seen in liver biopsy material (e-Fig. 19.4).

Hereditary Hemorrhagic Telangiectasia (Osler-Weber-Rendu Disease)

This autosomal dominant condition rarely affects the liver, with clinical liver disease uncommon (34). Dilated vascular channels in the portal tract and periportal region are seen (e-Fig. 19.5). There may be varying degrees of portal and periportal fibrosis, and fibrous septa can form, usually with-out regenerative nodules.

SINUSOIDS

Sinusoidal Dilatation

Sinusoidal dilatation occurs with or without accompanying liver plate atrophy, in various conditions. Most often zone 3 (centrolobular) conges-tion is seen (Fig. 19.3). This is typical in venous outflow obstruction, whether it is a result of congestive heart failure (e-Fig. 19.6), Budd–Chiari syndrome, or venoocclusive disease. Drugs can also cause zone 3 sinu-soidal dilatation; it is not uncommon in transplant patients treated with azathioprine. Zone 2 (midzonal) sinusoidal dilatation has been docu-mented as a paraneoplastic phenomenon (1).

Zone 1 (periportal) sinusoidal dilatation can be seen with long-term oral contraceptive pill usage (4,65). It is characteristic of eclampsia and

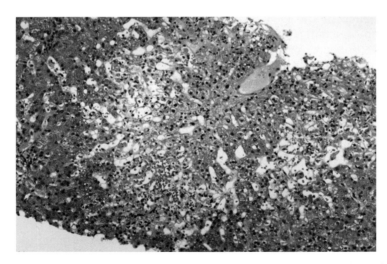

FIGURE 19.3 Zone 3 (centrolobular) congestion in a patient with congestive heart failure in whom serum aminotransferase values were elevated. Zone 3 sinusoids are dilated, and the terminal hepatic venule (central vein) is filled with blood (hematoxylin-eosin, original magni-fication ×200).

preeclampsia (12,47) in which sinusoidal fibrin thrombi (2) and ischemic necrosis may also be seen, and also typical of DIC (55).

Sinusoidal dilatation, generally irregularly distributed, has been seen after exposure to agents that also cause hepatic angiosarcoma, such as arsenic, vinyl chloride, and thorium dioxide (Thorotrast), and can also be seen in the vicinity of a space-occupying lesion (e-Fig. 19.7). The liver biopsy in acquired immunodeficiency syndrome can also show irregular sinusoidal dilatation. In pregnancy the sinusoidal dilatation may be predominantly periportal (17).

Sinusoidal dilatation is typically seen in sickle cell disease, in which the sinusoids are packed with the characteristic sickled erythrocytes (e-Fig. 19.8) (38,44). There is also marked enlargement of Kupffer cells, with siderosis and erythrophagocytosis. In Hodgkin lymphoma, sinusoidal dilatation may be prominent, although not diagnostic (8,9).

Peliosis Hepatis

The sinusoids are dilated and transformed into cystlike, blood-filled spaces (e-Figs. 19.9, 19.10) (60,64). Peliosis hepatis was first recognized in association with chronic debilitating conditions such as tuberculosis and malignancy. Many medications have been implicated, including oral contraceptives, anabolic steroids (3), corticosteroids, tamoxifen, danazol, azathioprine, as well as arsenic, vinyl chloride, and thorium dioxide (29,39,65,66). Peliosis can be scattered throughout the liver, and there is often nonpeliotic sinusoidal dilatation associated, with communications between the sinusoidal dilatation and the peliosis demonstrable. Bacillary angiomatosis strongly resembles peliosis hepatis (58).

Sinusoidal Thrombosis

Fibrin thrombi may form in sinusoids in DIC, in sickle cell disease, and in eclampsia (48).

Outflow Venous Disease

TERMINAL HEPATIC VENULES (CENTRAL VEINS)

Right Heart Failure

The hallmark of acute congestive heart failure is zone 3 (centrolobular) sinusoidal dilatation and congestion (e-Fig. 19.6) (15). Hepatocyte necrosis generally does not occur unless there is coincident left heart failure with systemic hypotension. With sustained heart failure, liver cell atrophy ensues and the Disse space becomes easily seen. In long-standing disease, zone 3 perivenular fibrosis develops with eventual linking of central areas by vascular fibrous septa (cardiac cirrhosis) (e-Fig. 19.11). True cirrhosis, with regenerative nodules and central-portal as well as central-central septa (see Chapter 20), is now uncommon. The terminal hepatic venules have thickened fibrotic walls and may show complete luminal obliteration (42).

Left Heart Failure and Systemic Hypotension

The hallmark of systemic hypotension (shock) is zone 3 (centrolobular) necrosis, which, if prolonged or severe, can involve zone 2 (e-Fig. 19.2) (5,30). Portal tracts and zone 1 hepatocytes usually are unremarkable, and there is usually little or no inflammation at first, with accumulations of polymorphonuclear leukocytes after a few days. There may be cholestasis.

Hepatic Venous Outflow Obstruction

Venous outflow may be impeded by congestive heart failure and primary and secondary neoplasms affecting the right heart. This section will concentrate on disorders of the hepatic vein and hepatic vein branches that contribute to impaired hepatic venous outflow.

BUDD–CHIARI SYNDROME. Budd–Chiari syndrome is a distinctive clinico-pathologic entity characterized by narrowing or occlusion of the hepatic veins (16,32,35,45) as a result of thrombus formation or nonthrombotic causes. Budd–Chiari is associated with (a) myeloproliferative disorders, such as polycythemia vera (63,64); (b) disorders of coagulation, including protein C deficiency; (c) several medications, including oral contraceptives (31); (d) pregnancy (26); and (e) neoplasms, either from direct invasion, as occurs with hepatocellular carcinoma, renal cell carcinoma, and adrenal cortical carcinoma, or from external compression. Uncommonly fibrous webs or membranes obstruct the hepatic vein (21,24). Uncommon causes include trauma, connective tissue disorders, and the use of cancer chemotherapeutic agents, as well as conditions affecting the heart primarily, such as constrictive pericarditis (59).

The classic clinical triad is of hepatomegaly, right upper quadrant abdominal pain, and ascites, with an insidious onset that may take many months to fully develop. Rarely, the onset may be acute (46).

Pathology. Variable changes can be seen (e-Figs. 19.12–19.23). Zone 3 sinusoidal congestion and dilatation may be the only finding in early Budd–Chiari (Fig. 19.4). Sometimes red blood cells appear to have replaced zone 1 hepatocytes within the liver cord (Fig. 19.4). Zone 3 hepatocytes then begin to atrophy (Fig. 19.5). With more severe and prolonged obstruction, hepatocytes may disappear completely with no inflammatory response. Occasionally true ischemic necrosis is seen. Thrombi can be seen in terminal hepatic venules, and, ultimately, there may be fibrous obliteration. Changes are not uniform throughout the liver, and areas of more severe and advanced change can alternate with relatively mildly affected regions.

After many weeks the centrolobular regions become fibrotic and central-central septa form. Fibrous obliteration of terminal hepatic venules, indistinguishable from the changes of VOD, can be seen. Liver plates can be thickened, and there may be associated nodular hyperplasia. True cirrhosis is rare and may be related to secondary thrombosis of the portal vein. It may be

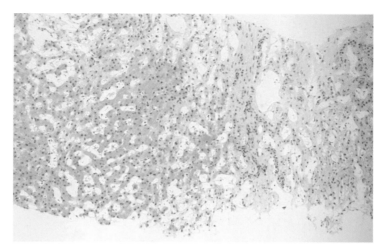

FIGURE 19.4   Budd–Chiari syndrome, early stage, showing zone 3 sinusoidal dilatation and early necrosis with red blood cells in liver cords (hematoxylin-eosin, original magnification ×200).

exceedingly difficult, solely on the basis of a single liver biopsy, to distinguish early Budd–Chiari syndrome from other causes of hepatic venous outflow obstruction.

VENOOCLUSIVE DISEASE. Budd–Chiari involves hepatic vein segments between the liver and the inferior vena cava. VOD, in contrast, affects smaller, intrahepatic portions of the hepatic vein system and the terminal hepatic venules (Fig. 19.6). The veins are occluded by fibrous tissue (e-Figs. 19.24–19.28) (49). This can be identified in biopsy samples, although

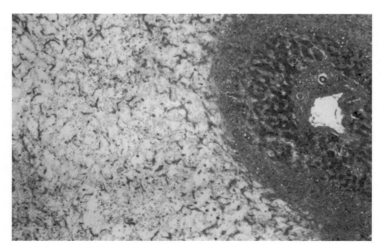

FIGURE 19.5   Budd–Chiari syndrome, late stage, showing atrophy of zone 2 and 3 hepatocytes (hematoxylin-eosin, original magnification ×100).

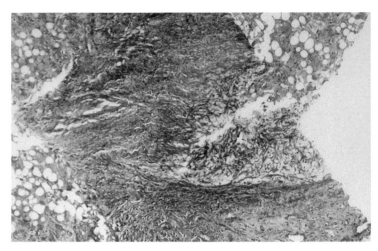

FIGURE 19.6   Venoocclusive disease, showing complete obliteration of hepatic vein lumen (trichrome, original magnification ×200).

it is generally not uniformly distributed throughout the liver and any one biopsy may not be helpful.

VOD is caused by (a) ingestion of pyrrolizidine alkaloids, which can be found in various herbal remedies; (b) several chemotherapeutic agents, including azathioprine and 6-mercaptopurine (4); (c) alkylating agents, particularly in bone marrow transplantation (36,56,57,64); (d) hepatic radiation (51); (e) hypervitaminosis A; (f) arsenic (28); and (g) thorium dioxide (13).

Pathology. Terminal hepatic venules show proliferation of loose connective tissue in the subintima leading to luminal narrowing (18). Connective tissue stains are particularly helpful. Surrounding liver shows changes of acute venous outflow obstruction, similar to Budd–Chiari syndrome and right heart failure, with congestion of zone 3 sinusoids and atrophy of hepatocytes. Thrombi are generally not seen, and inflammation is not prominent.

The subintimal lesions eventually become fibrotic, and perivenular fibrosis and central-central septa formation follow. Nodular hyperplasia and true regenerative nodules can occur, and cirrhosis may be the end result.

Fibrous obliteration of terminal hepatic venules can also be seen in alcoholic liver injury (10,11,40) (see Chapter 13) and in cirrhosis from almost any cause. The diagnosis of VOD should be based on both the vein changes and the histologic appearance of the zone 3 hepatocytes and sinusoids, as well as appropriate clinical factors.

REFERENCES

1. Aoyagi T, Mori I, Ueyma Y, et al. Sinusoidal dilatation of the liver as a paraneoplastic manifestation of renal cell carcinoma. Hum Pathol 1989;20:1193–1197.

2. Arias F, Mancilla-Jiminez R. Hepatic fibrinogen deposits in pre-eclampsia. N Engl J Med 1976;295:578–582.

3. Bagheri SA, Boyer JL. Peliosis hepatis associated with androgenic-anabolic steroid therapy. A severe form of hepatic injury. Ann Intern Med 1974;81:610–618.

4. Balás M. Sinusoidal dilatation of the liver in patients on oral contraceptives: electron microscopic study of 14 cases. Exp Pathol 1988;35:231–237.

5. Birgens HS, Henriksen J, Marzen P, et al. The shock liver. Clinical and biochemical findings in patients with centrolobular liver necrosis following cardiogenic shock. Acta Med Scand 1978;204:417–421.

6. Boyer JL, Hales MR, Klatskin G. "Idiopathic" portal hypertension due to occlusion of intrahepatic portal veins by organized thrombi. Medicine 1974;53:77–91.

7. Brown KM, Kaplan MM, Donowitz M. Extrahepatic portal venous thrombosis: frequent recognition of associated diseases. J Clin Gastroenterol 1985;7:153–159.

8. Bruguera M, Aranguibel F, Ros E, et al. Incidence and clinical significance of sinusoidal dilatation in liver biopsies. Gastroenterology 1978;75:474–478.

9. Bruguera M, Caballero T, Carreras E, et al. Hepatic sinusoidal dilatation in Hodgkin's disease. Liver 1987;7:76–80.

10. Burt AD, MacSween RNM. Hepatic vein lesions in alcoholic liver diseases: retrospective biopsy and necropsy study. J Clin Pathol 1986;39:63–67.

11. Caulet S, Fabre M, Schoevart D, et al. Quantitative study of centrolobular hepatic fibrosis in alcoholic disease before cirrhosis. Virchows Arch A Pathol Anat Histopathol 1989; 416:11–17.

12. Cohen J, Edelman RR, Chopra S. Portal vein thrombosis: a review. Am J Med 1992;92: 173–182.

13. Dejgaard A, Krogsgaard K, Jacobsen M. Veno-occlusive disease and peliosis of the liver after thorotrast administration. Virchows Arch A Pathol Anat Histopathol 1984;403: 87–94.

14. de la Monte S, Arcidi JM, Moore GW, et al. Midzonal necrosis as a pattern of hepatocellular injury after shock. Gastroenterology 1984;86:627–631.

15. Dunn GD, Hayes P, Breen KJ, et al. The liver in congestive heart failure: a review. Am J Med Sci 1973;265:174–189.

16. Farah S, Uthman S, Abyad A. Budd–Chiari syndrome: a review of ten cases. J Intern Med Res 1997;25:171–174.

17. Fisher MR, Neiman HL. Periportal sinusoidal dilatation associated with pregnancy. Cardiovasc Int Radiol 1984;7:299–302.

18. Goodman ZD, Ishak KG. Occlusive venous lesions in alcoholic liver disease. A study of 200 cases. Gastroenterology 1982;83:786–796.

19. Goritsas CP, Repanti M, Papadaki E, et al. Intrahepatic bile duct injury and nodular regenerative hyperplasia of the liver in a patient with polyarteritis nodosa. J Hepatol 1997;26:727–730.

20. Henrion J, Schapira M, Heller FR. Ischemic hepatitis: the need for precise criteria. J Clin Gastroenterol 1996;23:305.

21. Hoffman HD, Stockland B, von der Heyden U. Membranous obstruction of the inferior vena cava with Budd–Chiari syndrome in children: a report of nine cases. J Pediatr Gastroenterol Nutr 1987;6:878–881.

22. Horrocks P, Tapp E. Zahn's "infarcts" of the liver. J Clin Pathol 1966;19:475–478.

23. Jacobs MB. Hepatic infarction related to oral contraceptive use. Arch Intern Med 1984; 144:642–643.

24. Kage M, Arakawa M, Kojiro M, et al. Histopathology of membranous obstruction of the inferior vena cava in the Budd–Chiari syndrome. Gastroenterology 1992;102:2081–2090.

25. Kameda H, Yamazaki K, Imai F, et al. Obliterative portal venopathy: a comparative study of 184 cases of extrahepatic portal obstruction and 469 cases of idiopathic portal venous obstruction. J Gastroenterol Hepatol 1986;1:139–149.

26. Khuroo MS, Datta DV. Budd–Chiari syndrome following pregnancy. Report of 16 cases, with roentgenologic, hemodynamic and histologic studies of the hepatic outflow tract. Am J Med 1980;68:113–121.

27. Knochaert DC, Robaeys GK, Cox EJ, et al. Suppurative pylethrombosis: a changing clinical picture. Gastroenterology 1989;97:1028–1030.

28. Labadie H, Stoessel P, Callard P, et al. Hepatic venoocclusive disease and perisinusoidal fibrosis secondary to arsenic poisoning. Gastroenterology 1990;99:1140–1143.

29. Larrie D, Fréneaux E, Berson A, et al. Peliosis hepatis induced by 6-thioguanine administration. Gut 1988;29:1265–1269.

30. Lefkowitch JH, Mendez L. Morphologic features of hepatic injury in cardiac disease and shock. J Hepatol 1986;2:313–327.

31. Lewis JH, Tice HL, Zimmerman HJ. Budd–Chiari syndrome associated with oral contraceptive steroids. Review of treatment of 47 cases. Dig Dis Sci 1983;28:673–683.

32. Maddrey WC. Hepatic vein thrombosis (Budd–Chiari syndrome). Hepatology 1984;4: 44S–46S.

33. Maksoud JG, Mies S, da Costa Gayotto LC. Hepatoportal sclerosis in childhood. Am J Surg 1986;151:484–488.

34. Martini GA. The liver in hereditary haemorrhagic telangiectasia: an inborn error of vascular structure with multiple manifestations. A reappraisal. Gut 1978;19:531–537.

35. McDermott WV, Stone MD, Bothe A Jr, et al. Budd–Chiari syndrome. Historical and clinical review with an analysis of surgical corrective procedures. Am J Surg 1984;147:463–466.

36. McDonald GB, Hinds MS, Fisher LD, et al. Venoocclusive disease of the liver and multiorgan failure after bone marrow transplantation: a cohort study of 355 patients. Ann Intern Med 1993;118:255–267.

37. Mikkelson WP, Edmondson HA, Peters RL, et al. Extra- and intra-hepatic portal hypertension without cirrhosis (hepatoportal sclerosis). Ann Surg 1965;162:602–618.

38. Mills LR, Mwakyusa D, Milner PF. Histopathologic features of liver biopsy specimens in sickle cell disease. Arch Pathol Lab Med 1988;112:290–294.

39. Nadell J, Kosek J. Peliosis hepatis. Twelve cases associated with oral androgen therapy. Arch Pathol Lab Med 1977;101:405–410.

40. Nakano M, Worner TM, Lieber CS. Perivenular fibrosis in alcoholic liver injury: ultrastructure and histologic progression. Gastroenterology 1982;83:777–785.

41. Nakanuma Y, Ohta G, Kobayashi K, et al. Histological and histometric examination of the intrahepatic portal vein branches in primary biliary cirrhosis without regenerative nodules. Am J Gastroenterol 1982;77:405–413.

42. Nasrallah SM, Nassar VH, Galambos JT. Importance of terminal hepatic venule thickening. Arch Pathol Lab Med 1980;104:84–86.

43. Okuda K, Nakashima T, Okudaira M, et al. Liver pathology of idiopathic portal hypertension. Liver 1982;2:176–192.

44. Omata M, Johnson CS, Tong M, et al. Pathologic spectrum of liver diseases in sickle cell disease. Dig Dis Sci 1986;31:247–256.

45. Pati HP, Dayal S. Budd–Chiari syndrome: aetiology and geography. Q J Med 1996;89: 719–721.

46. Powell-Jackson PR, Melia W, Canalese J, et al. Budd–Chiari syndrome presenting as fulminant hepatic failure. Gut 1986;27:1101–1105.

47. Rolfes DB, Ishak KG. Liver disease in pregnancy. Histopathology 1986;10:555–570.

48. Rolfes DB. Ishak KG. Liver disease in toxemia of pregnancy. Am J Gastroenterol 1986;81: 1138–1144.

49. Rollins BJ. Hepatic veno-occlusive disease. Am J Med 1986;81:297–306.
50. Roughton BJ. Hepatic and portal vein thrombosis. Closely associated with chronic myeloproliferative disorders. Br Med J 1991;302:192–193.
51. Rowland R, Pieterse AS, Kimber RJ, et al. Radiation veno-occlusive liver disease. Aust N Z J Med 1981;11:534–538.
52. Seely TT, Blumenfeld CM, Ikeda R, et al. Hepatic infarction. Hum Pathol 1972;3:265–276.
53. Sekiya M, Sekigawa I, Hishikawa T, et al. Nodular regenerative hyperplasia of the liver in systemic lupus erythematosus. The relationship with anticardiolipin antibody and lupus anticoagulant. Scand J Rheumatol 1997;26:215–217.
54. Shimamatsu K, Wanless IR. Role of ischemia in causing apoptosis, atrophy, and nodular hyperplasia in human liver. Hepatology 1997;26:343–350.
55. Shimamura K, Oka K, Nakazawa M, et al. Distribution patterns of microthrombi in disseminated intravascular coagulation. Arch Pathol Lab Med 1983;107:543–547.
56. Shulman HM, Gown AM, Nujent DJ. Hepatic venoocclusive disease after bone marrow transplantation. Immunohistochemical identification of the material within occluded central venules. Am J Pathol 1987;127:549–558.
57. Shulman HM, Fisher LB, Schoch HG, et al. Venooclusive disease of the liver after marrow transplantation: histologic correlates of clinical signs and symptoms. Hepatology 1994;19:1171–1180.
58. Slater LN, Welch DF, Min K-W. *Rochalimaea henselae* causes bacillary angiomatosis and peliosis hepatis. Arch Intern Med 1992;152:602–606.
59. Tanaka M, Wanless IR. Pathology of the liver in Budd–Chiari syndrome: portal vein thrombosis and the histogenesis of veno-centric cirrhosis, veno-portal cirrhosis, and large regenerative nodules. Hepatology 1998;27:488–496.
60. Walter E, Möckel J. Images in medicine: peliosis hepatis. N Engl J Med 1997;337:1603.
61. Wanless IR. Micronodular transformation (nodular regenerative hyperplasia) of the liver: a report of 64 cases among 2,500 autopsies and a new classification of benign hepatocellular nodules. Hepatology 1990;11:787–797.
62. Wanless IR, Peterson P, Das A, et al. Hepatic vascular disease and portal hypertension in polycythemia vera and agnogenic myeloid metaplasis: a clinicopathologic study of 145 patients examined at autopsy. Hepatology 1990;12:1166–1174.
63. Watanabe K, Iwaki H, Satoh M, et al. Veno-occlusive disease of the liver following bone marrow transplantation: a clinical-pathological study of autopsy cases. Art Organs 1996; 20:1145–1150.
64. Wold LE, Ludwig J. Peliosis hepatis: two morphologic variants? Hum Pathol 1981;12: 388–389.
65. Zafrani ES, Pinaudeau Y, Dhumeaux D. Drug-induced vascular lesions of the liver. Arch Intern Med 1981;143:495–502.
66. Zafrani ES, Bernuau D, Feldmann G. Peliosis-like ultrastructural changes of the hepatic sinusoids in human chronic hypervitaminosis A. Hum Pathol 1984;15:1166–1170.

20

CIRRHOSIS, HEPATIC FIBROSIS, AND NONCIRRHOTIC PORTAL HYPERTENSION

The full understanding of cirrhosis requires that it be recognized as a pathophysiologic entity, rather than just a morphologic change. Cirrhosis is the clinical and pathologic constellation of portal hypertension, intrahepatic vascular shunting of blood, developing or developed hepatic dysfunction, and morphologic alterations of the liver itself. Fibrosis is not synonymous with cirrhosis (Table 20.1), although in many instances fibrosis precedes cirrhosis. The coarsely nodular liver of advanced syphilis (hepar lobatum) or the portal fibrosis of schistosomiasis is not cirrhosis. Portal hypertension may be present, but there is no hepatic dysfunction until late in the course of disease. Similarly, primary bile duct disorders, such as biliary atresia, primary biliary cirrhosis (PBC), and primary sclerosing cholangitis (PSC), may have significant portal hypertension, requiring liver transplantation, before there is evidence of a defect of synthetic or degradative function of the liver because the fibrosis that causes the portal hypertension is, at first, not accompanied by changes in liver plate architecture. In addition, the fibrous septa are portal to portal, and anastomotic connections between the portal vein and hepatic vein occur later.

A MORPHOLOGIC DEFINITION FOR THE PHYSIOLOGIC STATE OF CIRRHOSIS

Two key morphologic alterations, required for the clinical entity of cirrhosis, are seen: vascular septa and regenerative nodules (1,2,13,21,27,32,40) (Table 20.2).

Vascular septa (Fig. 20.1) bridge portal to central, normally connected only via the sinusoids. These septa are not simple areas of fibrosis or scarring but are dynamic alterations in the pattern of blood flow in the liver. Normally, blood flows into the liver via the portal vein and hepatic arteries and then traverses the sponge-like liver to reach the hepatic venous system and return to the general circulation. In cirrhosis, a considerable portion of

TABLE 20.1	**Examples of Noncirrhotic Hepatic Fibrosis**
	1. Schistosomiasis
	2. Tertiary syphilis
	3. Sarcoidosis
	4. Hypervitaminosis A
	5. Congenital hepatic fibrosis

the blood bypasses hepatocytes, passing almost directly from the hilum to the hepatic veins via the vascular septa (vascular shunting) (16,29). Since much of the liver's blood does not directly contact hepatocytes and does not participate in the usual physiologic activities of the liver, xenobiotics are incompletely removed from the circulation and, conversely, biosynthetic products, such as albumin and coagulation factors, do not enter the circulation. Vascular septa contribute to portal hypertension by increasing the resistance to blood flow through the liver (40). In the normal liver, the flow of blood from portal veins through sinusoids to hepatic veins is relatively unimpeded. The septa of cirrhosis are significantly less compliant than the sponge-like hepatic parenchyma.

The regenerative nodule (Fig. 20.2) is the second component of cirrhosis. After liver cell injury and/or necrosis, the liver regenerates. As the injured portion of the liver plate repairs, normal modulators of growth do not act and the usual one-cell-thick liver plate is replaced by liver plates two or more cells thick (1,2,24,32,37). Growth factors and cytokines can also cause even previously uninjured liver cells to proliferate leading to expansion of liver plates, so that most of the liver consists of liver plates containing two or more liver cells, with relative reduction of sinusoidal space. There is significantly less surface contact between blood and hepatocyte, further limiting the passage of chemical substances to and from the cell. In addition, expanding nodules compress the fibrous septa and the vessels within the septa, further contributing to portal hypertension (32,40).

The development of the vascular septa and the formation of regenerative nodules generally take place concurrently. However, in some

TABLE 20.2	**Key Features of Cirrhosis**
1. Vascular septa	
2. Regenerative nodules	
a. Thickened liver plates	
b. Development of sinusoidal basement membrane	
c. Tendency to progression	

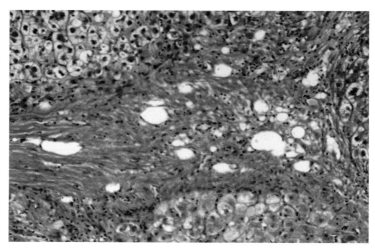

FIGURE 20.1 Septum from a cirrhotic liver showing multiple vascular channels (hematoxylin-eosin, original magnification ×100).

instances, particularly when the hepatic injury is primarily to portal tract structures, as in congenital biliary atresia and PBC, liver cell injury is a relatively late event and the liver plate and sinusoidal structure may be maintained in the face of extensive septum formation. Similarly, in chronic hepatitis regenerative nodules can be seen with relatively little fibrosis.

Hepatocyte pleomorphism and polyclonality are characteristic of the regenerative nodule. Different cell populations may be discerned. In a few cirrhotic livers, the degree of variation becomes sufficient to warrant the designation of dysplasia (3,5,6,10,19,20,26). The cells may be enlarged with

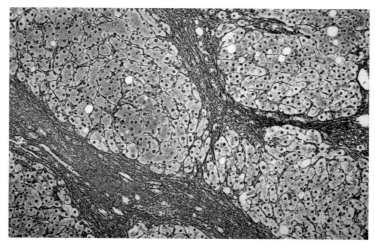

FIGURE 20.2 Regenerative nodules showing liver plates two or more cells thick (hematoxylin-eosin, original magnification ×100).

hyperchromatic, irregular nuclei having prominent nucleoli (large cell dysplasia) (e-Figs. 20.1–20.3), with relatively little increase in the nuclear/cytoplasmic ratio. This pattern is common in chronic hepatitis B infection and has been shown in experimental models of hepatocarcinogenesis (7,12). However, there is controversy about the relevance of large cell dysplasia in the development of hepatocellular carcinoma (HCC) in humans. Another form of dysplasia is characterized by cells that are equal in size to, or more often smaller than, the usual hepatocyte (small cell dysplasia) (e-Fig. 20.4), but having greatly increased nuclear/cytoplasmic ratio. This pattern is generally accepted to be a precursor to hepatocellular carcinoma in man (6,10).

The hepatocyte of the regenerative nodule may be markedly enlarged with marked eosinophilic granularity (oncocytic change) (e-Fig. 20.5). Various cell products can also be found in the hepatocytes of the cirrhotic liver, including Mallory hyalin, eosinophilic globules composed of α1-antitrypsin or fibrinogen, and, rarely, fat that may be present in only a few nodules. Bile is not usually seen in the hepatocyte of the regenerative nodule, and its presence in the absence of a cholestatic state may be indicative of HCC.

Macroregenerative nodules (MRNs) are 1 cm or more in diameter and can be exceedingly difficult to appreciate in the biopsy. They are more likely to be sites of liver cell dysplasia and HCC.

A third feature, difficult to appreciate in routine sections, is basement membrane development in the space of Disse (36) (Fig. 20.3) (capillarization), which contributes to impaired liver cell function. Sinusoids do not normally have a basement membrane. The sieve-like endothelial lining cells are highly permeable, allowing for relatively free passage of a large variety of substances. Capillarization further impairs hepatic function.

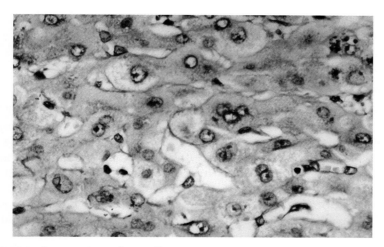

FIGURE 20.3 Basement membrane–like structure (capillarization) in the space of Disse in a cirrhotic liver (periodic acid–Schiff reaction, original magnification ×200).

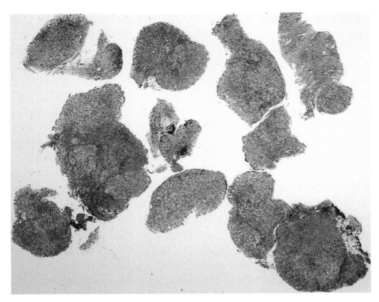

FIGURE 20.4 Fragmented cirrhosis biopsy, with regenerative nodules partially rimmed by vascular septa (hematoxylin-eosin, original magnification ×40).

A fourth key feature, not easily seen in biopsy, is that cirrhosis, when fully developed, it is almost always diffuse, although the degree may vary in parts of the liver. Exceptions are rare and generally pertain to the caudate lobe that, for reasons not always clear but possibly a result of blood vessel supply variability, can be relatively normal.

The last important feature of the cirrhotic nodule is its tendency to progress, the likely basis of the ultimate development of HCC in at least some instances of cirrhosis, when a specific oncogene is not active. Various cytokines, such as transforming growth factors, may be key.

DIAGNOSIS OF CIRRHOSIS

The histologic diagnosis of well-developed cirrhosis is not always straightforward (1,17,28,37). When an adequate sample is obtained, the diagnosis can be made on the basis of the hematoxylin-eosin-stained slide alone (Fig. 20.4, e-Fig. 20.6) or trichrome (e-Fig. 20.7). In this instance, well-defined nodules are surrounded by vascular septa. The diagnosis becomes more difficult when a suboptimal biopsy is obtained, either because of the inexperience of the individual performing the biopsy or, more often, because a needle providing a small sample is used (see Chapters 5 and 9). Fragmented biopsies suggest, but do not prove, cirrhosis unless there is demonstration of reticulin fibers encircling nodules (Fig. 20.5, e-Figs. 20.8, 20.9). The diagnosis can also be difficult when the cirrhosis is not fully developed and the features of cirrhosis are not well expressed in all areas of the liver (e-Fig. 20.10) (1,32,37,39).

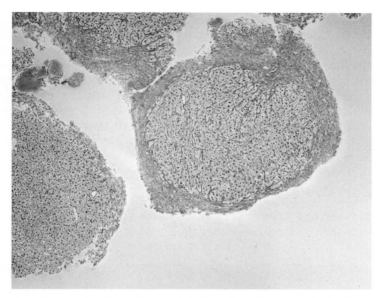

FIGURE 20.5 Fragmented biopsy from a cirrhotic patient showing reticulin fibers outlining a nodule (reticulin, original magnification ×200).

Generally, needle biopsy is more valuable than wedge biopsy in establishing the diagnosis of cirrhosis (17,37). The wedge obtains relatively peripheral, subcapsular liver tissue that may show misleading degrees of fibrosis often misinterpreted as cirrhosis (28).

The vascular septa contain portal tract structures. Degrees of inflammation and ductular reaction vary, depending on the cause (1,2,4,11, 31,32). Typically, septa are rich in elastic fibers, demonstrable with elastic stain, orcein stain, or Victoria blue (38) (Fig. 20.6). Ductular reaction can

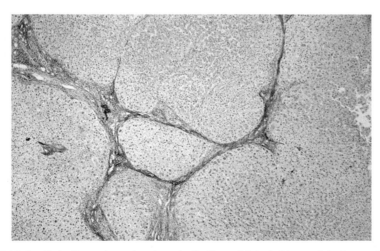

FIGURE 20.6 Cirrhotic septum showing elastic fibers (Victoria blue, original magnification ×100).

occur, to some degree, in any cirrhotic liver (1,2,22), tending to be more prominent in biliary/cholangiopathic disorders and after large duct obstruction.

Inactive cirrhosis refers to cases with relatively little inflammatory activity in the septa and little or no inflammation or necrosis within the lobule. In contrast, active cirrhosis has the features of chronic hepatitis, with interface hepatitis and varying degrees of necrosis in the lobule. Inflammation varies (1,2,4,11,31,32) and may be quite prominent, presumably contributing to further progression. There may be a discrepancy between the clinical and biochemical features and the morphologic features at any given time (31,34,36).

CAUSES OF CIRRHOSIS

Cirrhosis is the end stage of various disorders (Table 20.3). In a few cases, an etiologic factor cannot be established (cryptogenic).

TABLE 20.3 Causes of Cirrhosis	
Infections	Vascular disorders
Hepatitis B	Budd–Chiari syndrome
Hepatitis C	Venoocclusive disease
Hepatitis D	Chronic right heart failure
Autoimmune disorders	Other
Autoimmune hepatitis	Drugs and toxins
Primary biliary cirrhosis	Alcohol
Primary sclerosing cholangitis	Amiodarone
? Autoimmune cholangiopathy	Isoniazid
Metabolic disorders	Methyldopa
Wilson disease	Methotrexate
Hereditary hemochromatosis	Other
α1-Antitrypsin deficiency	Miscellaneous
Tyrosinemia	Indian childhood cirrhosis
Galactosemia	Post–intestinal bypass surgery
Glycogen storage diseases	Sarcoidosis
Long-term total parenteral nutrition	Cryptogenic disease
Other	
Large duct obstruction	
Congenital biliary atresia	
Gallstones	
Strictures	
Cystic fibrosis	

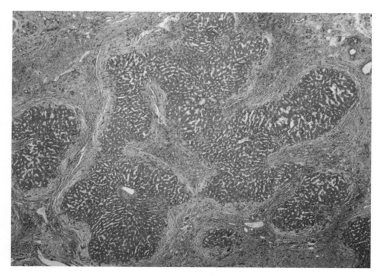

FIGURE 20.7   Primary sclerosing cholangitis showing swollen, pale hepatocytes (cholate stasis) at the periphery of the jigsaw-puzzle-shaped nodules, adjacent to the septum. This change is typical of chronic cholestasis (hematoxylin-eosin, original magnification ×200).

Morphologic Clues to the Pathogenesis of Cirrhosis

Cirrhosis can follow various injuries to the liver (Table 20.3). Etiologic factors can sometimes be determined with appropriate special studies, but often, clinical correlation is needed (e-Figs. 20.6–20.10). Except for the irregular ("jigsaw puzzle") nodules developing bile duct disorders (e-Fig. 20.11), it can be difficult to establish cause with hematoxylin-eosin sections alone.

Structural alterations are helpful. In adults, loss of interlobular bile ducts is often a result of PBC or PSC. Ductular reaction can be seen in any cirrhotic liver but is most suggestive of a primary biliary injury. Ductular reaction can be accentuated and can mimic either a benign bile duct tumor or even cholangiocarcinoma. Sclerosis of terminal hepatic venules (central veins) is often seen in alcoholic liver disease (9,25,30,33,45).

Nodules that form after the viral hepatitides tend to be round. Nodules of the cholangiopathic disorders, such as PBC, PSC, and congenital biliary atresia, tend to be highly irregular (jigsaw puzzle) (e-Fig. 20.6) because the injury initially leads to portal-to-portal fibrosis with irregular dissection of lobules. This characteristic pattern is difficult to see in the biopsy. Generally, however, chronic cholestasis changes, including marked swelling of the paraseptal hepatocytes (cholate stasis, feathery degeneration) and ductular reaction, typical of these disorders, can suggest the diagnosis (15) (Fig. 20.7). Regenerative activity may not develop until relatively late. Vascular occlusion is seen in venous outflow obstruction but it is not a specific finding and can also be seen in cirrhosis resulting from other causes (25). Progression of cirrhosis can lead to the formation of dysplastic MRNs and/or HCC (19,26,42,43) (Fig. 20.8).

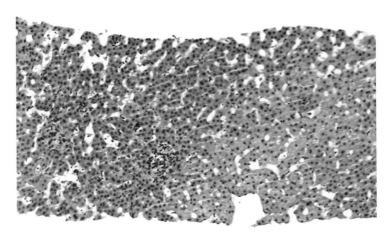

FIGURE 20.8 Small cell dysplasia occurring in a macroregenerative nodule, in a liver biopsy from a patient with chronic hepatitis C (hematoxylin-eosin, original magnification ×200).

Previously, the macroscopic pattern of cirrhosis was thought to be diagnostic of the cause, with terms such as "Laennec," "postnecrotic," and "posthepatitic" cirrhosis used. These terms are no longer used because they are not reliable indicators. As one example, Laennec pattern (now called "micronodular") was thought diagnostic of alcoholic liver disease. It is now clear that this pattern in alcoholic liver disease can progress from the Laennec pattern to the more irregular posthepatitic (macronodular) pattern, and other features (e.g., loss of bile ducts in PBC, ground-glass cells in HBV, stainable iron in hereditary hemochromatosis), as well as clinical information, are to be used in establishing cause.

INCOMPLETE SEPTAL FIBROSIS/CIRRHOSIS

In developing cirrhosis, nodularity may be indistinct without special stains, and the septa may not yet connect anatomic structures. Early septa appear as slender fibrous extensions that end blindly (39) (Fig. 20.9, e-Figs. 20.12, 20.13). Reticulin staining highlights the early regenerative change and extensions of fibrosis from portal tracts. The histologic picture of incomplete cirrhosis could be evidence of regression of cirrhosis (44). Regression of fibrosis has been recognized for many years in both experimental models and humans. It is not yet clear, however, that clinically manifest cirrhosis can regress (14).

NONCIRRHOTIC PORTAL HYPERTENSION

"Noncirrhotic portal hypertension" is the term for a distinct and rare condition with intrahepatic portal fibrosis associated with portal hypertension,

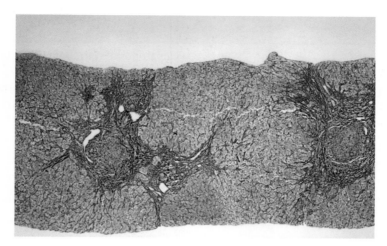

FIGURE 20.9   Incomplete septal cirrhosis, showing a slightly blunted, partial septum ending in the middle of the lobule and not connecting two architectural structures (hematoxylin-eosin, original magnification ×100).

without cirrhosis or extrahepatic portal obstruction, and without a recognizable cause (8,18,23,27,35,41). Noncirrhotic portal hypertension manifests as rapidly developing liver disease or even fulminant hepatic failure. The main histologic feature is the presence of paucicellular, dense portal tract fibrosis (Fig. 20.10, e-Fig. 20.14) and establishing the diagnosis requires exclusion of various clinically recognizable disorders that also contribute to portal hypertension in the absence of cirrhosis (Table 20.4) including true sclerosis of intrahepatic portal veins (see Chapter 1). Either

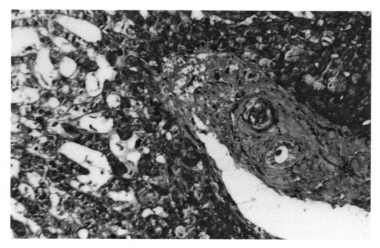

FIGURE 20.10   Portal fibrosis in a patient with idiopathic portal hypertension (Masson trichrome, original magnification ×10).

TABLE 20.4	Noncirrhotic Portal Hypertension	
Prehepatic	Hepatoportal (intrahepatic portal vein) sclerosis	
Idiopathic portal hypertension	Nodular regenerative hyperplasia	
Portal and/or splenic vein thrombosis	Partial nodular transformation	
Cavernous transformation of the portal vein	Congenital hepatic fibrosis	
Hepatic	Posthepatic	
Alcoholic hepatitis	Budd-Chiari syndrome	
Drug or toxin-induced hepatitis	Venoocclusive disease	
Hypervitaminosis A	Long-standing right heart failure	
Sarcoidosis		
Schistosomiasis		
Infiltrative disorders		
Gaucher		
Myeloproliferative		
Leukemia		
Noncirrhotic portal fibrosis		

injury or thrombosis of portal venous branches has been implicated in the pathogenesis of this condition. However, the obliterated veins may not be seen in biopsy material.

REFERENCES

1. Anthony PP, Ishak KG, Nayak NC, et al. The morphology of cirrhosis: definition, nomenclature, and classification. Bull WHO 1977;55:521–540.
2. Anthony PP, Ishak KG, Nayak NC, et al. The morphology of cirrhosis. Recommendations on definition, nomenclature, and classification by a working group sponsored by the World Health Organization. J Clin Pathol 1978;31:395–414.
3. Anthony PP, Vogel CL, Barker LF. Liver cell dysplasia: a premalignant condition. J Clin Pathol 1973;26:217–223.
4. Baggenstoss AH, Staufer MH. Posthepatitic and alcoholic cirrhosis: clinicopathologic study of 43 cases of each. Gastroenterology 1952;22:157–180.
5. Borzio M, Bruno S, Roncalli M, et al. Liver cell dysplasia and risk of hepatocellular carcinoma in cirrhosis: a preliminary report. Br Med J 1991;302:1312.
6. Crawford JM. Pathologic assessment of liver cell dysplasia and benign liver tumors: differentiation from malignant tumors. Semin Diagn Pathol 1990;7:115–128.
7. Cullen JM, Sandgren EP, Brinster RL, et al. Histologic characterization of hepatic carcinogenesis in transgenic mice expressing SV40 T-antigens. Vet Pathol 1993;30:111–118.
8. Eckhauser FE, Appleman HD, Knol JA, et al. Non-cirrhotic portal hypertension: different patterns of disease in children and adults. Surgery 1983;94:721–728.
9. Edmondson HA, Peters RL, Reynolds TB, et al. Sclerosing hyalin necrosis of the liver in the chronic alcoholic: a recognizable clinical syndrome. Ann Intern Med 1963;59:646–673.

10. Ferrell LD, Crawford JM, Dhillon AP, et al. Proposal for standardized criteria for the diagnosis of benign, borderline, and malignant hepatocellular lesions arising in chronic advanced liver disease. Am J Surg Pathol 1993;17:1113–1123.

11. Gall EA. Posthepatitis, postnecrotic and nutritional cirrhosis: a pathologic analysis. Am J Pathol 36:241–271.

12. Geller SA, Nichols WS, Kim S, et al. Hepatocarcinogenesis is the sequel to hepatitis in Z#2 alpha-1-antitrypsin transgenic mice: histopathological and DNA ploidy studies. Hepatology 1994;19:389–397.

13. Geller SA. Coming or going? What is cirrhosis? Arch Pathol Lab Med 2000;124:1587–1588.

14. Gerber MA, Popper H. Relation between central canals and portal tracts in alcoholic hepatitis: a contribution to the pathogenesis of cirrhosis in alcoholics. Hum Pathol 1972;3:199–207.

15. Gerber MA, Orr W, Denk H, et al. Hepatocellular hyalin in cholestasis and cirrhosis: its diagnostic significance. Gastroenterology 1973;64:89–98.

16. Gross G, Perrier CV. Intrahepatic portasystemic shunting in cirrhotic patients. N Engl J Med 1975;293:1046–1047.

17. Imamura H, Kawasaki S, Bandai Y, et al. Comparison between wedge and needle biopsies for evaluating the degree of cirrhosis. J Hepatol 1993;17:215–219.

18. Kage M, Arakawa M, Fukuda K, et al. Pathomorphologic study on the extrahepatic portal vein in idiopathic portal hypertension. Liver 1990;10:209–216.

19. Kondo F, Ebara M, Sugiura N, et al. Histological features and clinical course of large regenerative nodules: evaluation of their precancerous potentiality. Hepatology 1990;12:592–598.

20. Lefkowitch JH, Apfelbaum TF. Liver cell dysplasia and hepatocellular carcinoma in non-A, non-B hepatitis. Arch Pathol Lab Med 1987;111:170–173.

21. MacSween RNM, Scott AR. Hepatic cirrhosis: a clinicopathologic review of 320 cases. J Clin Pathol 1973;26:936–942.

22. Masuko K, Rubin E, Popper H. Proliferation of bile ducts in cirrhosis. Arch Pathol 1964;78:421–431.

23. Mikkelsen WP, Edmondson HA, Peters RL, et al. Extra- and intrahepatic portal hypertension without cirrhosis (hepatoportal sclerosis). Ann Surg 1965;162:602–618.

24. Morgan JD, Martcroft WS. Juvenile liver: age at which one-cell-thick liver plates predominate in the human liver. Arch Pathol 1961;77:86–88.

25. Nakanuma Y, Ohta G, Doishita K. Quantitation and serial section observations of focal venoocclusive lesions of hepatic veins in liver cirrhosis. Virchows Arch A Pathol Anat Histopathol 1985;405:429–439.

26. Nakanuma Y, Terada T, Ueda K, et al. Adenomatous hyperplasia of the liver as a precancerous lesion. Liver 1993;13:1–9.

27. Ohnishi K, Saito M, Sato S, et al. Portal hemodynamics in idiopathic portal hypertension (Banti's syndrome). Gastroenterology 1987;92:751–758.

28. Petrelli M, Scheuer PJ. Variation in subcapsular liver structure and its significance in the interpretation of wedge biopsies. J Clin Pathol 1967;20:743–748.

29. Popper H, Elias H, Petty DE. Vascular pattern of the cirrhotic liver. Am J Clin Pathol 1952;22:717–729.

30. Popper H, Szanto PB, Elias H. Transition of fatty liver into cirrhosis. Gastroenterology 1955;28:183–192.

31. Popper H, Rubin E, Krus S, et al. Postnecrotic cirrhosis in alcoholics. Gastroenterology 1960;39:669–685.

32. Popper H. Pathologic aspects of cirrhosis. Am J Pathol 1977;87:228–259.

33. Reynolds TB, Hidemura R, Michel H, et al. Portal hypertension without cirrhosis in alcoholic liver disease. Ann Intern Med 1969;70:497–506.

34. Rubin E, Krus S, Popper H. Pathogenesis of postnecrotic cirrhosis in alcoholics. Arch Pathol 1962;73:288–289.

35. Sarin SK. Non-cirrhotic portal fibrosis. Gut 1989;30:406–415.

36. Schaffner F, Popper H. Capillarization of hepatic sinusoids in man. Gastroenterology 1963;44:239–242.

37. Scheuer PJ. Liver biopsy in the diagnosis of cirrhosis. Gut 1970;11:275–278.

38. Scheuer PJ. Hepatic fibrosis and collapse: histological distinction by orcein staining. Histopathology 1980;4:487–490.

39. Sciot R, Staessen D, Van Damme B, et al. Incomplete septal cirrhosis: histopathological aspects. Histopathology 1988;13:593–603.

40. Shibayama Y. On the pathogenesis of portal hypertension in cirrhosis of the liver. Liver 1988;8:95–99.

41. Tandon BN, Lakshminarayanan R, Bhargava S, et al. Ultrastructure of the liver in non-cirrhotic portal fibrosis with portal hypertension. Gut 1970;11:905–910.

42. Terada T, Terasaki S, Nakanuma Y. A clinicopathologic study of adenomatous hyperplasia of the liver in 209 consecutive cirrhotic livers examined by autopsy. Cancer 1993;72:1551–1556.

43. Theise ND, Schwartz M, Miller C, et al. Macroregenerative nodules and hepatocellular carcinoma in forty-four sequential adult liver explants with cirrhosis. Hepatology 1992;16:949–955.

44. Wanless IR, Nakashima E, Sherman M. Regression of human cirrhosis. Morphologic features and the genesis of incomplete septal cirrhosis. Arch Pathol Lab Med 2000;124:1599–1607.

45. Worner TM, Lieber CS. Perivenular fibrosis as precursor lesion of cirrhosis. JAMA 1985; 254:627–630.

21

THE LIVER IN SYSTEMIC DISORDERS

Systemic disorders often affect the liver, and morphologic changes and the clinical presentation are usually mild. Some typical biopsy changes can be seen, however (22).

DIABETES MELLITUS

Morphologic changes are common in diabetes mellitus (DM), although clinical manifestations relating to the liver are quite rare (10).

Histopathologic Findings

Glycogenated (glycogen) nuclei, occurring especially in zone 1, and variable degrees of steatosis are the most common changes. Glycogenated nuclei are optically clear nuclei with a denser-than-usual nuclear membrane (Fig. 21.1, e-Figs. 21.1, 21.2). This phenomenon, whose pathogenesis is not clear, is presumed to reflect cytoplasmic accumulation of glycogen as a large vacuole that protrudes into the nucleus. In contrast with the usual ultrastructural rosette-like appearance of intracytoplasmic glycogen, the glycogen of the glycogenated nucleus appears dispersed. Glycogenated nuclei may be seen many years before the clinical onset of DM (10).

Glycogenated nuclei can also be present in Wilson disease (see Chapter 16), but are also present in otherwise normal adolescents and elderly patients.

Nonalcoholic Fatty Liver Disease (NAFLD)

Nonalcoholic fatty liver disease (NAFLD), including the nonalcoholic steatohepatitis (NASH), occurs in patients with DM and must be differentiated from true alcoholic steatohepatitis (ASH) (Chapter 13). Macrovesicular steatosis is common in DM and generally not zonal (Fig. 21.2, e-Figs. 21.3–21.5). In some cases the steatosis is mixed, microvesicular and macrovesicular.

Although there is still some disagreement in how to apply these terms, we use NAFLD as a comprehensive term that includes a spectrum of histopathologic changes ranging from steatosis, mild or marked, without obvious evidence of liver injury, NASH characterized by marked steatosis,

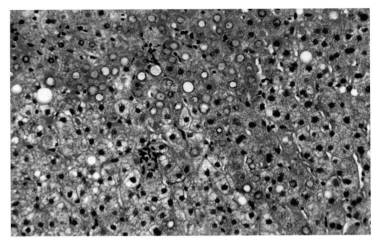

FIGURE 21.1 Diabetes mellitus. Glycogenated nuclei are seen as optically clear with denser than usual nuclear membrane (hematoxylin-eosin, original magnification ×400).

ballooned hepatocytes, sometimes with polymorphonuclear leukocyte (PMN) infiltration and accumulations of Mallory hyalin, and fibrosis/cirrhosis (Fig. 21.3, e-Figs. 21.6, 21.7). Mallory material is generally not as abundant as in ASH, is generally not as strongly eosinophilic, and is predominantly periportal. Portal tracts contain mild to moderate inflammatory cell infiltrate, mostly lymphocytes with some plasma cells and PMNs. Glycogenated nuclei, often seen in NAFLD, are not particularly prominent in ASH.

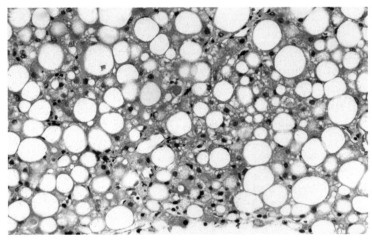

FIGURE 21.2 Diabetes mellitus. Severe steatosis (hematoxylin-eosin, original magnification ×40).

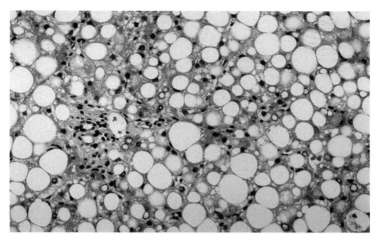

FIGURE 21.3   Diabetes mellitus with nonalcoholic steatohepatitis, showing marked steatosis with acute inflammatory cells and Mallory hyalin (hematoxylin-eosin, original magnification ×200).

NAFLD may progress to fibrosis and cirrhosis. Collagenization of the space of Disse, with deposition of type IV collagen, may precede the development of cirrhosis and has been described as a part of the spectrum of diabetic microangiopathy (Fig. 21.4, e-Fig. 21.8) (10,11,50).

The understanding of NAFLD/NASH has increased greatly with various morphologically based definitions and staging systems in the recent literature (13,16,47).

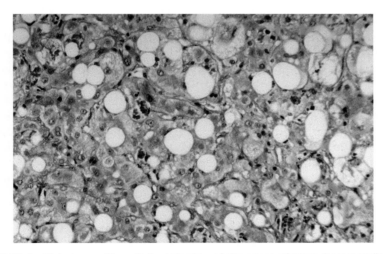

FIGURE 21.4   Diabetes mellitus. Collagenization of the space of Disse (hematoxylin-eosin, original magnification ×200).

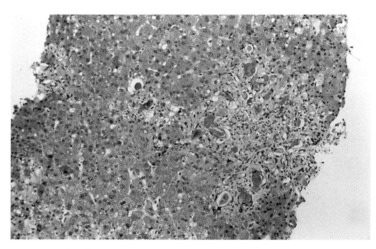

FIGURE 21.5 Sepsis. There is ductular proliferation, and the dilated ductules contain inspissated bile. Surrounding ducts and ductules are polymorphonuclear leukocytes (hematoxylin-eosin, original magnification ×100).

Other Conditions

Hepatic adenoma (29), nodular hyperplasia (100), and primary sclerosing cholangitis (PSC) (2) have been reported in association with DM.

SEPSIS

The liver is often affected in sepsis, but biopsy is rarely obtained, except in the setting of liver transplantation (see Chapter 25) (8).

Histopathologic Findings

Three sepsis patterns have been recognized: (a) perivenular canalicular cholestasis with mild steatosis, associated prominence of Kupffer cells, and nonspecific portal inflammatory infiltrate; (b) marked bile ductular reaction/proliferation with the perivenular canalicular cholestasis (Fig. 21.5) and ductular proliferation at the margin of the portal tracts, with ductules dilated and filled with inspissated bile (52), along with periductal and periductular infiltration with PMNs (pericholangitis) with secondary, reactive epithelial injury; and (c) nonbacterial cholangitis, most commonly associated with toxic shock syndrome (40). This variant may be a result of circulating staphylococcal toxin. PMNs are seen in the bile duct lumen, with necrosis of the epithelium.

HUMAN IMMUNODEFICIENCY VIRUS AND ACQUIRED IMMUNE DEFICIENCY SYNDROME (HIV/AIDS)

A wide spectrum of liver diseases occur in patients infected with human immunodeficiency virus (HIV) (Table 21.1) (7,25,32,41,49,61,70,83,87,

TABLE 21.1	Hepatic Involvement in HIV/AIDS
Hepatic parenchymal disease	
Cytomegalovirus (CMV)	
Mycobacterium avium complex (MAI)	
Cryptococcosis	
Candidiasis	
Aspergillosis	
Coccidioidomycosis	
Hepatitis B virus (HBV)	
Hepatitis C virus (HCV)	
Drug toxicity	
Biliary disease	
Cytomegalovirus cholangitis	
Cryptosporidium cholangitis	
Kaposi sarcoma	
Lymphoproliferative process	

105). The liver changes are secondary and do not reflect primary liver disease, although hepatitis primarily associated with HIV infection may occur in children and adults (66). The most frequently encountered features in both HIV-positive patients and patients with acquired immune deficiency syndrome (AIDS) are variable degrees of bile duct injury (AIDS cholangiopathy), prominence of Kupffer and sinusoidal endothelial cells, often with hemosiderosis, and steatosis (Fig. 21.6) (32,71).

Bile Duct Injury and AIDS Cholangiopathy

Bile duct injury varies from mild epithelial damage to changes that mimic bile duct obstruction with significant cholestasis and bile ductular proliferation (Fig. 21.7, e-Figs. 21.9, 21.10) (61). Sometimes significant periductal fibrosis is seen, indistinguishable from PSC (36,57). These changes also seen with either cryptosporidiosis or cytomegalovirus (CMV) infection affecting the biliary tree (61).

HIV gag protein p24 can be detected in sinusoidal endothelial and Kupffer cells but not in hepatocytes (Fig. 21.8). There is little evidence that HIV has a direct cytopathic effect in the liver (38), although propagation of HIV virus is feasible in vitro in hepatoma cell lines (95).

Many HIV patients also have hepatitis B or C chronic hepatitis (17,71). Granulomas, without an identifiable cause, are seen in 20% of patients, and 15% show nonspecific reactive changes. Cirrhosis, of varying causes, can also be seen. Peliosis hepatis and bacillary angiomatosis occur. Opportunistic infections affecting the liver are relatively uncommon. Kaposi sarcoma occurs sporadically.

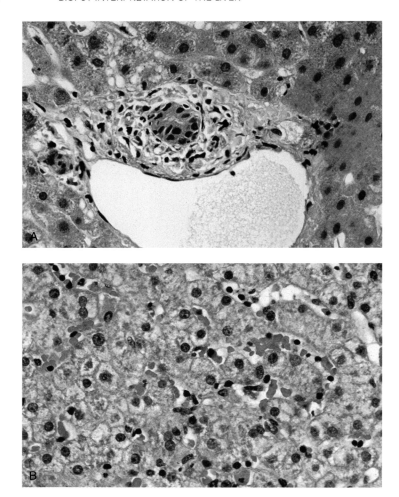

FIGURE 21.6   **A** and **B**. Acquired immune deficiency syndrome. Bile ducts show mild injury, and there is prominence of sinusoidal endothelial and Kupffer cells (hematoxylin-eosin, original magnification ×200).

Opportunistic Infections

Poorly formed microgranulomas should raise suspicion for *Mycobacterium avium-intracellulare* (MAI) infection (e-Fig. 21.11). Spindle cell proliferation can be prominent (pseudosarcoma), with the spindle cells containing innumerable acid-fast bacilli (37,75). *Mycobacterium tuberculosis* var. hominis, including miliary dissemination, also occurs in AIDS, with caseating or noncaseating granulomas.

Fungal Infections

Fungal infections occur usually with widespread dissemination. Special stains (periodic acid–Schiff, Gomori methenamine silver) highlight organisms,

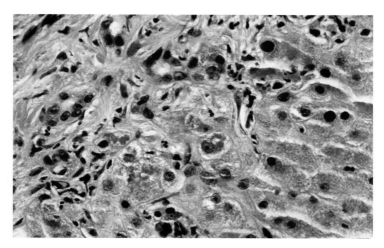

FIGURE 21.7   Acquired immune deficiency syndrome. Bile duct injury is moderately severe, and there is ductular proliferation and cholestasis suggesting large duct obstruction (hematoxylin-eosin, original magnification ×200).

including *Candida albicans*, *Histoplasma capsulatum*, *Cryptococcus neoformans*, and *Coccidioides immitis*. Blastomycosis, aspergillosis, and kala azar are rarely seen (26,76,87,110).

Protozoal Infections

Cryptosporidium can infect the biliary tree, with an associated cholangiopathy, but is rarely seen in biopsy samples (35). Hepatitis caused by microsporidia has been described (73,98).

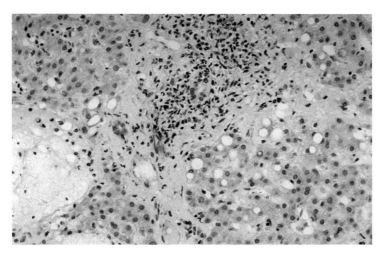

FIGURE 21.8   Acquired immune deficiency syndrome. Human immunodeficiency virus gag protein p24 is present in sinusoidal endothelial and Kupffer cells. (immunoperoxidase, anti-p24, original magnification ×100).

Cytomegalovirus

CMV infection was, prior to the development of effective antiviral therapy, frequently seen in AIDS patients. Characteristic intranuclear inclusions are generally easily seen, but in situ hybridization may be necessary (35,47).

VASCULAR DISORDERS

HIV-Associated Peliosis

HIV-associated peliosis of the liver is indistinguishable from peliosis hepatis seen in immunocompetent patients. Cystically dilated sinusoidal spaces are partially lined by nonneoplastic endothelial cells and filled with blood (Fig. 21.9, e-Figs. 21.13, 21.14) (21,70,90).

Bacillary Angiomatosis

Bacillary angiomatosis is a distinct lesion associated with HIV infection (30,51,70,90,96,104). It affects various organs, including the spleen and liver. In most cases there are cystically dilated spaces filled with blood, with variable surrounding fibrous and fibromyxoid stroma alternating with angioproliferative spindle cells. Clusters of lymphocytes and PMNs are admixed with blood and adjacent fibrous stroma and endothelial cells (Fig. 21.10, e-Figs. 21.15–21.18). Rod-shaped bacillary organisms (*Rochalimaea henselae*) can be demonstrated with Warthin-Starry silver stain (93,104). The organism is sensitive to erythromycin, and the lesion can resolve completely.

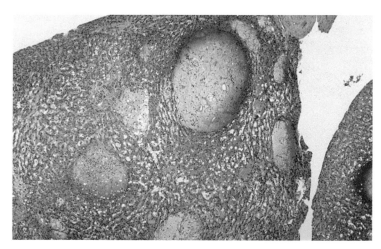

FIGURE 21.9 Peliosis hepatis in a patient with human immunodeficiency virus infection (hematoxylin-eosin, original magnification ×100).

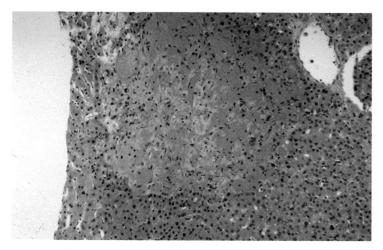

FIGURE 21.10   Bacillary angiomatosis in a patient with acquired immune deficiency syndrome showing cystically dilated vascular spaces with spindle cell proliferation (hematoxylin-eosin, original magnification ×100).

Kaposi Sarcoma (Kaposi Angioproliferative Lesion)

Kaposi sarcoma is generally seen as a disseminated malignancy and often affects the liver (90,96). The lesions are usually only a few millimeters in diameter and may not always appear in biopsy, despite being abundant in the liver. The angioproliferative lesion has irregular fascicles of spindle cells with extravasated red blood cells (Fig. 21.11, e-Figs. 21.19–21.24).

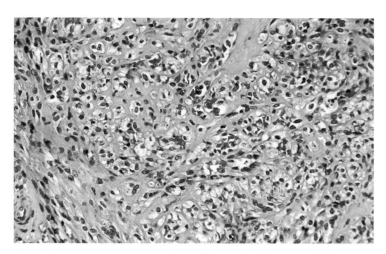

FIGURE 21.11   Kaposi sarcoma in a patient with acquired immune deficiency syndrome, showing tightly packed spindle cells and extravasated red blood cells (hematoxylin-eosin, original magnification ×100).

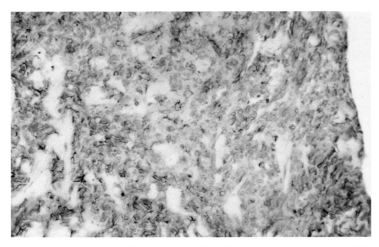

FIGURE 21.12   Reactivity of proliferating spindle cells in acquired immune deficiency syndrome to antibody directed against CD34 (hematoxylin-eosin, original magnification ×200).

Extracellular hemosiderin is seen, as well as intracellular eosinophilic globules of uncertain origin. Lymphocytes and plasma cells may be present. The proliferated spindle cells are most likely of endothelial cell origin, either vascular or lymphatic, with reactivity to antibodies routinely used for other neoplasms of endothelial cell origin, CD31 and CD34 (Fig. 21.12) (91).

Lymphoproliferative Disorders

The incidence of lymphoproliferative disorders is increased in AIDS. The liver is affected in approximately 25% of patients, as either a solitary mass or as multiple nodules. Lymphoma rarely involves bile ducts, primarily, clinically resembling PSC.

Most HIV-associated lymphomas are of the non-Hodgkin B-cell type. They are usually high grade, with either a predominantly large cell immunoblastic population or a Burkitt type, with small noncleaved cells (33,48).

In contrast with the posttransplantation immunocompromised patients, only half of AIDS-associated lymphoproliferative disorders are Epstein-Barr virus (EBV) associated (77,92). A c-myc gene rearrangement is more commonly seen in these patients (92).

Viral Hepatitides in AIDS

As many as 75% of AIDS patients have serologic evidence of HBV infection (32,71). The effect of HBV on the progression of HIV infection is controversial. Coinfection with HCV and HIV is also common (71). HIV adversely affects chronic HCV infection, leading to more severe and rapidly progressive disease (e-Figs. 21.22–21.26) (71,86). HCV infection can affect the progression of HIV in a similar fashion (56,71,72), to some extent dependent on the HCV genotype (94).

Drug Toxicity in Immunocompromised Patients

Drugs used for treatment of patients with AIDS may be hepatotoxic. These include antifungal agents, such as ketoconazole and fluconazole, as well as antimycobacterial drugs, such as rifampicin and isoniazid. The histologic distinction between viral and drug-induced hepatitides may be particularly difficult (71). Some antiretroviral drugs (e.g., dideoxyinosine) cause fulminant liver failure (71).

PREGNANCY

Benign Recurrent Cholestasis

The pathogenesis of benign recurrent cholestasis is not entirely clear but may be related to elevated estrogen levels. Histologically, perivenular intracanalicular cholestasis is seen without significant inflammation or liver cell necrosis (81,101). Recognition of the clinical setting is obviously helpful in differentiating this type of cholestasis from sepsis or drug-induced cholestasis.

Acute Fatty Liver of Pregnancy

Acute fatty liver of pregnancy is a serious condition associated with high mortality (68,81,82). The fat may be zonal, mostly involving zones 3 (perivenular) and 2, or diffuse, affecting the entire acinus (e-Figs. 21.27, 21.28). Steatosis is generally microvesicular, sometimes difficult to recognize on routine paraffin sections, but easily seen in cryostat-sectioned liver stained for fat. Zone 3 intracanalicular cholestasis and portal and lobular lymphocytic inflammatory infiltrate are usually seen (81,101). The portal infiltrate can be prominent, suggesting acute viral hepatitis. When only zone 3 fat is seen, tetracycline-induced toxicity (which can also be seen during pregnancy) must be considered.

Preeclampsia and Eclampsia

Preeclampsia is characterized by hypertension, proteinuria, and peripheral edema (82,85). If uncontrolled, it can lead to the convulsive, hyperreflexive condition of eclampsia. Liver biopsy is only rarely obtained. Parenchymal hemorrhage and necrosis are seen. Sinusoids may contain fibrin, evidence of intravascular coagulation, and fibrin thrombi can form, particularly in zone 1 (Figs. 21.13, 21.14, e-Figs. 21.29–21.32). With progression, fibrin thrombi are seen in many sinusoids and even arterioles (Fig. 21.15).

HELLP Syndrome

HELLP syndrome (hemolysis, elevated liver function tests, and low platelets) can be morphologically indistinguishable from, and may represent

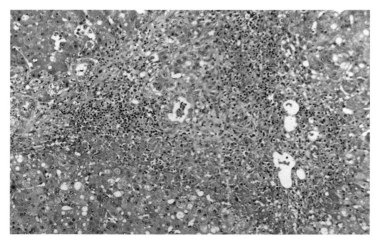

FIGURE 21.13 Eclampsia, showing deposition of fibrin in periportal sinusoids, with associated hepatocellular necrosis (hematoxylin-eosin, original magnification ×100).

a mild form of, eclampsia (e-Figs. 21.33, 21.34) (6,9,88). Sometimes the liver shows nonspecific changes, including portal inflammatory infiltrate, focal lobular necrosis, and glycogenated nuclei.

HEMATOLOGIC DISORDERS

The liver is often affected in hematologic disorders, including lymphoproliferative and myeloproliferative conditions (67,106,109). Kupffer cell

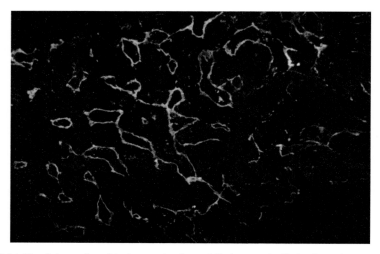

FIGURE 21.14 Eclampsia, with demonstration of fibrinogen in fibrin deposits (peroxidase-antiperoxidase, original magnification ×100).

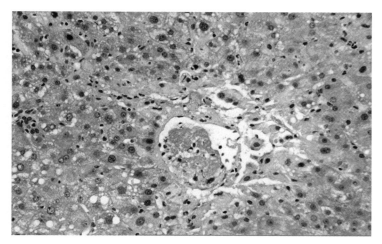

FIGURE 21.15 Eclampsia with demonstration of intravascular thrombus formation (Masson trichrome, original magnification ×100).

hyperplasia with associated hemosiderosis is commonly seen, usually attributable to multiple blood transfusions. Patients with hemophilia have a higher risk of infection with HBV and HCV, as well as HIV.

Anemia

Various nonspecific changes are seen with long-standing anemia, including mild macrovesicular steatosis and secondary hemosiderosis (Fig. 21.16). Chronic hemolysis can also lead to gallstones and changes of large duct obstruction (see Chapter 18).

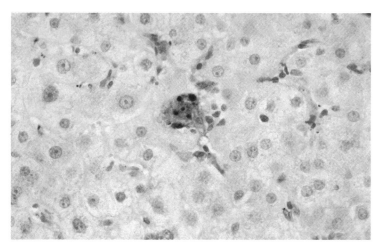

FIGURE 21.16 Secondary hemosiderosis, with demonstration of iron in Kupffer cells, in hemolytic anemia (Perls, original magnification ×200).

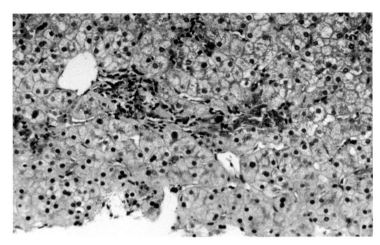

FIGURE 21.17   Sickle cell disease, showing clumped sickle-shaped red blood cells distending sinusoids (hematoxylin-eosin, original magnification ×200).

In sickle cell anemia, sinusoidal aggregation of sickle-shaped cells, with associated sinusoidal dilatation and congestion, and eventual liver cell necrosis is seen, in addition to secondary hemosiderosis. These changes are typical of patients in crisis (54) and only rarely encountered in biopsy samples (Fig. 21.17, e-Figs. 21.35, 21.36) (97).

Large vein thrombosis, affecting portal and/or hepatic veins, occurs in patients with paroxysmal nocturnal hemoglobinuria (55,97).

Lymphoproliferative Disorders

Liver involvement by lymphoid leukemias, non-Hodgkin lymphoma, and Hodgkin lymphoma is generally not clinically dominant. Liver biopsy is often performed to either identify the cause of associated fever or, particularly in Hodgkin lymphoma, for staging purpose. Rarely, massive infiltration by lymphoid cells contributes to fulminant failure (e-Figs. 21.37–21.40) (67,105,109).

LYMPHOID LEUKEMIA.   Infiltration in the lymphoid leukemias tends to be primarily portal (109). This is particularly prominent in lymphoblastic leukemia, in which the lymphoid cells are relatively primitive (e-Figs. 21.41, 21.42) (109).

HAIRY CELL LEUKEMIA.   The characteristic monocytoid hairy cells usually infiltrate sinusoids in a linear pattern. Other findings include dilated sinusoids and angiomatous (peliosis-like) lesions surrounded by rings of leukemic cells (15,108).

NON-HODGKIN LYMPHOMA.   Liver involvement is common in non-Hodgkin lymphoma, and the biopsy shows diffuse lymphoid infiltration (Fig. 21.18) (108).

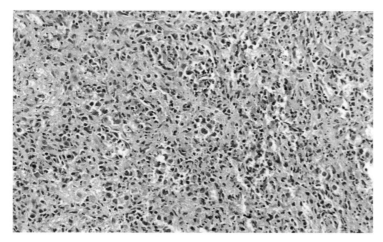

FIGURE 21.18   Non-Hodgkin lymphoma, with replacement of hepatic parenchyma by sheets of lymphoid cells (hematoxylin-eosin, original magnification ×100).

HODGKIN LYMPHOMA. When Hodgkin lymphoma involves the spleen, the liver is almost always involved. However, the characteristic Hodgkin lymphoma infiltrate is seen in only 15% of biopsies. Classic Reed-Sternberg cells are rarely seen (e-Fig. 21.43). Usually, a mixed inflammatory cell infiltrate, not specifically diagnosable as Hodgkin disease, is seen (Fig. 21.19). As many as 10% of biopsies show noncaseating epithelioid granulomas, similar to those of sarcoidosis. Sinusoidal dilatation and peliosis hepatis are seen (15). In some patients the only finding is intrahepatic cholestasis (53). Uncommonly, a lesion resembling PSC may be

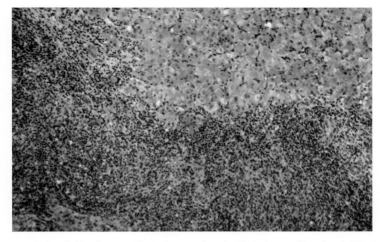

FIGURE 21.19   Hodgkin disease. There is an extensive lymphoproliferative infiltrate in this biopsy performed for acute liver failure (hematoxylin-eosin, original magnification ×100).

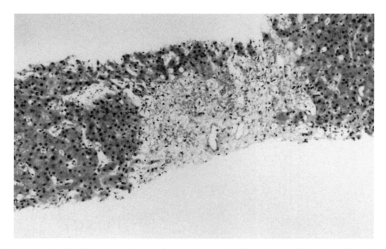

FIGURE 21.20 Budd-Chiari syndrome in a patient with lymphoproliferative disorder, showing characteristic atrophy and necrosis of zone 3 hepatocytes (hematoxylin-eosin, original magnification ×100).

seen (39), and the clinical and pathologic syndrome of vanishing bile duct syndrome can develop (39).

Myeloproliferative Disorders

All of the myeloproliferative disorders, including the myelogenous leukemias, polycythemia vera, myeloid metaplasia and myelofibrosis, and essential thrombocythemia, can affect the liver. In myelogenous leukemia the infiltrating cells are seen in both sinusoids and portal tracts.

The most common finding in the liver in the nonleukemia myeloproliferative disorders is infiltration of sinusoids by hematopoietic cells

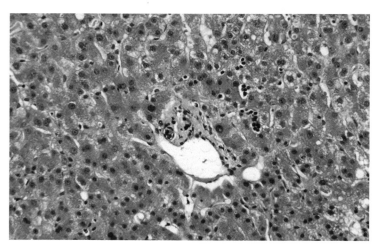

FIGURE 21.21 Extramedullary hematopoiesis in a patient with myelofibrosis (hematoxylin-eosin, original magnification ×200).

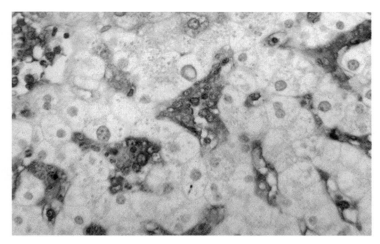

FIGURE 21.22   Multiple myeloma. There is deposition of light-chain immunoglobulins in the space of Disse (immunoperoxidase, anti–kappa light chain, original magnification ×200).

originating from all three hematopoietic lineages (24,69), sometimes causing portal hypertension. Sinusoidal dilatation from increased hepatic blood flow is often seen. Budd-Chiari syndrome occurs in myeloproliferative disorders (Fig. 21.20) (18,24). Nodular regenerative hyperplasia develops either secondary to ischemia or as a result of drug-induced hepatotoxicity (24). Extramedullary hematopoiesis is seen, particularly in myeloid metaplasia and myelofibrosis (Fig. 21.21).

Isolated circulating megakaryocytes can also be seen in sinusoids as a manifestation of stress and not necessarily as a component of a myeloproliferative disorder (e-Figs. 21.44, 21.45).

MYELOMA.   The liver is variably involved in myeloma. There may be sinusoidal and parenchymal infiltration by plasma cells or there may be tumorlike replacement. In myeloma, as well as in Waldenström's macroglobulinemia, there may be portal hypertension, nodular regenerative hyperplasia, and peliosis hepatis, as well as deposition of light chain immunoglobulins or macroglobulins in the space of Disse (Fig. 21.22) (99,102).

EPSTEIN-BARR VIRUS–RELATED DISORDERS

Infectious Mononucleosis

Infectious mononucleosis can be complicated by EBV-associated hepatitis. Sinusoidal infiltration with lymphoid cells almost always includes immunoblastic forms (Fig. 21.23). Kupffer cells are usually hyperplastic. There is little or no hepatocellular injury or necrosis. Small microgranulomas may also be present. Differential diagnosis includes leukemia and extramedullary hematopoiesis. Diagnosis is generally established after correlating serologic and histopathologic findings (44).

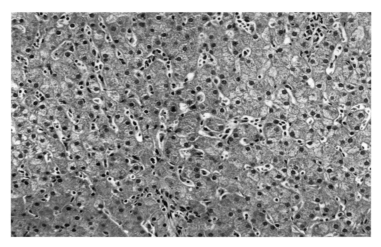

FIGURE 21.23 Infectious mononucleosis, showing sinusoidal infiltration by lymphoid cells, some of which are slightly immature and atypical (hematoxylin-eosin, original magnification ×200).

Viral-Associated Hemophagocytic Syndrome

Viral-associated hemophagocytic syndrome is a systemic viral infection generally associated with infection with either EBV or CMV and characterized by progressive, often profound, anemia (28). Histiocytes show phagocytosed hematopoietic cells. Most Kupffer cells contain red blood cells (Fig. 21.24). The Kupffer cells can be markedly hyperplastic and can resemble the infiltrate of malignant histiocytosis; with appropriate immunohistochemical studies, however, differentiation is generally easy (60).

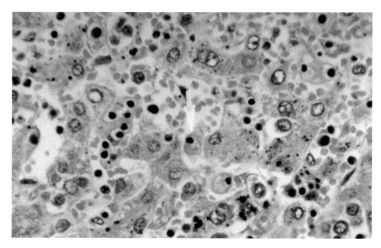

FIGURE 21.24 Viral-associated hemophagocytic syndrome. Kupffer cells contain phagocytosed red blood cells (hematoxylin-eosin, original magnification ×100).

Chronic Granulomatous Disease

Chronic granulomatous disease (CGD) is a result of impaired hydrogen peroxide production leading to failure of the myeloperoxidase–H_2O_2–halide killing system. Chronic granulomatous disease is an inherited, generally X-linked disease of male children and infants, characterized by recurrent infections and death at an early age, most often because of infection by catalase-positive organisms such as *Staphylococcus aureus*. Adults are rarely affected. Poorly formed necrotizing granulomas are seen in the parenchyma. Histiocytes surrounding the area of necrosis contain dusty brown lipofuscin pigment. Pigment-laden histiocytes are also in portal tracts with other inflammatory cells, particularly lymphocytes. Other infectious causes or drug-induced granulomas have to be excluded (63).

Reye Syndrome

Reye syndrome typically occurs in children treated with aspirin (103). Aspirin toxicity mimics Reye syndrome. Although histopathologic changes may be similar, ultrastructurally they appear to be unrelated. In Reye syndrome, hypoglycemia is often profound and is typically followed by the rapid development of encephalopathy and coma.

The characteristic histopathologic feature is diffuse microvesicular steatosis without significant inflammation, necrosis, or cholestasis (e-Figs. 21.47–21.49) (14,79). Fat droplets can be difficult to appreciate in routine histologic sections, and frozen sections stained with a fat stain (oil red O or Sudan IV) may be required. Fat droplets are generally smallest in zone 3 (Fig. 21.25). Alternatively, formalin-fixed wet tissue can be postfixed with osmium tetroxide to retain the fat (e-Fig. 21.50). The ultrastructural changes are

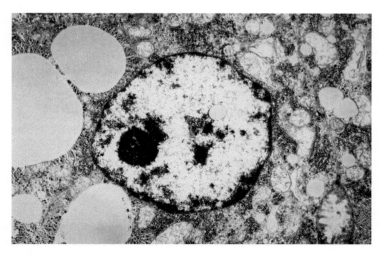

FIGURE 21.25   Reye syndrome. Zone 3 hepatocytes show microvesicular steatosis electron microscopy.

virtually diagnostic. Mitochondria are enlarged with decreased matrix density and fragmentation of the cristae (58). The enlargement of mitochondria correlates with the stage of encephalopathy.

Acute fatty liver of pregnancy, exposure to certain drugs (e.g., tetracycline, aflatoxin, and valproic acid), Jamaican vomiting sickness caused by ingestion of the unripe fruit of the ackee tree, defects of the urea cycle, and systemic carnitine deficiency are histologically similar, but clinical circumstances are different.

PARAPROTEIN DISORDERS

Amyloidosis

Amyloidosis is a systemic disease with at least four recognized forms: (a) primary or myeloma-related amyloidosis, associated with plasma cell dyscrasias, multiple myeloma, B-cell malignancies, and Waldenström disease, in which amyloid type A is found (19,46); (b) secondary or reactive amyloidosis, associated with long-standing chronic inflammatory diseases (27,31), Hodgkin lymphoma, and other malignant tumors, with amyloid A (AA) composed of apolipoprotein AA (17,23,26); (c) heredofamilial amyloidosis, inherited as an autosomal dominant disorder, with the protein component consisting of various transthyretins; and (d) a fourth form seen in renal patients on long-term hemodialysis, b2-microglobulinemia. The liver is usually involved in the first three forms. Approximately 20% of patients have hepatomegaly. Some develop jaundice and portal hypertension (19).

Amyloid is seen on routine hematoxylin-eosin–stained sections as pale eosinophilic or amphophilic, smudgy, amorphous, acellular material, usually deposited in the perisinusoidal space of Disse, in the vascular wall, or in the portal tract (Fig. 21.26, e-Figs. 21.51, 21.52). The characteristic apple-green birefringence after Congo red staining and polarization confirms the diagnosis (e-Fig. 21.53). With time, hepatocytes become compressed and atrophic.

Globular Amyloidosis

Pale eosinophilic amyloid globules deposit under the lining epithelium of large hepatic ducts, in the peribiliary glands, and on portal tract corrective tissue (Fig. 21.27, e-Figs. 21.54, 21.55) (42). Cholestasis and symptoms of large bile duct obstruction can ensue. Immunohistochemical stain for P component or immunofluorescent stain for thioflavine T can also be used.

Light-Chain Disease

Nonamyloid light-chain disease associated with plasma cell dyscrasias is seen in patients presenting with renal failure. Hepatomegaly with associated cholestasis can be seen. Light chain deposits are in the space of Disse and in portal tracts. These deposits generally do not stain with Congo red. Immunohistochemical studies show light chains, and sometimes heavy

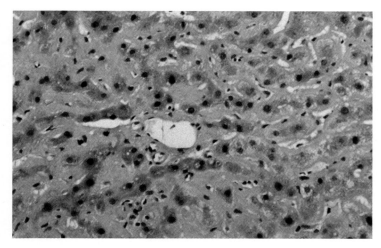

FIGURE 21.26 Amyloidosis, with amyloid deposited in the space of Disse (hematoxylin-eosin, original magnification ×100).

chains, as well as increased collagen type I and IV and fibronectin. Ultrastructurally, granular nonfibrillar material appears in the space of Disse.

THYROID DISORDERS

The liver synthesizes thyroid-binding protein, metabolizes thyroid hormones, and is the major site for conversion of thyroxine to 3,5,38-triiodothyronine. Consequently, abnormalities of thyroid function are sometimes seen with various acute and chronic hepatic disorders.

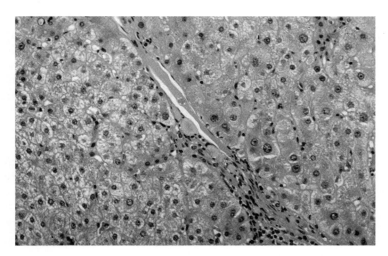

FIGURE 21.27 Globular amyloidosis. showing pale eosinophilic globules in a portal tract (hematoxylin-eosin, original magnification ×100).

Hyperthyroidism

Nonspecific changes can be seen, including mild macrovesicular steatosis, Kupffer cell hyperplasia, nuclear anisocytosis, and variable degrees, generally mild, of portal tract chronic inflammatory cell infiltration (6,68,74).

Hypothyroidism

Cholestasis has been described (4,5). Chronic autoimmune thyroiditis can be associated with primary biliary cirrhosis (see Chapter 17).

AUTOIMMUNE AND RELATED DISORDERS

Rheumatoid Arthritis

Generally only nonspecific changes are present, including steatosis, lipogranulomas, and fibrosis, perhaps related to treatment with corticosteroids and antimetabolites such as methotrexate (78). Sinusoidal dilatation and nodular hyperplasia are often seen in patients with Felty syndrome (rheumatoid arthritis, splenomegaly, and neutropenia) (12,20,34, 80,107). Spontaneous rupture of the liver has been described with rheumatoid vasculitis, but this will not likely be an issue of liver biopsy interpretation (34,80,107). Rheumatoid nodules are exceedingly rare and virtually never found in liver biopsy. In juvenile rheumatoid arthritis (Still disease), the liver biopsy shows only mild, nonspecific changes, although there may be significant elevation of serum transaminase values.

Systemic Lupus Erythematosus

Liver involvement is uncommon in systemic lupus erythematosus (SLE), with fewer than 10% of patients demonstrating elevations of serum transaminase values. Histologic changes are exceedingly rare and not consistent. There may be mild portal tract nonspecific chronic inflammation, occasional lobular granulomas, sinusoidal congestion, peliosis hepatis, nodular regenerative hyperplasia, PSC, and local hepatic infarction (2,43, 59,85). Macrovesicular steatosis can be seen after the treatment with corticosteroids. There is no association between antinuclear antibody–associated autoimmune hepatitis and SLE (see Chapter 10) (59).

Progressive Systemic Sclerosis

Chronic hepatitis has been described in some patients with progressive systemic sclerosis (scleroderma), as has nodular regenerative hyperplasia, PSC, PBC, and various changes secondary to vasculitis.

Polyarteritis Nodosa

The small branches of hepatic arteries can show typical vasculitis (e-Figs. 21.56, 21.57), with associated microscopic areas of infarction. Immune complexes containing HBV surface antigen have been demonstrated.

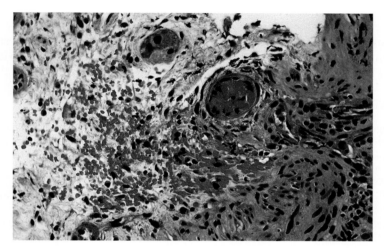

FIGURE 21.28   Cryoglobulinemia showing intravascular coagulation. Cryoglobulins were confirmed with immunofluorescence (hematoxylin-eosin, original magnification ×200).

Cryoglobulinemia

Chronic hepatitis due to HCV can lead to the development of essential (type II) mixed cryoglobulinemia. Patients generally present with the manifestations of cryoglobulinemia before liver disease is recognized (1). Cryoglobulin is demonstrable in hepatic vascular spaces. Immune complexes containing HCV antigen are also demonstrable (Fig. 21.28) (1,65).

Calcinosis, Raynaud Phenomenon, Esophageal Motility Disorders, Sclerodactyly, and Telangiectasia (CREST) Syndrome

Changes of PBC can be seen in patients with CREST syndrome.

Mixed Connective Tissue Disease

Mixed connective tissue disease is a rare disorder characterized by features of systemic lupus erythematosus, progressive systemic sclerosis, and polymyositis. It is associated with high titers of antibodies to the ribonucleoprotein fraction of extractable nuclear antigens and may also be associated with chronic hepatitis. Budd-Chiari syndrome has also been reported (62).

Polymyalgia Rheumatica

Granulomas may be seen in polymyalgia rheumatica. However, the findings are usually nonspecific, including macrovesicular steatosis and nodular regenerative hyperplasia.

Polymyositis

PBC can occur in patients with polymyositis (64,89).

Weber-Christian Disease

Macrovesicular steatosis, both without inflammation as well as with steato-hepatitis, is seen in patients with Weber-Christian disease (45). Mallory hyalin is observed in zone 1 (periportal) hepatocytes.

REFERENCES

1. Agnello V, Chung RT, Kaplan LM. Hepatitis C virus infection in type II cryoglobuline-mia. N Engl J Med 1992;327:1490–1495.
2. Albert-Flor JJ, Jeffers L, Schiff ER. Primary sclerosing cholangitis occurring in a patient with systemic lupus erythematosus and diabetes mellitus. Am J Gastroenterol 1984;79:889–891.
3. Al-Dalaan, Al-Balaa S, Ali MA, et al. Budd-Chiari syndrome in association with Behçet's disease. J Rheumatol 1991;18:622–626.
4. Ariza CR, Frate AC, Sierra I. Hypothyroidism-associated cholestasis. JAMA 1984;252:2392.
5. Babb RR. Association between diseases of the thyroid and the liver. Am J Gastroenterol 1984;79:421–423.
6. Baca L, Gibbons RB. The HELLP syndrome: a serious complication of pregnancy with hemolysis, elevated levels of liver enzymes, and low platelet count. Am J Med 1988;85:590–591.
7. Bach N, Theise ND, Schaffner F. Hepatic histopathology in the acquired immunodefi-ciency syndrome. Semin Liver Dis 1992;12:205–212.
8. Banks JG, Foulis AK, Ledingham IM, et al. Liver function in septic shock. J Clin Pathol 1982;35:1249–1252.
9. Barton JR, Riely CA, Adamec TA, et al. Hepatic histopathologic condition does not cor-relate with laboratory abnormalities in HELLP syndrome (hemolysis, elevated liver enzymes, and low platelet count). Am J Obstet Gynecol 1992;167:1538–1543.
10. Batman PA, Scheuer PJ. Diabetic hepatitis preceding the onset of glucose intolerance. Histopathology 1985;9:237–243.
11. Bernauau D, Guillot R, Durand AM, et al. Ultrastructural aspects of the liver perisinu-soidal space in diabetic patients with and without cholangiopathy. Diabetes 1982;31:1061–1067.
12. Blendis LM, Ansell ID, Lloyd-Jones K, et al. Liver in Felty's syndrome. Br Med J 1970;1:131–135.
13. Bondini S, Kleiner DE, Goodman ZD, et al. Pathologic assessment of non-alcoholic fatty liver disease. Clin Liver Dis 2007;11:17–23.
14. Brown RE, Ishak KG. Hepatic zonal degeneration and necrosis in Reye's syndrome. Arch Pathol Lab Med 1976;100:123–126.
15. Bruguera M, Caballero T, Carreras E, et al. Hepatic sinusoidal dilatation in association with Hodgkin's disease. Liver 1987;7:76–80.
16. Brunt EM, Janney CG, Di Bisceglie AM, et al. Nonalcoholic steatohepatitis: a proposal for grading and staging the histological lesions. Am J Gastroenterol 1999;94:2467–2474.
17. Castillo I, Bartolome J, Medejon A, et al. Hepatitis delta virus RNA detection in chronic HBsAg carriers with and without HIV infection. Digestion 1991;48:149–156.
18. Chesner IM, Muller S, Newman J. Ulcerative colitis complicated by Budd-Chiari syn-drome. Gut 1986;27:1096–1100.
19. Chopra S, Rubinow A, Koff RS, et al. Hepatic amyloidosis. A histopathologic analysis of primary (AL) and secondary (AA) forms. Am J Pathol 1994;115:186–193.

20. Cohen MD, Ginsburg WW, Allen GL. Nodular regenerative hyperplasia of the liver and bleeding esophageal varices in Felty's syndrome: a case report and literature review. J Rheumatol 1982;9:716–728.

21. Czapar CA, Weldo-Linne CM, Moore DM, et al. Peliosis hepatis in the acquired immunodeficiency syndrome. Arch Pathol Lab Med 1986;110:611–613.

22. De la Monte SM, Arcide JM, Moore GW, et al. Midzonal necrosis as a pattern of hepatocellular injury after shock. Gastroenterology 1984;86:627–631.

23. Devaney K, Goodman ZD, Epstein MS, et al. Hepatic sarcoidosis. Clinicopathologic features in 100 patients. Am J Surg Pathol 1993;17:1272–1280.

24. Dubois A, Dauzat M, Pignodel C, et al. Portal hypertension in lymphoproliferative and myeloproliferative disorders: hemodynamic and histologic correlation. Hepatology 1993;17:246–250.

25. Duffy LF, Daum F, Kahn E, et al. Hepatitis in children with acquired immunodeficiency syndrome. Histopathologic and immunocytologic features. Gastroenterology 1986;90: 173–181.

26. Falk S, Helm EB, Hubner K, et al. Disseminated visceral leishmaniasis (kala azar) in acquired immunodeficiency syndrome (AIDS). Pathol Res Pract 1988;183:253–255.

27. Fausa O, Nygaard K, Elgjo K. Amyloidosis and Crohn's disease. Scand J Gastroenterol 1977;12:657–662.

28. Favara BE. Hemophagocytic lymphohistiocytosis: a hemophagocytic syndrome. Semin Diagn Pathol 1992;9:63–74.

29. Foster JH, Donohue TA, Berman MM. Familial liver cell adenomas and diabetes mellitus. N Engl J Med 1978;299:239–241.

30. Garcia-Tsao G, Panzini L, Yoselevitz M, et al. Bacillary peliosis hepatis as a cause of acute anemia in a patient with the acquired immunodeficiency syndrome. Gastroenterology 1992;102:1065–1070.

31. Gitkind MJ, Wright SC. Amyloidosis complicating inflammatory bowel disease; a case report and review of the literature. Dig Dis Sci 1990;35:906–908.

32. Gordon SC, Reddy KR, Gould EE, et al. The spectrum of liver disease in the acquired immune deficiency syndrome (AIDS). Liver 1986;6:158–166.

33. Guarner J, del Rio C, Carr D, et al. Non-Hodgkin's lymphomas in patients with human immunodeficiency virus infection: presence of Epstein-Barr virus in situ hybridization, clinical presentation, and follow-up. Cancer 1991;68:2460–2465.

34. Harris M, Rash RM, Dymock IW. Nodular non-cirrhotic liver associated with portal hypertension in a patient with rheumatoid arthritis. J Clin Pathol 1974;27:963–966.

35. Hasan AF, Jeffers JL, Dickinson G, et al. Hepatobiliary cryptosporidiosis and cytomegalovirus infection mimicking metastatic cancer of the liver. Gastroenterology 1991;110:1743–1747.

36. Hay JE, Wiesner RH, Shorter RG, et al. Primary sclerosing cholangitis and celiac disease; a novel association. Gastroenterology 1988;94:A545.

37. Horsburgh CR Jr. *Mycobacterium avium* complex infection in the acquired immunodeficiency syndrome. N Engl J Med 1991;324:1332–1338.

38. Housset C, Lamas E, Courgnaud V, et al. Presence of HIV-1 in human parenchymal and non-parenchymal cells in vivo. J Hepatol 1993;19:252–258.

39. Hubscher SG, Lumley MA, Elias E. Vanishing bile duct syndrome: a possible mechanism for intrahepatic cholestasis in Hodgkin's lymphoma. Hepatology 1993;17:70–77.

40. Ishak KG, Rogers WA. Cryptogenic acute cholangitis: association with toxic shock syndrome. Am J Clin Pathol 1981;76:619–626.

41. Kahn E, Greco MA, Daum F, et al. Hepatic pathology in pediatric acquired immunodeficiency syndrome. Hum Pathol 1991;22:1111–1118.

42. Kanel GC, Uchida T, Peters RL. Globular hepatic amyloid: an unusual morphologic presentation. Hepatology 1981;1:647–652.

43. Khoury G, Tobi M, Oren M, et al. Massive hepatic infarction in systemic lupus erythematosus. Dig Dis Sci 1990;35:1557–1560.

44. Kilpatrick ZM. Structural and functional abnormalities of liver in infectious mononucleosis. Arch Intern Med 1966;117:47–53.

45. Kimura H, Kako M, Yo K, et al. Alcoholic hyalins (Mallory bodies) in a case of Weber-Christian disease: electron microscopic observation of liver involvement. Gastroenterology 1986;78:807–812.

46. Kirkpatrick CJ, Curry A, Galle J, et al. Systemic kappa light chain deposition and amyloidosis in multiple myeloma: novel morphological observations. Histopathology 1986;5:178–185.

47. Kleiner DE, Brunt EM, Van Natta M, et al. Design and validation of a histological scoring system for nonalcoholic fatty liver disease. Hepatology 2005;41:1313–1321.

48. Knowles DM, Chamulak GA, Subar M, et al. Lymphoid neoplasia associated with the acquired immunodeficiency syndrome. Ann Intern Med 1988;108:744–753.

49. Lai KK, Gang DL, Zawacki JK, et al. Fulminant hepatic failure with 28,38-dideoxyinosine (ddI). Ann Intern Med 1991;115:283–284.

50. Latry P, Bioulac-Sage P, Echinard E, et al. Perisinusoidal fibrosis and basement membrane-like material in the livers of diabetic patients. Hum Pathol 1987;18:775–780.

51. Leboit PE, Berger TC, Egbert BM, et al. Bacillary angiomatosis: the histopathology and differential diagnosis of a pseudoneoplastic infection in patients with human immunodeficiency virus disease. Am J Surg Pathol 1989;13:909–920.

52. Lefkowitch JH. Bile ductular cholestasis: an ominous histopathologic sign related to sepsis and "cholangitis lenta." Hum Pathol 1982;13:19–24.

53. Lefkowitch JH, Fakow S, Whitlock RT. Hepatic Hodgkin's disease simulating cholestatic hepatitis with liver failure. Arch Pathol Lab Med 1985;109:424–426.

54. Lefkowitch JH, Mendez L. Morphological features of hepatic injury in cardiac disease and shock. J Hepatol 1986;2:313–327.

55. Leibowitz AI, Hartman RC. The Budd-Chiari syndrome and paroxysmal nocturnal hemoglobinuria. Br J Hematol 1981;48:1–6.

56. Lesens O, Deschenes M, Steben M, et al. Hepatitis C virus is related to progressive liver disease in HIV-positive hemophiliacs and should be treated as an opportunistic infection. J Infect Dis 1999;179:1254–1258.

57. Ludwig J, Braham SS, LaRusso NF, et al. Morphological features of chronic hepatitis associated with primary sclerosing cholangitis and chronic ulcerative colitis. Hepatology 1981;1:632–640.

58. Maccini DM, Berg JC, Bell GA. Budd-Chiari syndrome and Crohn's disease. An unreported association. Dig Dis Sci 1989;34:1933–1936.

59. Mackay IR. The hepatitis–lupus connection. Semin Liver Dis 1991;11:234–240.

60. Mahmond H, Gaber O, Wang W, et al. Successful orthotopic liver transplantation in a child with Langerhans cell histiocytosis. Transplantation 1991;51:278–280.

61. Margulis SJ, Honig CL, Siave R. Biliary tract obstruction in the acquired immunodeficiency syndrome. Ann Intern Med 1986;105:207–210.

62. Marshall JB, Ravendran N, Sharp GC. Liver disease in mixed connective tissue disease syndrome. Arch Intern Med 1983;143:1817–1818.

63. McMaster KR, Hennigar GR. Drug-induced granulomatous hepatitis. Lab Invest 1981;44:61–73.

64. Milosevic M, Adams PC. Primary biliary cirrhosis and polymyositis. J Clin Gastroenterol 1990;12:332–335.

65. Misiani R, Bellavita P, Fenili D, et al. Hepatitis C virus infection in patients with essential mixed cryoglobulinemia. Ann Intern Med 1992;117:573–577.
66. Molina JM, Welker Y, Ferchal F, et al. Hepatitis associated with primary HIV infection. Correspondence. Gastroenterology 1992;102:739.
67. Nizalik E, Zayed E, Foyle A. Malignant lymphoma presenting as fulminant hepatic failure. Can J Gastroenterol 1989;3:111–114.
68. Ochmer SA, Brunt EM, Cohn S, et al. Fulminant hepatic failure caused by acute fatty liver of pregnancy treated by orthotopic liver transplantation. Hepatology 1990;11:59–64.
69. Pereira A, Bruguera M, Cervantes F, et al. Liver involvement at diagnosis of primary myelofibrosis: a clinicopathological study of twenty cases. Eur J Hematol 1988;40: 355–361.
70. Perkocha LA, Geaghan SM, Yen TSB, et al. Clinical and pathological features of bacillary peliosis hepatis in association with human immunodeficiency virus infection. N Engl J Med 1990;323:1581–1586.
71. Petrovic LM. HIV/HCV co-infection: histopathologic findings, natural history, fibrosis and impact of antiretroviral treatment. Liver Int 2007;27(5):598–606.
72. Piroth L, Duong M, Quantin C, et al. Does hepatitis C virus co-infection accelerate clinical and immunological evolution of HIV-infected patients? AIDS 1998;12:381–388.
73. Pol S, Romana C, Richard S, et al. Microsporidia infection in patients with the human immunodeficiency virus and unexplained cholangitis. N Engl J Med 1993;328:95–99.
74. Pollock DJ. The liver in celiac disease. Histopathology 1977;1:421–430.
75. Pottipati AR, Dave PB, Gumaste V, et al. Tuberculous abscess of the liver in acquired immunodeficiency syndrome. J Clin Gastroenterol 1991;13:549–553.
76. Pursell KJ, Telzak EE, Armstrong D. *Aspergillus* species colonization and invasive disease in patients with AIDS. Clin Infect Dis 1992;14:141–148.
77. Randhawa PS, Markin RS, Starzl TE, et al. Epstein-Barr virus-associated syndromes in immunosuppressed liver transplant patients. Am J Surg Pathol 1990;14:538–547.
78. Rau R, Karger T, Herborn G, et al. Liver biopsy findings in patients with rheumatoid arthritis undergoing long-term treatment with methotrexate. J Rheumatol 1989;16: 489–493.
79. Reye RDK, Morgan G, Baral J. Encephalopathy and fatty degeneration of the viscera, a disease entity in childhood. Lancet 1963;2:749–752.
80. Reynolds WJ, Wanless IR. Nodular regenerative hyperplasia of the liver in a patient with rheumatoid vasculitis: a morphometric study suggesting a role of hepatic arteritis in the pathogenesis. J Rheumatol 1984;11:838–842.
81. Riely CA. Acute fatty liver of pregnancy. Semin Liver Dis 1987;7:47–54.
82. Rolfes DB, Ishak KG. Liver disease in pregnancy. Histopathology 1986;10:555–570.
83. Rolfes DB, Ishak KG. Liver disease in toxemia of pregnancy. Am J Gastroenterol 1986;81:1138–1144.
84. Ross JS, Del Rosario A, Bui HX, et al. Primary hepatic leiomyosarcoma in a child with the acquired immunodeficiency syndrome. Hum Pathol 1992;23:69–72.
85. Runyon BA, LeBrecqui DR, Anuras S. The spectrum of liver disease in systemic lupus erythematosus: report of 33 histologically proved cases and review of the literature. Am J Med 1980;69:187–194.
86. Sabin CA, Telfer P, Phillips AN, et al. The association between hepatitis C virus genotype and HIV disease progression in a cohort of hemophiliac men. J Infect Dis 1997;175:164–168.
87. Sachs JR, Greenfield SM, Sohn M, et al. Disseminated *Pneumocystis carinii* infection with hepatic involvement in a patient with the acquired immune deficiency syndrome. Am J Gastroenterol 1991;86:82–85.

88. Saint-Marc, Girardin M-F, Zafrani ES, et al. Hepatic granulomas in Whipple's disease. Gastroenterology 1984;86:753–756.
89. Sattar MA, Guindi RT, Khan RA, et al. Polymyositis and hepatocellular carcinoma. Clin Rheumatol 1988;7:538–542.
90. Scoazec JY, Marche C, Girad PM, et al. Peliosis hepatis and sinusoidal dilatation during infection with the human immunodeficiency virus (HIV). Am J Pathol 1991;130:38–47.
91. Scully PA, Steinman HK, Kennedy C, et al. AIDS-related Kaposi's sarcoma displays differential expression of endothelial surface antigens. Am J Pathol 1988;130:244–251.
92. Shiramizu B, Herndier B, Meeker T, et al. Molecular and immunophenotypic characterization of AIDS-associated Epstein-Barr virus–negative, polyclonal lymphoma. J Clin Oncol 1992;10:383–389.
93. Slater LN, Welch DF, Min KW. *Rochalimaea henselae* causes bacillary angiomatosis and peliosis hepatis. Arch Intern Med 1992;152:602–606.
94. Soto B, Sanchez-Quijano A, Rodrigo L, et al. HIV infection modifies the natural history of chronic parenterally acquired hepatitis C with an unusual rapid progression to cirrhosis. A multicenter study on 547 patients. J Hepatol 1997;26:1–5.
95. Steffan A-M, Lafon M-E, Gendrault J-L, et al. Primary cultures of endothelial cells from the human liver sinusoid are permissive for human immunodeficiency virus type 1. Proc Natl Acad Sci U S A 1992;12:197–204.
96. Steeper TA, Rosenstein H, Weiser J, et al. Bacillary epithelioid angiomatosis involving the liver, spleen, and skin in an AIDS patient with concurrent Kaposi's sarcoma. Am J Clin Pathol 1992;97:713–718.
97. Sty JR. Hepatic vein thrombosis in sickle cell anemia. Am J Pediatr Hematol Oncol 1982;4:213–215.
98. Terada S, Reddy KR, Jeffers LJ, et al. Microsporidian hepatitis in the acquired immunodeficiency syndrome. Ann Intern Med 1987;107:61–62.
99. Thiruvengadam R, Penetranti R, Grolsky HJ, et al. Multiple myeloma presenting as space-occupying lesion of the liver. Cancer 1990;65:2784–2786.
100. Thung SN, Gerber MA, Bodenheimer HC Jr. Nodular regenerative hyperplasia of the liver in a patient with diabetes mellitus. Cancer 1982;49:543–546.
101. Vanjak D, Moreau R, Roche-Sciot J, et al. Intrahepatic cholestasis of pregnancy and acute fatty liver of pregnancy. An unusual but favorable association? Gastroenterology 1991;100:1123–1125.
102. Voinchet O, Degott C, Scoazec J-Y, et al. Peliosis hepatis, nodular regenerative hyperplasia of the liver, and light chain deposition in patient with Waldenström's macroglobulinemia. Gastroenterology 1988;95:482–486.
103. Waldman RJ, Hall WN, McGee H, et al. Aspirin as a risk factor in Reye's syndrome. JAMA 1990;150:456–459.
104. Welch DF, Pickett DA, Salter LN, et al. *Rochalimaea henselae* sp., a cause of septicemia, bacillary angiomatosis, and parenchymal peliosis. J Clin Microbiol 1992;30:275–280.
105. Witzleben CL, Marshall GS, Wenner W, et al. HIV as a cause of giant cell hepatitis. Hum Pathol 1988;19:603–605.
106. Woolf GM, Petrovic LM, Rojter SE, et al. Acute liver failure due to lymphoma: a diagnostic concern when considering liver transplantation. Dig Dis Sci 1994;39:1351–1358.
107. Young ID, Segura J, Ford PM, et al. The pathogenesis of nodular regenerative hyperplasia of the liver associated with rheumatoid vasculitis. J Clin Gastroenterol 1992;14:127–131.
108. Zafrani ES, Degos F, Guigui B, et al. The hepatic sinusoid in hairy cell leukemia: an ultrastructural study of 12 cases. Hum Pathol 1987;18:801–807.
109. Zafrani ES, Gaulard P. Primary lymphoma of the liver. Liver 1993;13:57–61.
110. Zimmerli W, Bianchi L, Gudat F, et al. Disseminated herpes simplex type 2 and systemic Candida infection in a patient with previous asymptomatic HIV infection. J Infect Dis 1988;157:597–598.

22

BACTERIAL, SPIROCHETAL, RICKETTSIAL, CHLAMYDIAL, PROTOZOAL, AND HELMINTHIC CAUSES OF HEPATITIS

Nonviral infectious agents can affect the liver, contributing to a hepatitis-like picture clinically and morphologically. These conditions are rarely encountered by a pathologist not practicing in respective endemic areas. However, in the era of modern travel as well as changing responses to therapy, they can occasionally be seen anywhere (42). Many infectious disorders occur as complications of acquired immunodeficiency syndrome (AIDS) or in other immunocompromised conditions, causd by chemotherapy or in the setting of organ transplantation.

BACTERIAL CAUSES OF HEPATITIS

Typhoid Fever

Typhoid fever, caused by *Salmonella typhi*, is rare in Western countries, except when acquired abroad (42). Early, the liver shows nonspecific reactive changes including lymphocytosis, focal hepatocyte necrosis, and Kupffer cell hypertrophy. Erythrophagocytosis can sometimes be seen, as can small nonnecrotizing epithelioid granulomas and microvesicular steatosis. In the symptomatic stage (fastigium) hepatosplenomegaly is present, sometimes with jaundice. Granulomas, when present, can enlarge and become necrotic (e-Figs. 22.1, 22.2). Bacilli are generally not demonstrable with Gram's stain, although they are readily recoverable from the bile and gallbladder. Cholangitis is rare.

Brucellosis

Humans can be infected with *Brucella* through occupational exposure or ingestion of milk products (17). Brucellosis mimics many clinical conditions. The infective agent is difficult to culture, and serologic tests establish the diagnosis. A nonspecific hepatitis, with nonnecrotizing granulomas, is seen (13). Cirrhosis is unusual.

Melioidosis

Burkholderia pseudomallei, the cause of melioidosis, occurs in tropical zones and only rarely in the Western hemisphere (7). Approximately 10% of Americans who served in the Vietnam War had antibodies, but there were only 300 cases and 50 deaths documented (41). Hepatosplenomegaly and jaundice are common. In acute stages abscesses of varying sizes are seen with bacilli demonstrable with Gram's or Giemsa stain. Necrotic granulomas then form; they either resemble typical tuberculosis granulomas or show stellate appearance, similar to those seen in *Yersinia* infections or cat-scratch disease.

Listeriosis

Listeria monocytogenes affects pregnant women and can be transmitted transplacentally (11). It also occurs in immunosuppressed individuals and only rarely in immunocompetent adults (12). Microabscesses are seen in the liver, with abundant Gram-negative rods. Granulomas can also be seen. In some cases, however, the biopsy can show features resembling viral hepatitis.

Cat-Scratch Disease

The liver is rarely involved in cat-scratch disease without clinically demonstrable lymphadenopathy (20). Characteristic granulomas of cat-scratch disease are described as stellate, usually with central necrosis. Bacilli are generally not demonstrable with Gram's stain but can be seen with silver impregnation methods. Bile ducts can be involved.

Actinomycosis

Actinomycosis of the liver is usually secondary to intra-abdominal infection, with transmission via the portal vein or thoracic infection. There are often multiple hepatic abscesses, which contain colonies of *Actinomyces*.

SPIROCHETAL CAUSES OF HEPATITIS

Syphilis
      Hepatic syphilis is exceedingly rare. The liver is typically not involved in primary syphilis.

Secondary Syphilis

In secondary syphilis, spirochetes become widely disseminated. Hepatitis can clinically be documented (6,37). There is often focal necrosis of hepatocytes, with portal inflammation and periductal inflammatory infiltrate rich in polymorphonuclear leukocytes and sometimes granulomas. Portal vessels can show vasculitis (51,53).

Tertiary Syphilis

The gumma is the characteristic lesion of tertiary syphilis. It can be quite large and clinically mistaken for a tumor. Gummas are giant cell granulomas with central necrosis, similar to those of tuberculosis. In contrast to caseation, the outlines of cellular architecture are not completely effaced. Plasma cells are usually prominent and an associated obliterative endarteritis may be present. Healing by fibrosis distorts the liver into nodule-like divisions of varying size (hepar lobatum) (53) (e-Figs. 22.3, 22.4). There is portal hypertension.

Congenital Syphilis

Congenital syphilis can manifest early during pregnancy or can be neonatal. Multiple, tiny, miliary-like foci of necrosis with giant cell response and associated portal inflammation are seen (e-Figs. 22.5, 22.6). Silver impregnation demonstrates numerous spirochetes when necrosis is prominent. Progressive pericellular fibrosis with liver plate atrophy and, ultimately, hepar lobatum may be seen.

Leptospirosis (Weil Disease)

Leptospira icterohemorrhagica is acquired from animals, but severe hepatorenal disease can be caused by various *Leptospira* serotypes. Biopsy shows severe cholestasis, most prominent in zones 3 and 2, with varying degrees of regenerative activity, including binucleate forms and mitoses (10). Extensive hepatocyte apoptosis is seen, with viral replication within hepatocytes (54), but balloon cells are relatively uncommon. Portal and lobular inflammation are not prominent. There is little or no steatosis.

Borreliosis (Relapsing Fever)

Liver biopsy, which is rarely performed in borreliosis because of the typical coagulopathy, shows multifocal liver cell necrosis with hemorrhage. Lymphocytes and polymorphonuclear leukocytes infiltrate sinusoids, with prominent Kupffer cells and erythrophagocytosis (34).

Lyme Disease

Lyme disease is a multisystem infection, with both acute and chronic phases. Liver involvement is usually not dominant (25,29). Acutely, mild portal tract inflammation is seen. In recurrent disease, hepatitis is more prominent, with prominent sinusoidal infiltration by lymphocytes and polymorphonuclear leukocytes. Hepatocytes are ballooned, with mitoses, and there is microvesicular steatosis and Kupffer cell hyperplasia.

MYCOBACTERIAL CAUSES OF HEPATITIS

Tuberculosis

Tuberculosis remains a disease of major importance worldwide, with frequent involvement of the liver (16). Typically, caseating granulomas can be seen in the lobule or portal tracts. Bacilli can be few or even undetectable, although molecular techniques, such as polymerase chain reaction, can establish the diagnosis (3,56).

Early, the lesion resembles a typical bacterial microabscess; this stage is exceedingly transient and rarely seen in the biopsy material. Granulomas sometimes have a relatively modest epithelioid and giant cell reaction, and the dominant feature may be central fibrinoid necrosis in which acid-fast bacilli are generally easily demonstrated (immature granuloma) (e-Figs. 22.7, 22.8).

In immunosuppressed individuals, innumerable acid-fast bacilli may be seen, with a picture resembling that of *Mycobacterium avium-intracellulare* (MAI) complex infection.

Leprosy

Liver involvement is uncommon (15). In lepromatous patients, abundant foamy macrophage clusters are distributed randomly throughout the liver, with acid-fast bacilli easily demonstrable. A polymorphonuclear neutrophilic reaction is seen at this stage (36). In the tuberculoid stage, granulomas are seen but acid-fast bacilli are scanty or absent. Amyloidosis can also be seen in the liver biopsy in patients with long-standing disease.

RICKETTSIAL AND CHLAMYDIAL CAUSES OF HEPATITIS

Q Fever

Q fever, caused by *Coxiella burnetti*, is transmitted by inhalation. Next to fever, hepatic involvement is the most common clinical feature. The typical lesion is a fibrin-ring granuloma, with a peripheral rim of epithelioid histiocytes with lymphocytes and occasional Langhans giant cells, within which there is a fibrin layer (Fig. 22.1) (5,32,47). The fibrin-ring granuloma characteristically surrounds an empty space that is usually about the size of a large fat vesicle (e-Figs. 22.9–22.13). Tuberculoid granulomas with central necrosis are also seen. The fibrin-ring granuloma is not pathognomonic for Q fever and can be seen in other infections (39,44,45).

Boutonneuse Fever

In boutonneuse fever, liver inflammation occurs without clinical evidence of hepatitis. Usually there is focal liver cell necrosis without granulomas, often accompanied by a lymphocytic infiltrate but with unremarkable portal tracts (26,31,58). Immunohistochemical reactions demonstrate rickettsial antigen in sinusoidal endothelial cells.

Chlamydial Infection

The liver can be involved in psittacosis and in genital infection. In psittacosis, there may be jaundice and hepatomegaly. The liver shows focal hepatocyte necrosis and Kupffer cell hypertrophy (60). In genital

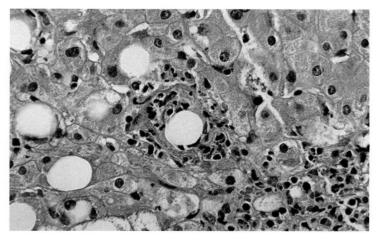

FIGURE 22.1   Fibrin-ring granuloma in Q fever (hematoxylin-eosin, original magnification ×200).

chlamydial infection (*Chlamydia trachomatis*) there may be an associated perihepatitis (Fitz-Hugh and Curtis syndrome) (60).

PROTOZOAL CAUSES OF HEPATITIS

Malaria

The characteristic feature of malaria in the liver is malarial pigment (a molecule consisting of iron and a protein moiety) in erythrocytes and Kupffer cells during the stage of parasitemia and later in portal macrophages (Fig. 22.2, e-Figs. 22.13, 22.14). Sinusoids are distended by red blood cells in which parasites are often visible. Lobular or portal inflammation is generally mild (19,21,33). Liver cells may show glycogen depletion. With shock there may be zone 3 necrosis and cholestasis. Malarial antigen can be demonstrated within liver cells (23).

Amebiasis

The hallmark of liver involvement is the amebic abscess, usually in the right lobe and often multiple. The diagnosis should be considered in any case of liver abscess (30). Prior to the development of an abscess, the amebic trophozoites can be found in the sinusoids, with associated edema and focal coagulative necrosis and only a mild polymorphonuclear leukocyte response (2) (e-Fig. 22.15). The trophozoites resemble macrophages but tend to have a somewhat bluer cytoplasm. Erythrophagocytosis is common. The organisms can be highlighted with trichrome stain and periodic acid–Schiff reaction, and demonstrated immunohistochemically. With increasing lysis, the central, necrotic portion of the abscess enlarges. Older lesions become fibrotic. The surrounding liver is often edematous, showing

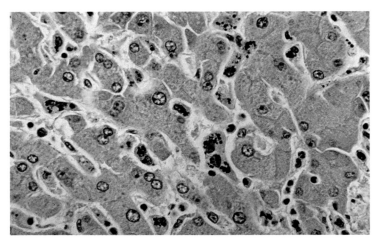

FIGURE 22.2   Malarial pigment in Kupffer cells (hematoxylin-eosin, original magnification ×400).

the changes typical of space-occupying lesions. There may be marked cholestasis (46).

Leishmaniasis

Visceral leishmaniasis (kala azar) is caused by several species of *Leishmania* and is seen in AIDS (9). Kupffer cells are prominent, and there is a diffuse sinusoidal and portal chronic inflammation with many plasma cells (Fig. 22.3). Parasites are generally demonstrable in both portal macrophages and Kupffer cells and, rarely, in hepatocytes (22). In

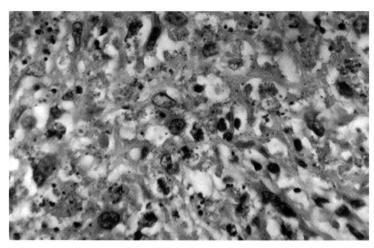

FIGURE 22.3   Leishmaniasis in a patient with acquired immune deficiency syndrome (hematoxylin-eosin, original magnification ×400).

another form of hepatic leishmaniasis, macrophage clusters are seen within the parenchyma containing only rare parasites. Epithelioid granulomas, with varying degrees of central necrosis, may be seen, and fibrin-ring granulomas, similar to those of Q fever, have been described (44). Steatosis is common, and there may be jaundice. Sometimes there may be hemorrhagic necrosis, perhaps a result of shock.

Balantidiasis

Balantidium coli is a rare cause of dysentery and, as with amebiasis, can cause liver abscess.

Toxoplasmosis

Congenital toxoplasmosis may present as giant cell hepatitis. More often the liver biopsy shows multiple foci of necrosis, with enlarged sinusoidal cells in which the parasites can be demonstrated. In acquired toxoplasmosis there can be a severe hepatitis with foci of necrosis and cholestasis (56). Nonnecrotizing giant and epithelioid cell granulomas can also be seen (59).

Babesiosis

In babesiosis, transmitted by ticks, the liver shows parasite-containing erythrocytes distending sinusoids, with Kupffer cell hyperplasia and zone 3 ischemic necrosis.

HELMINTHIC CAUSES OF HEPATITIS

Ascariasis

The *Ascaris* worms fill and distend the grossly visible bile ducts, causing liver biopsy changes similar to those of any large duct obstruction (28,35). (e-Figs. 22.16–2.18)

Schistosomiasis

In the early stages of schistosomiasis, eggs become trapped in portal vein radicles where they elicit an eosinophilic reaction; sometimes this results in an eosinophilic abscess with abundant fibrin deposition (24,48). Subsequently, an epithelioid and giant cell granuloma forms (12). Schistosomal pigment, indistinguishable from malarial pigment, is present in portal macrophages and Kupffer cells. Portal fibrosis eventually develops, leading to portal hypertension and the characteristic pipe stem pattern of fibrosis seen microscopically (24) (e-Fig. 22.19).

Echinococcosis

The larval forms of *Echinococcus granulosus* and *Echinococcus multilocularis* cause hydatid disease of the liver. Liver biopsy can be dangerous, potentially leading to dissemination through the abdominal cavity.

E. granulosus forms a spherical cyst with a complex wall consisting of an outer acellular laminated membrane and an inner transparent germinal membrane to which the budding protoscolices attach. Host reaction is modest with some granulation tissue. Eosinophils are usually not prominent.

In *E. multilocularis* there is no fibrous rim and the cyst wall is relatively thin. The wall is laminated, but there is no germinal layer and protoscolices are not seen. The membranes invade necrotic liver tissue, and there is a variable, generally mild, host response (e-Fig. 22.20).

Clonorchiasis

The liver fluke *Clonorchis sinensis*, found principally in the Far East, is acquired by the ingestion of uncooked freshwater fish (38). The worms thrive in the distal bile ducts, but in severe cases they can be found in the proximal bile ducts and the gallbladder. The liver biopsy initially shows dilated interlobular bile ducts and ascending cholangitis, and sometimes abscess formation, with subsequent chronic inflammation, including many eosinophils, and fibrosis. Worms are generally not seen in the interlobular bile ducts. The larger bile ducts show epithelial hyperplasia. Multicentric, mucin-secreting cholangiocarcinoma may develop (8,27).

Opisthorchiasis

Infection with *Opisthorchis* species flukes occurs less frequently than with *Clonorchis*, but the manifestations are essentially the same, including the development of cholangiocarcinoma.

Enterobiasis

Rarely *Enterobius vermicularis* can manifest as nodules of the liver (enterobioma) (18,43). A necrotic center is surrounded by a granulomatous reaction, which becomes fibrotic.

Strongyloidiasis

The larvae of *Strongyloides vermicularis* are present in small portal vessels and in sinusoids, often without significant inflammation. There may be a chronic inflammatory cell infiltrate, often with multinucleated giant cells (49).

Capillariasis

Adult worms and eggs of *Capillaria hepatica* can be seen in the liver, with marked infiltration by eosinophils and a granulomatous reaction.

Toxocariasis (Visceral Larva Migrans)

Visceral larva migrans is primarily a disease of children (52). The liver shows small foci of necrosis, with many eosinophils and variable numbers of histiocytes and giant cells (55). The granulomas are often somewhat cylindrical and elongated, representing long tracts of tissue destruction.

Fascioliasis

Humans are only occasionally infected as a result of eating contaminated watercress. The fluke migrates to the large bile ducts and the gallbladder (38). As the fluke migrates through the liver, an inflammatory tract develops marked necrosis and eosinophilia, with eventual fibrosis. Bile duct dilatation occurs, as in clonorchiasis, with inflammatory and proliferative changes of the bile duct epithelium (1,17,51). Cholangiocarcinoma has not been reported.

REFERENCES

1. Acosta-Ferreira W, Vercelli-Hetta J, Falconi LM. Fasciola hepatica human infection. Virchows Arch A 1979;383:319–327.
2. Adams EB, MacLeod IN. Invasive amebiasis. II. Amebic liver abscess and its complications. Medicine 1977;56:325–334.
3. Akcan Y, Tuncer S, Hayran M, et al. PCR on disseminated tuberculosis in bone marrow and liver biopsy specimens: correlation to histopathological and clinical diagnosis. Scand J Infect Dis 1997;29:271–274.
4. Andrade ZA, Peixoto E, Guerret S, et al. Hepatic connective tissue changes in hepatosplenic schistosomiasis. Hum Pathol 1992;23:566–673.
5. Atienza P, Raymond M-J, Degott C, et al. Chronic Q fever hepatitis complicated by extensive fibrosis. Gastroenterology 1988;95:478–481.
6. Baker AL, Kaplan MM, Wolfe HJ, et al. Liver disease associated with early syphilis. N Engl J Med 1971;284:1422–1423.
7. Barnes OF, Appleman MD, Cosgrove MM. A case of melioidosis originating in North America. Am Rev Respir Dis 1986;134:170–171.
8. Belamaric J. Intrahepatic bile duct carcinoma and *C. sinensis* infection in Hong Kong. Cancer 1973;31:468–473.
9. Berenguer J, Moreno S, Cercenado E, et al. Visceral leishmaniasis in patients infected with human immunodeficiency virus (HIV). Ann Intern Med 1989;111:129–132.
10. Bhamarapravati N, Boonyapaknavig V, Viarnuvatti V, et al. Liver changes in leptospirosis: a study of needle biopsies in 22 cases. Am J Proctol 1966;17:480–487.
11. Bourgeois N, Jacobs F, Tavares ML, et al. *Listeria monocytogenes* in a liver transplant recipient: case report and review of the literature. J Hepatol 1993;18:284–289.
12. Brito JM, Borojevic R. Liver granulomas in schistosomiasis: mast cell–dependent induction of SCF expression in hepatic stellate cells is mediated by TNF-alpha. J Leukoc Biol 1997;62:389–396.
13. Cervantes F, Carbonell J, Bruguera M, et al. Liver disease in brucellosis. A clinical and pathologic study of 40 cases. Postgrad Med J 1982;58:346–350.
14. Chen MG, Mott KE. Progress in assessment of morbidity due to Fasciola hepatica infection. Trop Dis Bull 1990;87:R1–R37.
15. Chen TSN, Drutz DJ, Whelan GE. Hepatic granulomas in leprosy. Arch Pathol Lab Med 1976;100:182–185.
16. Cook GC. Liver involvement in systemic infection. Eur J Gastroenterol Hepatol 1997;9:1239–1247.
17. Corbel MJ. Brucellosis: an overview. Emerg Infect Dis 1997;3:213–221.
18. Daly JJ, Baker GF. Pinworm granuloma of the liver. Am J Trop Med Hyg 1984;33:62–64.
19. de Brito T, Barone AA, Faria RM. Human liver biopsy in *P. falciparum* and *P. vivax* malaria: a light and electron microscopy study. Virchows Arch A 1969;348:220–229.

20. Delbeke D, Sandler MP, Shaff MI, et al. Cat-scratch disease: report of a case with liver lesions and no lymphadenopathy. J Nucl Med 1988;29:1454–1456.
21. Deller JJ, Cifarelli PS, Berque S, et al. Malaria hepatitis. Milit Med 1967;132:614–620.
22. Duarte MIS, Mariano ON, Corbett CEP. Liver parenchymal cell parasitism in human visceral leishmaniasis. Virchows Arch A 1989;415:1–6.
23. Duarte MI, Boulos M, Segurado AA, et al. Hyperreactive malarious splenomegaly: immunohistochemical demonstration of Plasmodium falciparum antigen in liver cells. Trans R Soc Trop Med Hyg 1997;91:429–430.
24. Dunn MW, Berkowitz FE, Miller JJ, et al. Hepatosplenic cat-scratch diseases and abdominal pain. Pediatr Infect Dis J 1997;16:269–72.
25. Duray PH. Clinical pathologic correlations of Lyme disease. Rev Infect Dis 1989;11 (Suppl 6):S1487–S1493.
26. Ferreira VA, Vianna MR, Yasuda PH, et al. Detection of leptospiral antigen in the human liver and kidney using an immunoperoxidase staining procedure. J Pathol 1987;151:125–131.
27. Flavell DJ. Liver-fluke infection as an aetiological factor in bile-duct carcinoma of man. Trans R Soc Trop Med Hyg 1981;75:814–824.
28. Gayotto LCDC, Muszkar RML, Souza IV. Hepatobiliary alterations in massive miliary ascariasis. Histopathological aspects of an autopsy case. Rev Inst Med Trop Sao Paulo 1990;32:91–95.
29. Goellner MH, Agger WA, Burgess JH, et al. Hepatitis due to recurrent Lyme disease. Ann Intern Med 1988;108:707–708.
30. Greenstein AJ, Lowenthal BA, Hammer GF, et al. Continuing patterns of disease in pyogenic abscess: a study of 38 cases. Am J Gastroenterol 1984;79:217–226.
31. Guardia J, Martinez-Vazquez JM, Moragas A. The liver in boutonneuse fever. Gut 1974; 15:549–551.
32. Hofmann CE, Heaton JW Jr. Q fever hepatitis: clinical manifestations and pathological findings. Gastroenterology 1982;83:474–479.
33. Joshi YK, Tandon SK, Acharya SK, et al. Acute hepatic failure due to *Plasmodium falciparum* liver injury. Liver 1986;6:357–360.
34. Judge DM, Samuel I, Perine PL, et al. Louse-born relapsing fever in man. Arch Pathol Lab Med 1974;97:136–140.
35. Khuroo M, Zarger SA, Mahajan R. Hepatobiliary and pancreatic ascariasis in India. Lancet 1990;1:1503–1503.
36. Kramarsky B, Edmondson HA, Peters RL, et al. Lepromatous leprosy in reaction. Arch Pathol Lab Med 1968;85:516–531.
37. Lee RV, Thornton GF, Conn HO. Liver disease associated with secondary syphilis. N Engl J Med 1972;284:1423–1425.
38. Liu LX, Harinasuta KT. Liver and intestinal flukes. Gastroenterol Clin North Am 1996; 25:627–636.
39. Lobdell DH. "Ring" granulomas in cytomegalovirus hepatitis. Arch Pathol Lab Med 1987;11:880–882.
40. Maincent G, Labadie H, Fabre M, et al. Tertiary hepatic syphilis. A treatable cause of multilobular liver. Dig Dis Sci 1997;42:447–450.
41. McCormick JB, Sexton DJ, McMurray JG, et al. Human-to-human transmission of Pseudomonas pseudomallei. Ann Intern Med 1973;83:512–513.
42. Mermin JH, Townes JM, Gerber M, et al. Typhoid fever in the United States, 1985–1994: changing risks of international travel and increasing antimicrobial resistance. Arch Intern Med 1998;158:633–638.
43. Mondou EN, Gnepp DR. Hepatic granuloma resulting from *Enterobius vermicularis*. Am J Clin Pathol 1989;91:97–100.

44. Moreno A, Marazuela M, Yerba M, et al. Hepatic fibrin-ring granulomas in visceral leishmaniasis. Gastroenterology 1988;95:1123–1126.

45. Murphy E, Griffiths MR, Hunter JA, et al. Fibrin-ring granulomas: a non-specific reaction to liver injury? Histopathology 1991;19:91–93.

46. Nigam P, Gupta AK, Kapoor KK, et al. Cholestasis in amoebic liver abscess. Gut 1985;26: 140–145.

47. Pellegrin M, Delsol G, Aubergant JC, et al. Granulomatous hepatitis in Q fever. Hum Pathol 1980;11:51–57.

48. Pereira LM, McFarlane BM, Massarolo P, et al. Specific liver autoreactivity in schistosomiasis mansoni. Trans R Soc Trop Med Hyg 1997;91:310–314.

49. Poltera AA, Katsimbura N. Granulomatous hepatitis due to Strongyloides stercoralis. J Pathol 1974;113:241–246.

50. Rizkallah MF, Meyer L, Ayoug EM. Hepatic and splenic abscesses in cat-scratch disease. Pediatr Infect Dis J 1988;7:191–195.

51. Romeu J, Rybak B, Dave P, et al. Spirochetal vasculitis and bile ductular damage in early hepatic syphilis. Am J Gastroenterol 1980;74:352–354.

52. Schantz PM. *Toxocara* larva migrans now. Am J Trop Med Hyg 1989;41(Suppl):21–34.

53. Sobel HJ, Wolf EH. Liver involvement in early syphilis. Arch Pathol Lab Med 1972;93: 565–568.

54. Sun HC, Deng PF, Wang CJ, et al. Liver involvement in epidemic haemorrhagic fever: in-situ hybridization, immunohistochemical and pathological studies. J Gastroenterol Hepatol 1997;12:540–546.

55. Taylor MRH, Keane CT, O'Connor P, et al. The expanded spectrum of toxocaral disease. Lancet 1988;1:692–695.

56. Tiwari I, Rolland CF, Popple AW. Cholestatic jaundice due to toxoplasma hepatitis. Postgrad Med J 1982;58:299–300.

57. Vago L, Barberis M, Gori A, et al. Nested polymerase chain reaction for *Mycobacterium tuberculosis* IS6110 sequence on formalin-fixed paraffin-embedded tissues with granulomatous diseases for rapid diagnosis of tuberculosis. Am J Clin Pathol 1998;109: 411–415.

58. Walker DH, Staiti A, Mansueto G, et al. Frequent occurrence of hepatic lesions in boutonneuse fever. Acta Trop 1986;43:175–181.

59. Weitberg AB, Alper JC, Diamond I, et al. Acute granulomatous hepatitis in the course of acquired toxoplasmosis. N Engl J Med 1979;300:1093–1096.

60. Wollner-Hanssen P, Weström L, Märdh P-A. Perihepatitis and chlamydial salpingitis. Lancet 1980;1:901–904.

61. Yow EM, Brennan JC, Preston J, et al. The pathology of psittacosis: a report of two cases with hepatitis. Am J Med 1959;27:739–747.

23

BENIGN TUMORS AND TUMOR-LIKE CONDITIONS

Benign proliferative and neoplastic processes arise from hepatocytes, biliary epithelium, stromal (mesenchymal) elements, or combinations of those elements (Tables 23.1 and 23.2). These tumors are relatively rare. Mesenchymal tumors, such as lipoma and leiomyoma, resemble those at other sites and will not be discussed in great detail.

BENIGN HEPATOCELLULAR TUMORS AND TUMOR-LIKE CONDITIONS

Benign hepatocellular tumors are uncommon. In the past, most were diagnosed incidentally, when they reached significant dimensions, or at autopsy. Liver cell adenomas became more common with the widespread use of oral contraceptives. Increasing awareness of benign liver tumors and sophisticated imaging techniques allow for detection of small tumors. However, it is still difficult for the pathologist to establish the correct diagnosis for these processes, especially when only a core biopsy is available.

Hepatocellular Adenoma

Prior to the introduction of contraceptive pills, hepatocellular adenoma was one of the rarest of human tumors (54,55,86). The estimated incidence is 3 to 4 cases per 100,000 (41,54,63,68). Anabolic steroids (9,54) and other medications (59) have been associated, as have metabolic diseases, including glycogenosis I (18,50,84), glycogenosis IV (3), tyrosinemia (115), diabetes mellitus (34), galactosemia (27), and thalassemia (16). Rarely, adenomas develop spontaneously (39,117). Adenomas developing in the setting of a metabolic disease have an increased incidence of hepatocellular carcinoma (HCC) (9,39,41,54,56,66).

Patients may be asymptomatic or can present with right upper quadrant abdominal pain. If the tumor is large, it may be palpable. Subcapsular adenomas can rupture with intraperitoneal hemorrhage and acute abdominal manifestations (45,55,84). Adenomas can

TABLE 23.1	**Benign Hepatocellular Tumors and Tumor-Like Conditions**

1. Hepatocellular adenoma
2. Multiple hepatocellular adenomatosis
3. Macroregenerative nodules
4. Focal nodular hyperplasia
5. Nodular hyperplasia
6. Partial nodular transformation

TABLE 23.2	**Mesenchymal Tumors and Tumor-Like Conditions of the Liver**

A. Mixed epithelial and mesenchymal tumors
   1. Mesenchymal hamartoma (2,22,60,92)
   2. Mixed hamartoma (mixed adenoma) (53)
B. Vascular
   1. Infantile hemangioendothelioma (19,50,53,117)
   2. Cavernous hemangioma (50,53,88)
   3. Lymphangioma and hepatic lymphangiomatosis (104)
   4. Hereditary hemorrhagic telangiectasia (67,109)
C. Lipomatous
   1. Lipoma (50,53)
   2. Pseudolipoma (50,53)
   3. Angiomyolipoma (angiomyelolipoma, myelolipoma) (35,45,103)
   4. Focal fatty change (50,95)
D. Fibrous
   1. Fibroma (50,53)
   2. Inflammatory pseudotumor (5,10,47,57,63)
E. Myomatous
   1. Leiomyoma (42)
F. Neural
   1. Neurofibromatosis (62)
   2. Schwannoma (49)
G. Chondroid
   1. Chondroma (33)

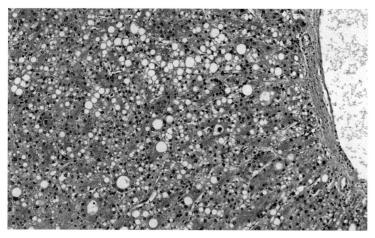

FIGURE 23.1   Liver cell adenoma. Bland hepatocytes arranged in two- or three-cell-thick liver plates (hematoxylin-eosin, original magnification ×100).

regress spontaneously (13,28) and after withdrawal of medications (13,28,54,82,86,93,102). Adenomas are usually single and most often right lobe, but can be multiple (6,16,52,71,89,90). They vary considerably in size and, with advanced imaging techniques, are detected when quite small (75,84,88).

PATHOLOGY. Liver cell adenomas consist of bland-appearing hepatocytes, arranged in two- and three-cell-thick liver plates (Figs. 23.1, 23.2,

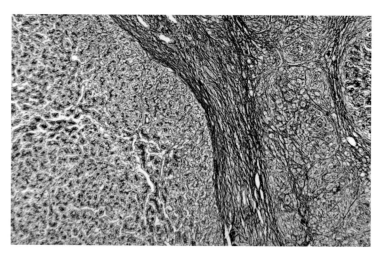

FIGURE 23.2   Liver cell adenoma. Reticulin silver preparation highlighting thickened liver cell plates (reticulin silver preparation, original magnification ×100).

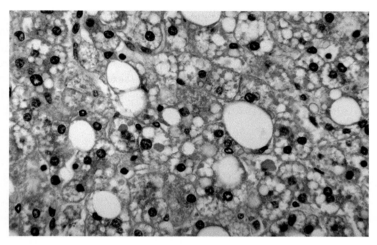

FIGURE 23.3 Liver cell adenoma. Giant mitochondria are present in some hepatocytes (hematoxylin-eosin, original magnification ×400).

e-Figs. 23.1–23.8). Bile-containing acinar structures can be seen. Liver cells can be either larger or smaller than the surrounding nonneoplastic hepatocytes and may have a relatively increased nuclear/cytoplasmic ratio, resembling well-differentiated hepatocellular carcinoma. Some adenomas express hormone receptors (70). Adenoma cells can also contain more glycogen than the surrounding liver and appear relatively pale. Various cytoplasmic materials and inclusions can be seen, including Mallory hyalin, lipofuscin, giant mitochondria, and oncocytic change (55,83,89) (Fig. 23.3). Mitotic figures are rare. Focal necrosis, with or without apoptosis, microgranulomas, and extramedullary hematopoiesis, may be seen (63,68,84). Some adenomas show focally atypical, pleomorphic cells, often with hyperchromatic nuclei, and as many as 10% have giant cell transformation (9,39,43,55,58,73). Fibrosis is not prominent. Vascular elements, particularly thick-walled arteries and arterioles, are seen at the periphery of the tumor. Thick-walled veins are seen as well as small-caliber, thin-walled vascular channels randomly distributed within the tumor. Sinusoidal endothelial cells and Kupffer cells are present (38,55).

DIFFERENTIAL DIAGNOSIS. Hepatic adenoma must be differentiated from well-differentiated HCC, focal nodular hyperplasia (FNH) (79), macroregenerative nodules (MRNs), nodular regenerative hyperplasia (NRH), multiple hepatocellular adenomatosis, focal steatosis, and sometimes even normal liver.

In HCC, the nuclear/cytoplasmic ratio is high and cellular atypia is usually more pronounced. There is usually only a scanty reticulin network in HCC in contrast with an adenoma in which the reticulin network is usually maintained. Adenoma is distinguished from FNH by the absence of portal tract structures and terminal hepatic venules (central veins), as well as lack of the central fibrotic zone characteristic of FNH. In biopsy material, however, differentiation can be exceedingly difficult. Recent studies have shown that based on molecular criteria, HNF1α and β-catenin mutations and the presence or absence of inflammation, liver cell adenomas can be distinguished from FNH (Table 23.3) (7).

TABLE 23.3	Histopathologic, Clinical, and Molecular Features of Benign Liver Lesions		
Pathology	Molecular Features	Clinical Relevance	Associations
Typical hepatic adenoma	Monoclonality	Bleeding risk	Focal nodular hyperplasia
Variant 1 Adenoma with clear cells and/or lipid	HNF 1α mutation	Bleeding risk	MODY3 diabetes, multiple colonic adenomas, younger
Variant 2 Adenoma/? HCC	B-catenin mutation	Bleeding risk? HCC sequel	Males > Females
Variant 3 "telangiectatic FNH"	No known mutation	Bleeding risk	Multiple adenomas Vascular/CNS disorders
Variant 4 No specific trait	No known mutation	Bleeding risk	
Typical FNH	Polyclonality inc apo1/apo2 ratio		Adenoma Hemangioma
Lack of one or more typical FNH features		Difficult to differentiate from adenoma	
Unusual features (e.g., steatosis)		Difficult to differentiate from adenoma	

Adapted from Bioulac-Sage P, Balaboud C, Bedossa P, et al. Pathological diagnosis of liver cell adenoma and focal nodular hyperplasia: Bordeaux update. J Hepatol 2007;46: 521–527.

MRNs in cirrhosis or after massive necrosis can be indistinguishable from liver cell adenoma. Cellular atypia is generally not seen. Adenomas rarely occur in cirrhosis, except in the metabolic disorders. NRH can involve the whole liver, and the nodules are quite small, representing exaggerated lobules, usually with surrounding compressed atrophic-appearing hepatocytes.

Multiple Hepatocellular Adenomatosis

Multiple hepatocellular adenomatosis is exceedingly rare (6,17,33,55, 63, 67,84). Adenomas may be clustered in one lobe but can be diffuse. The diagnosis is applied with four or more adenomas with unremarkable intervening liver parenchyma (5,6,88). Progressive hepatocellular proliferation develops as a response to chronic low-grade ischemia, similar to NRH and possibly partial nodular transformation (110,111). There is no proven association with contraceptive pills or anabolic steroids.

PATHOLOGY. Nodules consist of bland, benign hepatocytes, arranged in one- or two-cell-thick liver plates. Macrovesicular steatosis may be focally present. Areas of hemorrhage can also be present.

Macroregenerative Nodule

MRNs, defined as at least 0.8 cm in size, have been also called adenomatous hyperplasia, adenomatous regeneration, and large regenerative nodules (29,31,32,36). Some are most likely preneoplastic (29,36,61,76,80, 88,103), evidenced by their occurrence adjacent to HCC (29,76,88). MRNs usually occur in cirrhosis but also with submassive liver necrosis. MRNs can be multiple (103,109).

PATHOLOGY. MRN type I (ordinary or typical) is composed of liver cell plates that are two or three cells thick, similar to those in cirrhosis. Portal tracts are usually present. The liver cells are bland, with no significant cytologic atypia, and may contain various intracytoplasmic materials, including fat, hemosiderin, bile, and/or Mallory material (98,101,103,109) (Fig. 23.4, e-Fig. 23.9). In contrast, MRN type II (atypical MRN, atypical adenomatous hyperplasia, borderline lesions) has focal or multifocal small or large cell dysplasia, with altered architectural pattern and irregular liver cell plates, and there may be nodule-in-nodule formation and focal pseudoacinar formation (Fig. 23.5).

DIFFERENTIAL DIAGNOSIS. The distinction between MRN type II and HCC can be very difficult; MRN II nodules may represent true hepatocellular carcinoma in situ (32,61,88). Extensive loss of the underlying reticulin network, irregular thickness of the liver cell plates, and significant cytologic nuclear atypia are features favoring HCC.

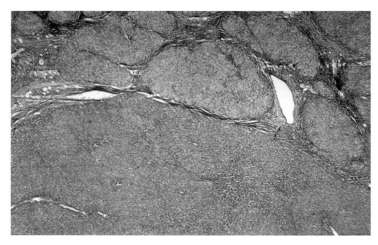

FIGURE 23.4 Macroregenerative nodule, type I. Note the relatively bland hepatocytes arranged in two- to three-cell-thick liver plates. Focal macrovesicular steatosis is present (hematoxylin-eosin, original magnification ×40).

Focal Nodular Hyperplasia

A benign pseudotumor, FNH is one of the most common benign liver lesions, occurring predominantly in young women (15,55,78,81,84,87). Although usually solitary, multiple lesions have been described (42,111). FNH can also be associated with other benign tumors, including adenomas and hemangiomas (20,39,46,71). Most cases are found incidentally,

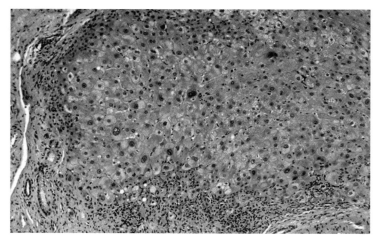

FIGURE 23.5 Macroregenerative nodule, type II (adenomatous hyperplasia). Note the nodule-in-nodule formation and liver cells with large cell dysplasia. This would qualify for so-called borderline lesion (hematoxylin-eosin, original magnification ×100).

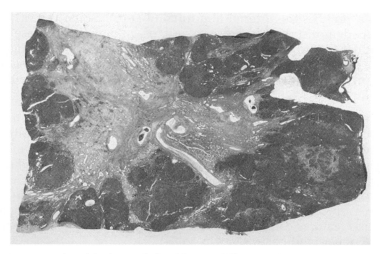

FIGURE 23.6   Focal nodular hyperplasia with central fibrovascular area (hematoxylin-eosin, original magnification ×40).

but a small proportion of patients present with abdominal pain or a palpable mass. FNH can be associated with oral contraceptive use (39,54,110, 112).

The most characteristic feature is the central, stellate fibrovascular zone, which has the historically entrenched name of "fibrous scar" or "scarlike fibrosis (Figs. 23.6 and 23.7, e-Figs. 23.10–23.15). Pathogenesis of FNH can, in many cases, be attributed to a hyperplastic response of the

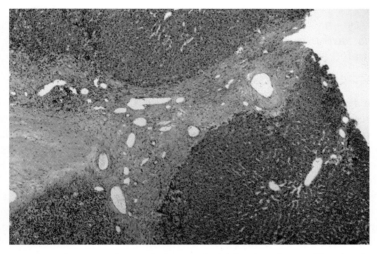

FIGURE 23.7   Focal nodular hyperplasia. Marginal bile ductular proliferation is present (hematoxylin–eosin, original magnification ×40).

liver to a pre-existing arterial abnormality (110). Some recent studies, however, demonstrated overexpression of glutamine synthase in the periportal areas in very early stages of FNH development, suggesting that the primary event is portal tract and portal vein injury, leading to formation of arteriovenous shunts, ductular reaction, and finally, scar formation (8).

PATHOLOGY. The diagnosis of FNH can be difficult in biopsy material. Hepatocytes surrounding the fibrovascular zone are cytologically bland but may show mild degenerative changes, focal steatosis, or increased glycogen. They are arranged in incomplete nodules or pseudonodules and are partially surrounded by slender fibrous septa extending from the central fibrotic zone. Focal thickening of liver cell plates is common. Portal structures or complete portal tracts are seen. Cholestasis and chronic cholestasis features can be seen, and zone 1 (periportal) hepatocytes can contain copper-binding protein (15,55,84).

The central fibrovascular zone contains mature collagen and numerous vascular channels, most of them medium and large thick-walled arteries. Arteries often show fibromuscular hyperplasia, myointimal proliferation, and myxomatous change, very often with significant lumen narrowing (55,84). Veins are unremarkable. True portal tracts, native interlobular or larger bile ducts are not seen within the central fibrovascular zone, but marginal bile ductular proliferation is common. A mild chronic inflammatory infiltrate, with occasional polymorphonuclear leukocytes, is common but nonspecific. Recently, new histologic forms of FNH have been recognized and a histologic scoring system proposed (30,78). Several recent findings pertinent to the pathogenesis have prompted an updated classification of FNH and liver cell adenoma and those findings are incorporated in Table 23.3 (7).

DIFFERENTIAL DIAGNOSIS. Differential diagnosis includes hepatocellular adenoma, cirrhosis, mixed hamartoma, bile duct adenoma (BDA), well-differentiated HCC, and the fibrolamellar variant of HCC (81,107).

Nodular Regenerative Hyperplasia

Nodular regenerative hyperplasia (NRH) is a benign regenerative lesion composed of hyperplastic hepatocytes forming small nodules not surrounded by fibrous tissue, eventually diffusely distributed. Relatively uncommon, it presents with noncirrhotic portal hypertension or its complications (e.g., ascites, variceal bleeding) (19,55,85,96,99). NRH can sometimes clinically mimic venoocclusive disease (74).

NRH is associated with various hematologic and immunologic diseases (55,74,75,84,85). Immunosuppressive drugs and toxins have also been implicated (74). NRH can be seen following liver transplantation. Recently, NRH has been recognized in patients with inflammatory bowel diseases treated with 6-thioguanine (91). Spontaneous regression of NRH may be seen. The pathogenesis is not entirely clear, but it is postulated that

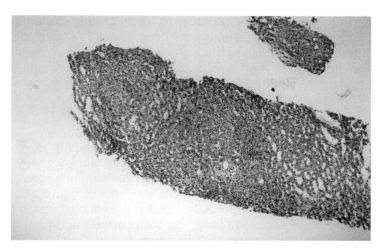

FIGURE 23.8   Nodular regenerative hyperplasia. Note the well-defined regenerative nodules of liver parenchyma without significant fibrosis (hematoxylin-eosin, original magnification ×100).

inadequate vascular supply and even local ischemic events play a role (96,111,113).

PATHOLOGY. NRH is best recognized at low magnification. Distinct contours of regenerative nodules, composed of unremarkable hepatocytes, are centered on generally unchanged portal tracts, rimmed by slightly or markedly atrophic hepatocytes at the periphery (Figs. 23.8 and 23.9, e-Figs. 23.16–23.22). Liver cell dysplasia is rare (92). Unremarkable sinusoidal

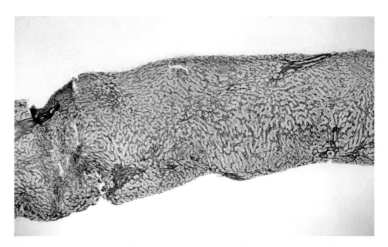

FIGURE 23.9   Nodular regenerative hyperplasia. Note the compression of underlying reticulin network at the periphery of the nodules (reticulin silver preparation, original magnification ×100).

endothelial and Kupffer cells are present. Vascular alterations have been described, including inconspicuous portal vein branches and hepatic artery inflammation (55,84). Reticulin silver preparation is helpful, particularly for the earliest detection of NRH (e-Fig. 23.23). A preserved reticulin network with one- and two-cell-thick liver plates is seen with a peripheral rim of compressed hepatocytes (Fig. 23.9).

Partial Nodular Transformation

Partial nodular transformation (PNT) is an exceptionally rare, benign, tumor-like solitary nodule, 3 to 40 mm in diameter, almost always arising in the hilum. Patients present with portal hypertension, portal vein thrombosis, ascites, and esophageal varices (25,55,92). Fewer than 20 cases have been reported. The pathogenesis is thought to be similar to that of NRH as a response to insufficient blood supply, as with portal vein thrombosis. The extrahepatic portal vein frequently shows evidence of old thrombosis. A hypercoagulable state may contribute to portal vein thrombosis.

PATHOLOGY. The features of PNT are subtle, with regenerative and incomplete liver nodules and slender fibrous septa that partially circumscribe the nodules. Portal tracts are at the periphery (Fig. 23.10). Bile ductule proliferation is not seen. Portal vein branches are inconspicuous, and occlusion or thrombosis is not usually evident. Sinusoidal dilatation may be seen. Liver plates are focally two to three cells thick, best seen with reticulin silver stain. The hepatocytes are generally bland.

DIFFERENTIAL DIAGNOSIS. Differential diagnosis includes NRH and FNH (Fig. 23.11).

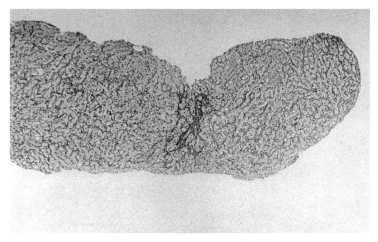

FIGURE 23.10 Partial nodular transformation. Paucicellular portal tract with a slender septum extending into the parenchyma (hematoxylin-eosin, original magnification ×100).

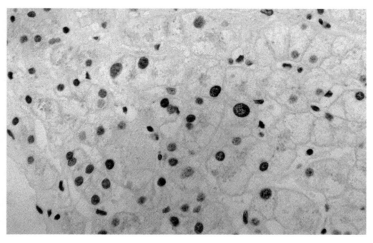

FIGURE 23.11 Proliferative activity in focal nodular hyperplasia, nodular regenerative hyperplasia, and liver cell adenoma (immunoperoxidase, avidin-streptavidin, antibody to proliferating cell nuclear antigen, original magnification ×200).

BENIGN BILIARY EPITHELIAL TUMORS

Bile Duct Adenoma

True bile duct adenoma (BDA) is exceedingly rare and usually incidentally discovered. A few millimeters to 2 cm, tumors are well-circumscribed, pale tan, sometimes easily seen on the capsular surface or in the immediate subcapsular region (2). They may be multiple (55).

PATHOLOGY. BDA consists of numerous small, relatively uniform bile duct–like structures that are not cystically dilated. A small amount of bland, paucicellular collagen is between ducts, which are sharply demarcated from the surrounding liver parenchyma (Fig. 23.12, e-figs. 23.24, 23.25). The epithelium is benign but can show hyperchromatic, enlarged nuclei and less cytoplasm than the biliary epithelium of interlobular bile ducts. Mitoses are not seen. A few inflammatory cells, including lymphocytes and polymorphonuclear leukocytes, may be present.

DIFFERENTIAL DIAGNOSIS. Differential diagnosis includes benign biliary (microbiliary) hamartoma (von Meyenburg complex, microhamartoma), biliary adenofibroma, cholangiocarcinoma, and metastatic adenocarcinoma. Bile duct hamartoma is a developmental malformation, part of the spectrum of fibropolycystic diseases of the liver, and may be single or multiple (14,25,55) (see Chapter 6). Distinctly tortuous, or angulated, focally cystically dilated ductlike structures, often filled with inspissated bile or dense eosinophilic proteinaceous acellular debris, are seen, and the surrounding stroma is fibrotic (Fig. 23.13). Bile duct hamartoma is often adjacent to or arises from existing portal tract structures. The epithelial

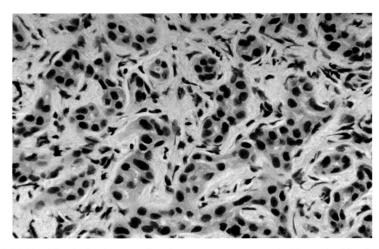

FIGURE 23.12 Bile duct adenoma showing numerous somewhat irregular bile duct structures embedded in a paucicellular fibrous stroma. Note that the epithelial cells lack any degree of atypia. The whole lesion is sharply demarcated from the surrounding liver parenchyma (hematoxylin-eosin, original magnification ×20).

cells in BDA show reactivity for both low and high molecular weight keratins (CAM5.2 and AE1/3), indicating that these cells may originate from either hepatocytes or biliary epithelium, or from a common stem cell. In contrast, bile duct hamartoma reacts strongly with high molecular weight keratin (AE1/3 or CK19). Biliary adenofibroma is similar to BDA but usually larger, with bile duct structures embedded in fibrous stroma. The epithelium may show focal apocrine metaplasia (104).

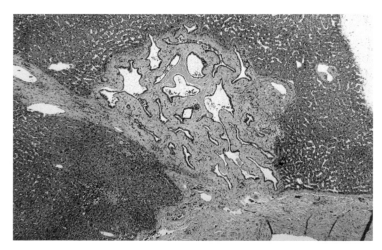

FIGURE 23.13 Von Meyenburg complex (microhamartoma) with cystically dilated ductlike structures, arising from or adjacent to the portal tract (hematoxylin-eosin, original magnification ×100).

Cholangiocarcinoma can develop in the background of BDA (14), as well as with multiple bile duct hamartomas (14,23,48). Differentiation of BDA from metastatic adenocarcinoma can be difficult in frozen section material.

Solitary Unilocular Bile Duct Cyst

Solitary unilocular bile duct cysts are lined by benign columnar or cuboidal biliary-type epithelium, surrounded by a variable amount of indistinct fibrous tissue (55). Mononuclear inflammatory cells can be seen (Fig. 23.14).

DIFFERENTIAL DIAGNOSIS. Diagnoses to consider are parasitic cysts, posttraumatic cysts, and healing abscess wall. Posttraumatic cysts and healing abscess do not have true epithelial lining.

Ciliated Foregut Cyst

This develops from embryonic foregut with differentiation to respiratory-type (bronchial) structures, often with four distinct layers including pseudostratified respiratory-type epithelium, subepithelial tissue, smooth muscle layer, and fibrous capsule (55,100). The ciliated foregut cyst is almost invariably unilocular.

Biliary Cystadenoma

Biliary cystadenoma is a relatively rare lesion. It is usually single and multiloculated with a predilection for the right lobe of the liver (1,53,114). The tumor can be as large as 25 to 30 cm and may replace almost the entire liver lobe. A smooth inner epithelial lining is present.

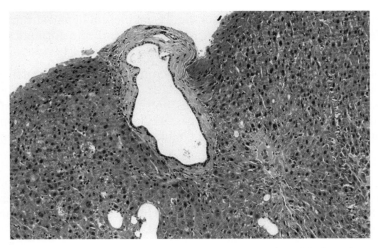

FIGURE 23.14 Solitary, simple cyst lined by flattened cuboidal epithelium (hematoxylin-eosin, original magnification ×100).

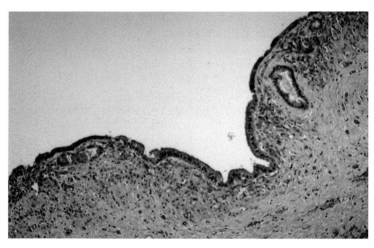

FIGURE 23.15   Biliary cystadenoma with mesenchymal ovarian-like stroma. The epithelium is nonciliated, columnar, and mucin producing with no cytologic atypia (hematoxylin-eosin, original magnification ×100).

PATHOLOGY. The cysts are lined by mucin-producing, nonciliated columnar or cuboidal focally flattened epithelium (Fig. 23.15, e-Fig. 23.26). In women, a mesenchymal ovarian-like stroma is usually seen, suggesting that these tumors arise from intrahepatic ectopic ovarian tissue (53,114). Cholesterol crystals, as well as hemosiderin-laden and ceroid-laden macrophages, may be prominent. When the fluid is blood tinged, malignancy should be suspected. Three types have been recognized: (a) hepatobiliary cystadenoma with mesenchymal stroma, (b) hepatobiliary cystadenoma without mesenchymal stroma, and (c) intraductal polypoid hepatobiliary cystadenoma. In men there is no mesenchymal stroma. If not completely excised, the tumor may recur. Malignant transformation is relatively common (53,116,116,118).

DIFFERENTIAL DIAGNOSIS. Diagnoses to consider are ciliated foregut cyst, intrahepatic choledochocyst, and parasitic cysts. Intrahepatic choledochocyst occurs in the hilum and does not exhibit mesenchymal stroma. Parasitic cysts usually have fibrous capsule, often with calcifications and without identifiable lining epithelium, and often with identifiable parasites.

Biliary Papillomatosis

Biliary papillomatosis is an unusual, multifocal, histopathologically benign lesion that is relentlessly progressive in growth and ultimately fatal (72,108). Patients are usually male adults who present with symptoms and signs of biliary obstruction.

PATHOLOGY. Intrahepatic and extrahepatic bile ducts are dilated and contain exaggerated papillary growth of the biliary epithelium with supporting fibrovascular stroma. The epithelial cells are in most cases bland, columnar, with mucin-containing cytoplasm and basally located nuclei. Focal inflammation and ulceration may also be seen, and necrotic cellular debris admixed with inflammatory cells may fill the lumen. Complications include bacterial cholangitis, sepsis, and liver failure. Malignant transformation has been reported (77).

BENIGN MESENCHYMAL TUMORS

Benign mesenchymal tumors can be divided into several groups according to their origin. These relatively rare tumors are listed in Table 23.2.

Mixed Epithelial and Mesenchymal Tumors

MESENCHYMAL HAMARTOMA. This uncommon childhood tumor has a male predominance and comprises approximately 5% of pediatric liver tumors. The tumor results from malformation of primitive hepatic mesenchyme. Children present with a painless abdominal mass, with a characteristic imaging appearance. The tumor is usually solitary and large, with a right lobe predilection (22,24,35,62,94).

Pathology. Solid tumor areas have a mixture of hepatic and mesenchymal cells, often with vascular proliferation, bile ducts or duct–like structures, and cystically dilated spaces (Fig. 23.16, e-Figs. 23.27–23.30). Scattered stellate mesenchymal cells are embedded in edematous collagenous or myxoid stroma. Cystically dilated spaces represent distended bile duct–like structures. Bile ducts often are at the periphery, with atrophic epithelium and focal acute inflammation. Entrapped hepatocytes in abundant mesenchymal stroma

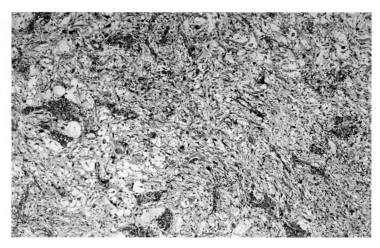

FIGURE 23.16 Mesenchymal hamartoma composed of a mixture of epithelial (liver and bile duct) cells and embedded in the edematous myxoid stroma (hematoxylin-eosin, original magnification ×100).

show reactive and regenerative changes. Foci of hematopoiesis are occasionally seen. Thick-walled blood vessels may be at the periphery (26,66).

Differential Diagnosis. Differential diagnosis includes embryonal (undifferentiated) sarcoma and infantile hemangioendothelioma. Differentiation from embryonal sarcoma is particularly important, since both lesions may exhibit loose, edematous, myxoid stroma. In most embryonal sarcomas, the cellularity is readily evident, and neoplastic cells show distinctive cytologic features of highly malignant cells.

MIXED HAMARTOMA. Mixed hamartoma is an exceedingly rare solitary tumor usually diagnosed in infants to teenagers (55). Also called mixed adenoma because of the epithelial components, it has bile ductular structures and hepatocytes embedded in dense fibrous stroma lacking vascular structures and portal tracts.

Pathology. The tumor is pseudonodular, with benign hepatocyte nests surrounded by dense fibrous tissue Proliferated bile ductules and thick-walled arterial vessels are at the interface with the fibrous tissue.

Differential Diagnosis. The principal diagnosis to consider is FNH. The central fibrovascular scar of FNH is virtually diagnostic. The diffuse, uniform nodularity of mixed hamartoma, easily recognized in a resected specimen, may not be obvious in biopsy material. Mixed hamartoma has a cirrhosis-like pattern but is focal.

Benign Vascular Tumors

INFANTILE HEMANGIOENDOTHELIOMA. Infantile hemangioendothelioma (IH) can be single, most commonly in the right lobe, or multifocal. Size may vary from a few millimeters to more than 20 cm. Multiple tumors impart a spongiform appearance to the liver. Larger tumors are well circumscribed but not encapsulated and are variegated, often with scattered calcifications (52,54,55,57).

Pathology. The tumor consists of small vessels with plump endothelial cells. Type I IH contains stroma composed of unremarkable collagen and reticulin fibers (20) (Fig. 23.17, e-Figs. 23.31, 23.32). Foci of hematopoiesis are frequently seen. Type II IH is an aggressive variant with multilayered endothelial cells and occasional tufting (119). Type II IH has variable degrees of nuclear pleomorphism, hyperchromasia, and mitoses and may metastasize. Typical angiosarcoma may develop (60,95).

CAVERNOUS HEMANGIOMA. This most common benign tumor, uncommon in children, can be solitary or multiple, often only a few millimeters in size. Hemangiomas can also be extremely large, replacing considerable portions of liver parenchyma (52,55,90). Hemangioma can be multiple and can occur with FNH.

Pathology. Cavernous spaces are lined by a single layer of benign endothelial cells (Fig. 23.18). Antibodies, including factor VIII, CD31, and

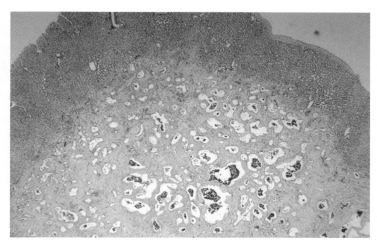

FIGURE 23.17 Hemangioma with cavernous spaces lined by a single layer of endothelial cells (hematoxylin-eosin, original magnification ×40).

CD34, can be used but are generally not necessary. Fibrosis and calcifications are common. Sclerosis is seen with larger lesions, with extensive fibrosis, hyalinization, and narrowing; sometimes complete obliteration of vascular spaces occurs.

LYMPHANGIOMA AND HEPATIC LYMPHANGIOMATOSIS. Multiple hepatic lymphangiomatosis is exceedingly rare (106). Solitary lymphangiomas in the liver are even rarer, and their existence is controversial. A systemic form of lymphangiomatosis occurs in children, affecting multiple organs, the

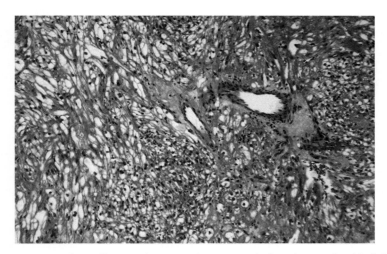

FIGURE 23.18 Angiomyolipoma. The tumor is composed of a mixture of epithelioid cells, with smooth muscle differentiation, variable amount of fat, and thick-walled blood vessels (hematoxylin-eosin, original magnification ×100).

skeleton, lymph nodes, soft tissue, and the retroperitoneum, with potentially poor prognosis. Multiple hepatic lymphangiomatosis is seen as clustered multiple soft white-tan tumors with cystically dilated spaces that expel milky fluid when punctured (106). Benign flattened endothelial cells line irregular spaces. The surrounding fibrous stroma shows focal calcifications, and adjacent hepatocytes may be compressed and atrophic.

HEREDITARY HEMORRHAGIC TELANGIECTASIA (OSLER-WEBER-RENDU DISEASE). Telangiectasias can be seen in any part of the liver, including lobules and portal tracts. The primary abnormality is thought to be a dilatation of intrahepatic arteries. Dilated vascular spaces lined by unremarkable endothelial cells are surrounded by fibrous stroma (70,111) (Fig. 23.19). NH can also be seen (111).

Benign Lipomatous Tumors

LIPOMA. Lipoma is one of the rarest benign liver tumors and usually incidental. Usually single and well demarcated, they range from a few millimeters to 2 cm (52,55). The cell of origin has not been identified. Portal tract structures are preserved, and many hepatocytes contain large fat droplets. Differential diagnosis includes pseudolipoma, liver cell adenoma with abundant fat, and so-called focal fatty change.

PSEUDOLIPOMA. Pseudolipoma is another rare, small, encapsulated lesion. It consists of mature lipocytes on the capsular surface or in the immediate subcapsular region, presumed to be from an adherent appendix epiploica, with varying degrees of degeneration, calcification, and occasionally true osseous metaplasia (52,55).

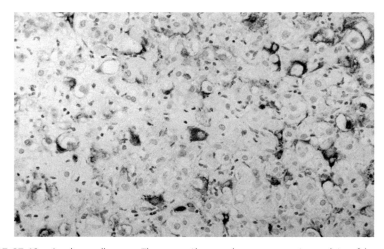

FIGURE 23.19 Angiomyolipoma. The smooth muscle component consists of bundles of epithelioid cells, strongly positive for smooth muscle actin and focal positivity for HMB45 (immunoperoxidase, avidin-streptavidin, original magnification ×100).

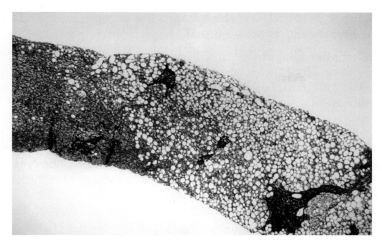

FIGURE 23.20   Focal fatty change. Localized macrovesicular steatosis involving only a portion of liver parenchyma. Surrounding liver is without significant histopathologic findings (hematoxylin-eosin, original magnification ×100).

ANGIOMYOLIPOMA. Angiomyolipoma is a rare benign lipomatous tumor resembling the more common renal angiomyolipomas. Patients are between 30 and 72 years of age (37). Tumors are usually solitary and may be as large as 20 cm.

Pathology. Three components occur in variable proportions: smooth muscle, blood vessels, and fat (Fig. 23.20, e-Figs. 23.33–23.36). The smooth muscle component is seen as sheets and bundles of spindle and epithelioid cells. Tortuous vascular channels with thick-walled vessels are particularly prominent at the periphery. Lipomatous tissue varies from as little as 5% to more than 90%. Hibernoma-like cells can be seen. Epithelioid cells have granular and eosinophilic cytoplasm, but many have clear glycogen-rich cytoplasm. Tumors with extensive extramedullary hematopoiesis have been termed "myelolipoma" or "angiomyelolipoma." Immunohistochemical analysis demonstrates diffuse reactivity for smooth muscle actin, focal reactivity for vimentin, and widespread reactivity for S-100 and HMB45. The expression of HMB45 is characteristic (e-Fig. 23.37) (37,47,105). The tumor is benign with a diploid DNA pattern (47). Malignant transformation has not been reported.

Differential Diagnosis. Differential diagnosis includes other benign lipomatous lesions, such as lipoma, pseudolipoma, and focal steatosis. The epithelioid smooth muscle cells may mimic hepatocytes and can be misinterpreted as HCC. Metastatic renal cell carcinoma also has to be excluded.

FOCAL FATTY CHANGE. Focal fatty change, or localized steatosis of the liver, can sometimes be misinterpreted as neoplastic growth on computed tomography scan (11,52,97). The lesion is not encapsulated, and the surrounding liver may be entirely normal.

Differential Diagnosis. In a biopsy, focal fatty change is indistinguishable from other forms of steatosis. Diabetics particularly show this change. The differential diagnosis includes steatotic liver cell adenoma, as well as subcapsular lipoma or pseudolipoma (57).

Benign Fibrous Tumors

FIBROMA. This exceedingly rare benign tumor arises from submesothelial connective tissue. It has also been called localized (solitary) mesothelioma, localized fibrous mesothelioma, and extraovarian fibrothecoma. No association has been made with asbestos exposure.

Pathology. The tumor is composed of bland bundles of fibrocytes, with varying degrees of cellularity. Fibrocytes alternate with dense collagen bands. There is strong immunohistochemical staining for vimentin (52,55).

Differential Diagnosis. The principal diagnoses to consider are fibrosarcoma and leiomyosarcoma when the cells are highly atypical with pleomorphic nuclei and increased numbers of mitoses.

INFLAMMATORY PSEUDOTUMOR. This rare inflammatory lesion presents as a localized parenchymal mass or at the hepatic hilum. Patients may be febrile but usually are asymptomatic (4,5,49,59,65).

Pathology. An abundant and mixed inflammatory infiltrate is seen, including spindle and foamy histiocytes, lymphocytes, and numerous plasma cells (e-Fig. 23.38) Hepatocytes may be entrapped in this infiltrate. The central portion of the lesion is fibroblastic/myofibroblastic, and the tumor is also called inflammatory myofibroblastic tumor. Vascular invasion can sometimes be seen (12).

Differential Diagnosis. Diagnosis is usually difficult. The differential includes both benign and malignant tumors, including lymphoproliferative disorders, histiocytosis X, and healing abscesses. Careful clinical history, imaging studies, and cultures for microorganisms can be helpful.

REFERENCES

1. Akwari OE, Tucker A, Seigler HF, et al. Hepatobiliary cystadenoma with mesenchymal stroma. Ann Surg 1990;211:18–27.
2. Allaire GS, Rabin L, Ishak KG, et al. Bile duct adenoma. A study of 152 cases. Am J Surg Pathol 1988;12:708–715.
3. Alshak NS, Cocjin J, Podesta L, et al. Hepatocellular adenoma in glycogen storage disease type IV. Arch Pathol Lab Med 1994;118:88–91.
4. Amankonah TD, Strom CB, Vierling JM, et al. Inflammatory pseudotumor of the liver as the first manifestation of Crohn's disease. Am J Gastroenterol 2001;96:2520–2522.
5. Anthony PP, Telesinghe PU. Inflammatory pseudotumor of the liver. J Clin Pathol 1986;39:761–768.

6. Arsenault TM, Johnson CD, Gorman B, et al. Hepatic adenomatosis. Mayo Clin Proc 1996;71:478–480.

7. Bioulac-Sage P, Balaboud C, Bedossa P, et al. Pathological diagnosis of liver cell adenoma and focal nodular hyperplasia: Bordeaux update. J Hepatol 2007;46:521–527.

8. Bioulac-Sage P, Laumonier H, Cubel G, et al. Overexpression of glutamine synthase in focal nodular hyperplasia: early stages in the formation support the hypothesis of a focal hyperarterialization with venous (portal and hepatic) and biliary damage. Comparative Hepatology 2009; 7:2–12.

9. Boyd PR, Mark GJ. Multiple hepatic adenomas and a hepatocellular carcinoma in a man on oral methyl testosterone for eleven years. Cancer 1977;40:1765–1770.

10. Bravo R, Macdonald-Bravo H. Changes in the nuclear distribution of cyclin (PCNA) but not its synthesis depend on DNA replication. EMBO J 1985;4:655–661.

11. Brawer MK, Austin GE, Lewin KJ. Focal fatty changes of the liver, a hitherto poorly recognized entity. Gastroenterology 1980;78:247–252.

12. Broughan TA, Fischer WL, Tuthill RJ. Vascular invasion by hepatic inflammatory pseudotumor. Cancer 1993;71:2934–2940.

13. Buckler H, Provino M, Akovbiantz A, et al. Regression of liver cell adenoma: a follow-up study of three consecutive patients after discontinuation of oral contraceptive use. Gastroenterology 1982;82:775–782.

14. Burns CD, Kuhns JG, Wieman J. Cholangiocarcinoma in association with multiple biliary microhamartomas. Arch Pathol Lab Med 1990;114:1287–1289.

15. Butron Villa MM, Haot J, Desmet VJ. Cholestatic features in focal nodular hyperplasia of the liver. Liver 1984;4:387–395.

16. Cannon RO III, Dusheiko GM, Long JA Jr, et al. Hepatocellular adenoma in a young woman with beta-thalassemia and secondary iron overload. Gastroenterology 1981;81:534–536.

17. Chen KT, Bocian JJ. Multiple hepatic adenomas. Arch Pathol Lab Med 1983;107:274–275.

18. Coire CI, Qizilbash AH, Castelli MF. Hepatic adenomata in type Ia glycogen storage disease. Arch Pathol Lab Med 1987;111:166–169.

19. Colina F, Alberti N, Solis JA, et al. Diffuse nodular regenerative hyperplasia of the liver (DNRH): a clinicopathologic study of 24 cases. Liver 1989;9:253–265.

20. De Carlis L, Pirotta V, Rondinara G, et al. Hepatic adenoma and focal nodular hyperplasia: diagnosis and criteria for treatment. Liver Transplant Surg 1997;3:160–165.

21. Dehner LP, Ishak KG. Vascular tumors of the liver in infants and children: a study of 30 cases and review of the literature. Arch Pathol 1971;92:101–111.

22. Dehner LP, Ewing SL, Sumner HW. Infantile mesenchymal hamartoma of the liver. Histologic and ultrastructural observations. Arch Pathol 1975;99:379–381.

23. Dekker A, Ten Kate FJW, Terpstra OT. Cholangiocarcinoma associated with multiple biliary microhamartomas. Arch Pathol Lab Med 1990;114:1287–1289.

24. De Maioribus CA, Lally KP, Sim K, et al. Mesenchymal hamartoma of the liver: a 35 year review. Arch Surg 1990;125:598–600.

25. Desmet VJ. Congenital diseases of intrahepatic bile ducts: variations on the theme "ductal plate malformation." Hepatology 1992;16:1069–1083.

26. Dick AP, Gresham GA. Partial nodular transformation of the liver presenting with ascites. Gut 1972;13:289–292.

27. Edmonds AM, Hennigar GR, Crook R. Galactosemia: report of a case with autopsy. Pediatrics 1952;10:40–47.

28. Edmondson HA, Reynolds TB, Henderson B, et al. Regression of liver cell adenomas associated with oral contraceptives. Ann Intern Med 1977;86:180–182.

29. Eguchi A, Nakashima O, Okudaira S, et al. Adenomatous hyperplasia in the vicinity of small hepatocellular carcinoma. Hepatology 1992;15:843–848.

30. Fabre A, Audet P, Vilgrain V, et al. Histologic scoring of liver biopsy in focal nodular hyperplasia with atypical presentation. Hepatology 2002;35:414–420.

31. Ferrell L, Crawford J, Dhillon A, et al. Proposal for standardized criteria for the diagnosis of benign, borderline and malignant hepatocellular lesions arising in chronic advanced liver disease. Am J Surg Pathol 1993;17:1113–1123.

32. Ferrell L, Wright T, Lake J, et al. Incidence and diagnostic features of macroregenerative nodules vs. small hepatocellular carcinoma in cirrhotic livers. Hepatology 1992;16:1372–1381.

33. Flejou J-F, Barge J, Menu Y, et al. Liver adenomatosis: an entity distinct from liver cell adenomas? Gastroenterology 1985;89:1132–1138.

34. Foster JH, Donohue TA, Berman MM. Familial liver-cell adenomas and diabetes mellitus. N Engl J Med 1978;299:239–241.

35. Fried RH, Wardzala A, Wilson RA, et al. Benign cartilaginous tumor (chondroma) in the liver. Arch Pathol Lab Med 1986;110:203–206.

36. Furuya K, Nakamura M, Yamamoto Y, et al. Macroregenerative nodule of the liver: a clinicopathologic study of 345 autopsy cases of chronic liver disease. Cancer 1988;61:99–105.

37. Goodman ZD, Ishak KG. Angiomyolipomas of the liver. Am J Surg Pathol 1984;8:745–750.

38. Goodman ZD, Mikel UV, Lubbers PR, et al. Kupffer cells in hepatocellular adenoma. Am J Surg Pathol 1986;11:191–196.

39. Grange J-D, Guechot J, Legendre C, et al. Liver adenoma and focal nodular hyperplasia in a man with high endogenous sex steroids. Gastroenterology 1987;93:1409–1413.

40. Grigioni WF, D'Errico A, Bacci F, et al. Primary liver neoplasms: evaluation of proliferative index using MoAb Ki67. J Pathol 1989;158:23–29.

41. Gyorffy EJ, Bredfeldt JE, Black WC. Transformation of hepatic cell adenoma to hepatocellular carcinoma due to oral contraceptive use. Ann Intern Med 1989;110:489–490.

42. Haber M, Reuben A, Burrell M, et al. Multiple focal nodular hyperplasia of the liver associated with hemihypertrophy and vascular malformations. Gastroenterology 1995;108:1256–1262.

43. Hall PA, Levison DA, Woods AL, et al. Proliferating cell nuclear antigen (PCNA) immunolocalization in paraffin sections: an index of cell proliferation with evidence of deregulated expression in some neoplasms. J Pathol 1990;162:285–294.

44. Hawkins EP, Jordan GL, McGavran MH. Primary leiomyoma of the liver. Am J Surg Pathol 1980;4:301–304.

45. Hayes D, Lamki H, Hunter IW. Hepatic-cell adenoma presenting with intraperitoneal hemorrhage in the puerperium. BMJ 1977;2:1394.

46. Herman P, Pugliese V, Machado MA, et al. Hepatic adenoma and focal nodular hyperplasia: differential diagnosis and treatment. World J Surg 2000;24:372–376.

47. Hoffman AL, Emre S, Verham RP, et al. Hepatic angiomyolipoma: two case reports of caudate-based lesions and review of the literature. Liver Transplant Surg 1997;3:46–54.

48. Honda N, Cobb C, Lechago J. Bile duct carcinoma associated with multiple von Meyenburg complexes in the liver. Hum Pathol 1986;17:1287–1290.

49. Horiuchi R, Uchida T, Kojima T, et al. Inflammatory pseudotumor of the liver. Clinicopathologic study and review of the literature. Cancer 1990;65:1583–1590.

50. Howell RR, Stevenson RE, Ben-Menchem Y, et al. Hepatic adenomata with type 1 glycogen storage disease. JAMA 1976;236:1481–1484.

51. Hytiroglou P, Linton P, Klion F, et al. Benign schwannoma of the liver. Arch Pathol Lab Med 1993;117:216–218.

52. Ishak KG. Mesenchymal tumors of the liver. In: Okuda K, Peters RL, eds. Hepatocellular carcinoma. New York: John Wiley and Sons, 1976:247–307.

53. Ishak KG, Willis GW, Cummins SD, et al. Biliary cystadenoma and cystadenocarcinoma. Report of 14 cases and review of the literature. Cancer 1977;29:322–338.
54. Ishak KG. Hepatic neoplasms associated with contraceptive and anabolic steroids. In: Lingeman C, ed. Recent advances in cancer research, vol 66. Berlin: Springer-Verlag, 1979:79–128.
55. Ishak KG. Benign tumors and pseudotumors of the liver. Appl Pathol 1988;6:82–104.
56. Janes CH, McGill DB, Ludwig J, et al. Liver cell adenoma at the age of 3 years and transplantation 19 years later after development of carcinoma: a case report. Hepatology 1993;17:583–585.
57. Karhunen PJ. Hepatic pseudolipoma. J Clin Pathol 1985;38:877–879.
58. Kawakita N, Seki S, Sakaguchi H, et al. Analysis of proliferating hepatocytes using a monoclonal antibody against proliferating cell nuclear antigen/cyclin in embedded tissues from various liver diseases fixed in formaldehyde. Am J Pathol 1992;140:513–520.
59. Kessler E, Turani H, Kayser S, et al. Inflammatory pseudotumor of the liver. Liver 1988;8:17–23.
60. Kirchner SG, Hellar RM, Kasselberg AG, et al. Infantile hemangioendothelioma with subsequent malignant degeneration. Pediatr Radiol 1981;11:42–45.
61. Kondo F, Hirooka N, Wada K, et al. Histological features and clinical course of large regenerative nodules: evaluation of their precancerous potentiality. Hepatology 1990;12:592–598.
62. Lack E. Mesenchymal hamartoma of the liver: a clinical and pathologic study of nine cases. Am J Pediatr Hematol Oncol 1986;8:91–98.
63. Le Bail B, Jouhanole H, Deugneier Y, et al. Liver adenomatosis with granulomas in two patients on long-term oral contraceptives. Am J Surg Pathol 1992;16:982–987.
64. Lederman SM, Martin EC, Laffey KT, et al. Hepatic neurofibromatosis, malignant schwannoma and angiosarcoma in von Recklinghausen's disease. Gastroenterology 1989;92:234–239.
65. Li GH, Li JQ, Lin YZ. Inflammatory pseudotumor of the liver. J Surg Oncol 1989;42:244–248.
66. Limmer J, Fleig WE, Leupold D, et al. Hepatocellular carcinoma in type I glycogen storage disease. Hepatology 1988;8:531–537.
67. Lui AFK, Hiratzka LF, Hirose FM. Multiple adenomas of the liver. Cancer 1980;45:1001–1004.
68. Maltjalian DA, Graham CH. Liver adenoma with granulomas. The appearance of granulomas in oral contraceptive–related hepatocellular adenoma and in the surrounding nontumorous liver. Arch Pathol Lab Med 1982;106:244–246.
69. Martini GA. The liver in hereditary hemorrhagic telangiectasia—an inborn error of vascular structure with multiple manifestations: a reappraisal. Gut 1978;19:531–537.
70. Masood S, West AB, Barwick KW. Expression of steroid hormone receptors in benign hepatic tumors. An immunohistochemical study. Arch Pathol Lab Med 1992;116:1355–1359.
71. Mathieu D, Bruneton JN, Droulliard J, et al. Hepatic adenomas and focal nodular hyperplasia: dynamic CT study. Radiology 1986;160:53–58.
72. Mercadier M, Bodard M, Fingerhut A, et al. Papillomatosis of the intrahepatic bile ducts. World J Surg 1984;8:30–35.
73. Miyachi K, Fritzler MJ, Tan EM. Autoantibody to a nuclear antigen in proliferating cells. J Immunol 1978;121:2228–2234.
74. Morales JM, Prieto C, Colina F, et al. Nodular regenerative hyperplasia of the liver in renal transplantation. Transplant Proc 1987;19:3694–3696.
75. Nakanuma Y, Ohta G, Sasaki K. Nodular regenerative hyperplasia of the liver associated with polyarteritis nodosa. Arch Pathol Lab Med 1984;108:133–135.

76. Nakanuma Y, Terada T, Terasaki S, et al. "Atypical adenomatous hyperplasia" in liver cirrhosis: low grade hepatocellular carcinoma or borderline lesion? Histopathology 1990;17:27–35.

77. Neuman RD, LiVolsi VA, Rosenthal NS, et al. Adenocarcinoma in biliary papillomatosis. Gastroenterology 1976;70:779–782.

78. Nhuyen BN, Flejou JF, Terris B, et al. Focal nodular hyperplasia of the liver. A comprehensive pathologic study of 305 lesions and recognition of new histologic forms. Am J Surg Pathol 1999;23:1441–1445.

79. Nokes SR, Baker ME, Spritzer CE, et al. Hepatic adenoma: MR appearance mimicking focal nodular hyperplasia. J Comput Assist Tomogr 1988;12:885–887.

80. Orsatti G, Theise ND, Thung SN, et al. DNA image cytometric analysis of macroregenerative nodules (adenomatous hyperplasia) of the liver: evidence in support of their preneoplastic nature. Hepatology 1993;17:621–627.

81. Pain JA, Gimson AES, Williams R, et al. Focal nodular hyperplasia of the liver: results of treatment and options in management. Gut 1991;32:524–527.

82. Parker P, Burr I, Slonim A, et al. Regression of hepatic adenoma in type Ia glycogen storage diseases with dietary therapy. Gastroenterology 1981;81:534–536.

83. Paulson EK, McClellan JS, Washington K, et al. Hepatic adenoma: MR characteristics and correlation with pathologic findings. AJR Am J Roentgenol 1994;163:113–116.

84. Petrovic LM. Benign hepatocellular tumors and tumor-like lesions. In: Ferrell L, ed. Diagnostic problems in liver pathology. Philadelphia: Hanley & Belfus, 1994:119–141.

85. Reynolds WJ, Wanless IR. Nodular regenerative hyperplasia of the liver in a patient with rheumatoid vasculitis: a morphometric study suggesting a role for hepatic arteritis in the pathogenesis. J Rheumatol 1984;11:838–842.

86. Rooks JB, Ory HW, Ishak KG, et al. Epidemiology of hepatocellular adenoma: the role of oral contraceptive use. JAMA 1979;242:644–648.

87. Sadowski DC, Lee SS, Wanless IR, et al. Progressive type of focal nodular hyperplasia characterized by multiple tumors and recurrence. Hepatology 1995;21:970–975.

88. Sakamota M, Hirohashi S, Shimosato Y. Early stages of multistep hepatocarcinogenesis: adenomatous hyperplasia and early hepatocellular carcinoma. Hum Pathol 1991; 22:172–178.

89. Salisbury JR, Portmann BC. Oncocytic cell adenoma. Histopathology 1987;11:191–196.

90. Schwartz SI, Husser WC. Cavernous hemangioma of the liver: a single institution report of 16 resections. Ann Surg 1987;205:456–465.

91. Shastri S, Dubinsky M, Poordad F, et al. Nodular hyperplasia of the liver (Sabourin lesion) occurring with inflammatory bowel diseases in association with 6-thioguanine therapy. Am J Clin Pathol 2002;118:631.

92. Sherlock S, Feldman CA, Moran B, et al. Partial nodular transformation of the liver with portal hypertension. Am J Med 1966;40:195–203.

93. Steibrecher UP, Lsibona R, Huang SN, et al. Complete regression of hepatocellular adenomas after withdrawal of oral contraceptives. Dig Dis Sci 1981;26:1045–1050.

94. Stocker JT, Ishak KG. Mesenchymal hamartoma of the liver. Report of 30 cases and review of the literature. Pediatr Pathol 1983;1:245–267.

95. Strate SM, Rutledge JC, Weinberg AG. Delayed development of angiosarcoma in multinodular infantile hepatic hemangioendothelioma. Arch Pathol Lab Med 1984;108:943–944.

96. Stromeyer FW, Ishak KG. Nodular transformation (nodular "regenerative" hyperplasia) of the liver. A clinicopathologic study of 30 cases. Hum Pathol 1981;12:60–71.

97. Taylor CR, Taylor KJ, Belleza N. Focal fatty changes in the liver: academic or epidemic? J Clin Gastroenterol 1982;4:475–478.

98. Terada T, Hosos M, Nakanuma Y. Mallory body clustering in adenomatous hyperplasia in human cirrhotic livers: report of four cases. Hum Pathol 1989;20:886–890.

99. Terada T, Nakanuma Y. Cell proliferative activity in adenomatous hyperplasia of the liver and small hepatocellular carcinoma. An immunohistochemical study demonstrating proliferating cell nuclear antigen. Cancer 1981;70:591–598.

100. Terada T, Nakanuma Y, Kono N, et al. Ciliated hepatic foregut cyst. A mucus histochemical, immunohistochemical, and ultrastructural study in three cases in comparison with normal bronchi and intrahepatic bile ducts. Am J Surg Pathol 1990;14:356–363.

101. Terada T, Nakanuma Y. Iron-negative foci in siderotic macroregenerative nodules in human cirrhotic liver. A marker of incipient neoplastic lesions. Arch Pathol Lab Med 1989;113:916–920.

102. Tesluk H, Laurie J. Hepatocellular adenoma: its transformation to carcinoma in a user of oral contraceptives. Arch Pathol Lab Med 1981;105:296–299.

103. Theise ND, Schwartz M, Miller C, et al. Macroregenerative nodules and hepatocellular carcinoma in forty four sequential adult liver explants with cirrhosis. Hepatology 1992;16:949–955.

104. Tsui WMS, Loo KT, Chow LTC, et al. Biliary adenofibroma. A heretofore unrecognized benign biliary tumor of the liver. Am J Surg Pathol 1993;17:186–192.

105. Tsui WMS, Yuen AKT, Tse CCH. Hepatic angiomyolipoma with a deceptive trabecular pattern and HMB-45 reactivity. Histopathology 1992;21:569–571.

106. Van Steenbergen W, Joosten E, Marchal G, et al. Hepatic lymphangiomatosis. Report of a case and review of the literature. Gastroenterology 1985;88:1968–1972.

107. Vecchio FM, Fabrano A, Ghirlanda G, et al. Fibrolamellar carcinoma of the liver. The malignant counterpart of focal nodular hyperplasia with oncocytic change. Am J Clin Pathol 1984;81:521–526.

108. Veloso FT, Ribeiro AT, Teixeira A, et al. Biliary papillomatosis: report of a case with 5-year follow-up. Am J Gastroenterol 1983;78:645–648.

109. Wada K, Kondo F, Kondo Y. Large regenerative nodules and dysplastic nodules in cirrhotic livers: a histopathologic study. Hepatology 1988;8:1684–1688.

110. Wanless IR, Mawdsley C, Adams R. On the pathogenesis of focal nodular hyperplasia. Hepatology 1985;5:1194–1200.

111. Wanless IR, Gryfe A. Nodular transformation of the liver in hereditary hemorrhagic telangiectasia. Arch Pathol Lab Med 1986;110:331–335.

112. Wanless IR, Albrecht S, Bilbao J, et al. Multiple focal nodular hyperplasia associated with vascular malformations of various organs and neoplasia of the brain: a new syndrome. Mod Pathol 1989;2:456–462.

113. Washington K, Lane KL, Meyers WC. Nodular regenerative hyperplasia in partial hepatectomy specimens. Am J Surg Pathol 1993;17:1151–1158.

114. Weihing RR, Shintaku IP, Geller SA, et al. Hepatobiliary and pancreatic mucinous cystadenocarcinomas with mesenchymal stroma: analysis of estrogen and progesterone receptors and expression of tumor associated antigens. Mod Pathol 1997;10:372–379.

115. Weinberg AG, Mize CE, Worthem HG. The occurrence of hepatoma in the chronic form of tyrosinemia. J Pediatr 1976;88:434–438.

116. Wheeler DA, Edmondson HA. Cystadenoma with mesenchymal stroma (CMS) in the liver and bile ducts: a clinicopathologic study of 17 cases, 4 with malignant change. Cancer 1985;56:1434–1445.

117. Wheeler DA, Edmondson HA, Reynolds TB. Spontaneous liver cell adenoma in children. Am J Clin Pathol 1986;85:6–12.

118. Woods GL. Biliary cystadenocarcinoma. Case report of hepatic malignancy originating in benign cystadenoma. Cancer 1981;1:2936–2940.

119. Yasunaga C, Sueishi K, Ohgami H, et al. Heterogeneous expression of endothelial cell markers in infantile hemangioendothelioma. Immunohistochemical study of two solitary cases and one multiple one. Am J Clin Pathol 1989;91:673–681.

24

PRIMARY AND METASTATIC MALIGNANT TUMORS OF THE LIVER

Malignant neoplasms, both secondary and primary, are common in the liver. Metastases are far more common than primary liver malignancies.

PRIMARY EPITHELIAL TUMORS OF THE LIVER

Hepatocellular Carcinoma

Hepatocellular carcinoma (HCC), a common neoplasm worldwide with as many as one million new cases per year, is most common in Southeast Asia and Central Africa. In North America and Europe the incidence is rising. The most important risk factors are hepatitis B (HBV) and C (HCV) viral infection, hemochromatosis, cirrhosis of any cause including alcoholic liver disease, and many drugs and toxins (2,15,16,25,28,44,48,50,52,60,93, 98,100,103,158,169,181,189,199). Less common associations include metabolic and other disorders (1,27,31,39,71,77,90,95,99,108,113,118,130, 143,149,158,160,182,191).

HBV DNA is integrated into the host genome and likely promotes carcinogenesis (25,28,93,98,100). Repeated and persistent injury followed by inflammation and regeneration triggers the carcinogenic cascade of events leading to carcinogenesis with many factors contributing (42,64, 119,122,152,169,172,180,184,188). Chronic HCV is also associated with a high incidence of HCC. HCV is an RNA virus with a mode of replication different from that of HBV; it is not integrated into the host genome, and the mechanism of hepatocarcinogenesis is still poorly understood (37,58, 93,116,145,169,175,188,196).

CLINICAL FEATURES. Varied and nonspecific manifestations include abdominal pain, weight loss, and, with progression, hepatomegaly, jaundice, and signs of bile duct obstruction. Liver tests are abnormal but relatively nonspecific, often reflecting underlying chronic liver disease. Elevated serum α-fetoprotein (AFP) values, although not specific, can indicate development and growth of HCC. Imaging techniques can detect relatively early lesions, but small HCCs (less than 1.5 cm) are often not

344

TABLE 24.1	**Primary Epithelial Tumors of the Liver (Based on a Revised World Health Organization Classification)**

1. Hepatocellular carcinoma
2. Hepatoblastoma
3. Cholangiocarcinoma
4. Mixed hepatocholangiocarcinoma
5. Hepatobiliary cystadenocarcinoma

Reproduced with permission from Ishak KG, Anthony PP, Sobin LH. Histological typing of tumors of the liver. World Health Organization histological classification of tumors. 2nd Ed. Berlin: Springer-Verlag, 1994.

seen. The prognosis of larger (greater than 6 cm) tumors is poor. The fibrolamellar variant of HCC (FL-HCC) may have a somewhat better prognosis (33,80,81,135,138). HCC can be solitary or multinodular (79,80). In multinodular tumors, the question of multicentric origin versus intrahepatic metastases remains unresolved. As many as 90% of HCCs develop in the background of a cirrhotic liver, especially in high-incidence regions, but HCC also occurs in noncirrhotic liver (33,54,136,180).

HCC has a propensity for intravascular spread, most often to the portal vein system. Hepatic veins can also be involved, leading to venous outflow obstruction (Budd-Chiari syndrome). Tumor can extend to the inferior vena cava, the right atrium, and there may be gastric and esophageal varices (33). Direct extension into bile ducts can lead to hemobilia or symptoms of large bile duct obstruction. Spread to adjacent organs, such as stomach and duodenum, also occurs (33,80). Rarely, HCC undergoes spontaneous regression (59,69).

CLASSIFICATION. Numerous classifications and criteria have been proposed for the diagnosis of HCC (38,90). The World Health Organization (WHO) classification (Table 24.1), which emphasizes the importance of both architectural and cytologic features in establishing the diagnosis, is widely accepted (80).

PATHOLOGY: ARCHITECTURAL PATTERNS. Several patterns are seen. The most common is the trabecular or sinusoidal pattern, with exaggerated liver plates, sometimes 15 to 20 cells thick or more, separated by sinusoids that maintain endothelial lining cells confirmed with immunostains for factor VIII, CD31, and CD34 (Fig. 24.1, e-Figs, 24.1–24.3) (33,81). Kupffer cells are often present, in reduced numbers. Solid areas may be seen, and necrosis may be prominent.

The second common pattern is acinar or pseudoglandular. Gland-like structures, formed by hepatocytes, may contain fibrin, bile, and even

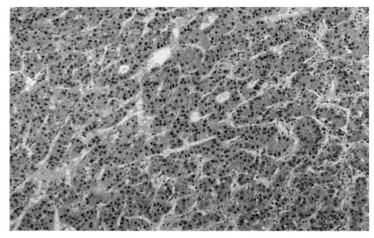

FIGURE 24.1 Hepatocellular carcinoma, trabecular pattern (hematoxylin-eosin, original magnification ×100).

histiocytes (Fig. 24.2, e-Figs. 24.4–24.6). Bile can be seen in the cytoplasm of tumor cells, most often the acinar variant, and is pathognomonic for HCC (e-Fig. 24.7). Many HCCs have mixed architecture, with both trabecular and acinar areas (Fig. 24.3, e-Figs. 24.8, 24.9).

A third pattern is solid, compact, or pelioid with thickened liver cell trabecula. Immunostains can demonstrate sinusoids, but they are

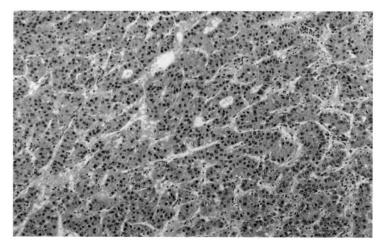

FIGURE 24.2 Hepatocellular carcinoma, predominantly acinar pattern. Note the presence of bile within the acinar lumina (hematoxylin-eosin, original magnification ×100).

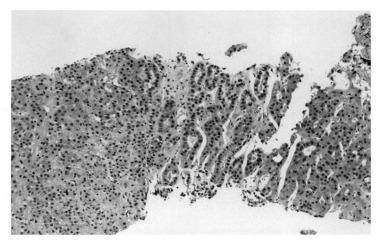

FIGURE 24.3   Hepatocellular carcinoma, mixed pattern, trabecular and acinar (hematoxylin-eosin, original magnification ×200).

compressed by the expanding liver plates, giving the impression of a solid neoplasm (e-Fig. 24.10). Large pseudovascular blood-filled spaces (vacular mimicry) (e-Fig. 24.11) similar to those of peliosis hepatis are often seen and may signify poorer prognosis. These tumors can rupture and cause hemoperitoneum.

Histologic Variants of HCC (Table 24.2)

In many well-differentiated HCCs, hepatocytes are quite bland with minimal cytologic atypia. Cells retain their polygonal shape and eosinophilic finely granular cytoplasm. Nuclei are usually round, and the early sign of atypia is nuclear enlargement with hyperchromasia, irregular nuclear contour, and irregular nuclear chromatin. Nuclei of dysplastic cells often show more cytologic atypia than the nuclei of well-differentiated HCC.

TABLE 24.2	**Histologic Variants of Hepatocellular Carcinoma (HCC)**
HCC of the usual type	
Sclerosing HCC	
Clear cell HCC	
Spindle cell (sarcomatoid) HCC	
Pleomorphic (giant cell anaplastic) HCC	
Fibrolamellar HCC	

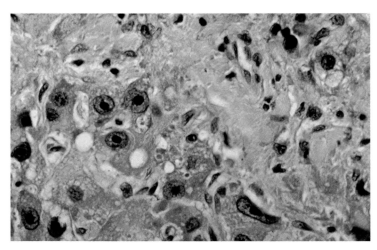

FIGURE 24.4 Hepatocellular carcinoma, intracytoplasmic inclusions (hematoxylin-eosin, original magnification ×400).

Eosinophilic nucleoli may be prominent. Individual cells may not be enlarged.

HEPATOCELLULAR CARCINOMA OF THE USUAL TYPE. HCC cells can be strikingly similar to benign, nonneoplastic hepatocytes, with somewhat more basophilic cytoplasm, and variable degrees of pleomorphism, arranged in several-cells-thick trabeculae.

Various intracytoplasmic inclusions can be seen including Mallory-like material, albumin, fibrinogen, pale bodies, and megamitochondria (33,74,80,140,142,164) (Fig. 24.4). Intranuclear eosinophilic pseudoinclusions, representing focal invaginations of the cytoplasm, are also seen. Mucin is not an HCC product, and its presence should suggest either metastatic adenocarcinoma or cholangiocarcinoma (CCa) (87,106,120,148,151). In HBV associated HCC, viral antigens are only rarely demonstrated in tumor cells (98).

Differential Diagnosis. Conditions to be distinguished in usual type HCC include macroregenerative nodules (MRNs), liver cell adenoma (LCA), CCa, and hepatoblastoma (HB). In some cases, liver cell dysplasia may be quite similar to HCC.

Distinguishing between HCC and MRNs with liver cell dysplasia can be problematic. Liver cells in a well-differentiated HCC can be very bland and resemble benign hepatocytes. In contrast, dysplastic liver cells often show prominent cytologic atypia. The architectural pattern may be similar in both conditions, although liver cell plates are usually thicker in HCC. The diagnosis of well-differentiated HCC can be exceedingly difficult, especially in biopsy samples, and reticulin silver preparation is usually helpful. In most HCCs, including well-differentiated ones, the reticulin network is

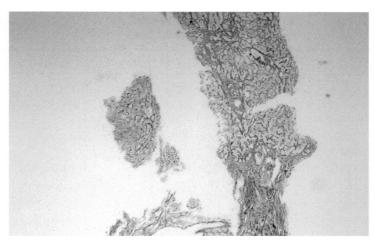

FIGURE 24.5   Hepatocellular carcinoma, trabecular pattern. Note attenuation and almost complete absence of underlying reticulin pattern (reticulin silver preparation, original magnification ×100).

significantly attenuated or even absent (Fig. 24.5, e-Fig. 24.11). Glypican-3 immunostain is often positive in HCC (e-Figs. 24.13, 24.14) and can be helpful. However, although sensitive, it is not completely specific. It can also be useful in aspirate samples (e-Fig. 24.15).

Differentiation of HCC from LCA can also be difficult. LCA arises in the noncirrhotic liver, whereas most HCCs are seen with cirrhosis. LCA is usually solid, although focal acinar pattern may also be seen. LCA does not have significant cytologic atypia, and there is no significant attenuation of reticulin network.

Differentiation between acinar HCC and CCa can also be problematic, particularly in biopsies (110). Intracytoplasmic mucin is strong evidence for CCa. In contrast, intracytoplasmic bile in tumor cells is diagnostic of HCC. Desmoplastic stromal reaction is more prominent in CCa but is not always helpful because it is also seen in sclerosing HCC.

Imunohistochemical markers are helpful in differentiating HCC from CCa (e-Figs. 24.16–24.18) (Table 24.3).

SCLEROSING HEPATOCELLULAR CARCINOMA. The sclerosing variant of HCC is associated with hypercalcemia (79,150). The tumor shows trabecular, acinar, or mixed trabecular-acinar architectural pattern. Malignant hepatocytes are embedded in abundant, relatively dense, hypocellular fibrous stroma (33,79). FL-HCC, CCa, and other metastatic adenocarcinomas can be similar.

The FL-HCC fibrous stroma is distinctly lamellar (Fig. 24.6, e-Figs. 24.19, 24.20). The hepatocytes are large, polygonal, and eosinophilic, with abundant intracytoplasmic pale bodies. Characteristically, FL-HCC occurs in younger patients in contrast with the sclerosing variant of HCC, which usually occurs in older patients.

TABLE 24.3   Immunohistochemical Markers Helpful in Differentiating HCC from Cholangiocarcinoma (Compiled Data)

	HCC	Cholangiocarcinoma
AFP	15%–70%	Negative >90%
CEA polyclonal (canalicular pattern)	50%–90%	Negative >90%
Hepar-1 (intracytoplasmic granular)	80%–90%	Negative
α1-antitrypsin	55%–90%	Negative >90%
CD10	~50%	Negative
CAM5.2	~40%	Negative .80%
CK8/18	~20%	(Poor prognosis)
CEA monoclonal (cytoplasmic/luminal)	Usually negative	80%–90%
MOC31	Negative >90%	Positive
CK7	Negative >70%	80%–90%
CK19	Negative >80%	80%–90%
CK20	Negative >90%	30%–70%
AE1/3	Negative >90%	>80%
EMA	Negative >90%	>70%
Keratin 903	Negative >90%	>80%
P53	<10% (focal)	>60%

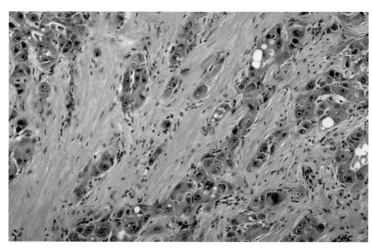

FIGURE 24.6   Fibrolamellar hepatocellular carcinoma (hematoxylin-eosin, original magnification ×200).

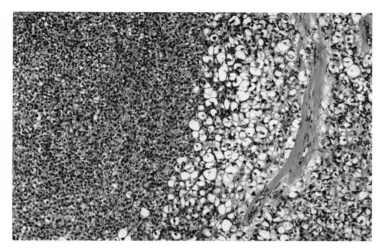

FIGURE 24.7   Hepatocellular carcinoma, clear cell variant (hematoxylin-eosin, original magnification ×200).

Metastatic adenocarcinomas, particularly those arising in the biliary tree and pancreas, can be quite desmoplastic, but the stroma is usually not as dense as in sclerosing HCC. Immunohistochemical studies can be helpful (109,159,190,197).

CLEAR CELL HEPATOCELLULAR CARCINOMA. In clear cell HCC, tumor cytoplasm is clear because of abundant glycogen. Clear cells alternate with tumor cells resembling nonneoplastic hepatocytes (Fig. 24.7, e-Fig. 24.21). Clear cell HCC can be associated with hypoglycemia, sometimes with hypercholesterolemia, and may have a somewhat better prognosis than usual HCC (22). Differentiation from other clear cell tumors, particularly metastatic renal cell carcinoma (RCC) or adrenocortical carcinoma (AdCC), can be difficult. Cirrhosis strongly favors the diagnosis of HCC. Vimentin and LeuM-1 immunostaining are characteristic of RCC, and AdCC shows synaptophysin, inhibin, and Melan-A, rare in HCC. Intracellular bile is diagnostic of HCC as is a canalicular pattern with polyclonal CEA (e-Fig. 24.) (33).

SPINDLE CELL (SARCOMATOID) HEPATOCELLULAR CARCINOMA. Spindle cell or sarcomatoid variant of HCC is rare. The tumor consists of spindle cells arranged in fascicles. An organoid pattern can also be seen. Multinucleated giant cells are common (92). Differentiation from true sarcomas, including leiomyosarcoma and fibrosarcoma, may be difficult, but true mesenchymal tumors can express vimentin.

PLEOMORPHIC (GIANT CELL, ANAPLASTIC) HEPATOCELLULAR CARCINOMA. The least common histologic variant of HCC is pleomorphic or giant cell variant, in which the tumor cells are arranged in solid sheets and most tumor cells

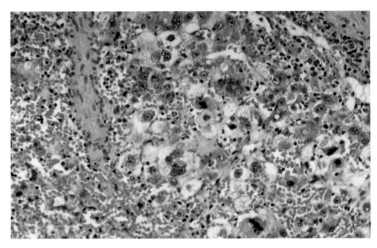

FIGURE 24.8   Pleomorphic (giant cell) variant of hepatocellular carcinoma (hematoxylin-eosin, original magnification ×200).

exhibit bizarre nuclear features. In addition, many cells may be multinucleated (33,76) (Fig. 24.8, e-figs 24.22–24.31).

FIBROLAMELLAR HEPATOCELLULAR CARCINOMA. FL-HCC is more often seen in younger adults, in the background of a noncirrhotic liver. Both sexes are equally affected. A generally better prognosis is attributed to patient's age, resectability of the tumor, and absence of cirrhosis (33,46,113,140). Tumor cells show abundant eosinophilic granular cytoplasm and are distinctly oncocytic (Fig. 24.6, e-Figs. 24.32–24.41). Sheets of oncocytic cells are separated by pale, paucicellular, lamellated fibrous stroma imparting the characteristic microscopic appearance. Tumor cells can produce bile. Pale bodies show reactivity with antibody for fibrinogen, demonstrable in frozen sections. Eosinophilic intracytoplasmic globules composed of C-reactive protein, fibrinogen or α1-antitrypsin are also seen (17,18,24). Most cases have copper and copper-binding protein.

Histologic Grading of Hepatocellular Carcinoma

In contrast with most other malignant tumors, histologic grading has not proven particularly useful in determining HCC prognosis. Edmondson and Steiner proposed four grades of HCC (47). Most HCCs are grade II or III. Well-differentiated HCC, grade I, may be difficult to distinguish from LCA or MRNs with dysplasia. Grade IV tumors may be indistinguishable from undifferentiated adenocarcinomas from other primary sites (33).

IMMUNOHISTOCHEMISTRY. There is no single reliable and specific immunohistochemical marker for HCC (110). Hepatocytes, both benign and malignant, generally show strong reactivity with low molecular weight keratin (CAM 5.2, CK8) but not with a high molecular weight keratin

(CK7, CK19). CCa, in contrast, can be positive for both. AFP is demonstrable in 10% to 70% of HCCs (Table 24.3) (78,91,109,120,151).

Antibodies helpful in establishing the diagnosis of HCC include hepatocyte paraffin 1 (hepar-1), α1-antitrypsin, demonstration of canalicular pattern with polyclonal CEA, and highlighting of the sinusoidal pattern with CD10, CD31, or CD34 (29,109,110,122,151,153). Neuroendocrine differentiation can sometimes be shown with chromogranin and synaptophysin (14). Human chorionic gonadotropin (HCG) and estrogen and progesterone receptors can also be demonstrated in some cases (137).

PROLIFERATION MARKERS. Various antibodies, including those for proliferating cell nuclear antigen and Ki-67 (Mib-1), may be useful in demonstrating the high level of cell proliferation within the tumor but are not useful in establishing the diagnosis (97,148).

FLOW CYTOMETRY AND IMAGE ANALYSIS. Flow cytometry and morphometric studies of HCC have shown conflicting results (40,57,138,139,152,180, 188). Image analysis may be useful as an adjunct tool in differentiating between dysplasia, well-differentiated HCC, and poorly differentiated HCC (9).

ELECTRON MICROSCOPY. Electron microscopy may be useful in some cases of HCC, but it is rarely used in routine practice (33).

MOLECULAR STUDIES. Molecular studies have shown significant differences in the expression of various oncogenes in nonneoplastic liver and HCC, including hepatocyte growth factor (HGF) and its receptors c-met and c-myc (122,131,154,156,172,175,183,189). For example, HGF RNA is not expressed in normal or cirrhotic liver tissue but is present in LCA and HCC. Its receptor c-met is also significantly up-regulated in LCA and HCC, as opposed to normal livers, and the expression of HGF and c-met is also associated with higher expression of c-myc protooncogene (122,183). The role of a putative stem cell in liver regeneration and carcinogenesis has been extensively studied in the last several years (178). A computer-assisted imaging neural network expert system can be a helpful adjunct tool in differentiating hepatocellular large cell dysplasia from HCC (9).

Premalignant Conditions

LIVER CELL DYSPLASIA. Liver cell dysplasia was described more than 20 years ago, but its nature and significance remains controversial (11,12). In large cell dysplasia (LCD), cells are large, with prominent hyperchromatic nuclei, often with intranuclear inclusions (10–12) (Fig. 24.9, e-Fig. 24.42). The number of affected cells in a regenerative nodule may be variable with single cells or groups, or LCD can occupy the entire nodule. LCD is more commonly seen in cirrhosis resulting from HBV or HCV but can be present in chronic hepatitis and cirrhoses of other causes (34,53,115,127,144, 152). LCD usually has an aneuploid DNA pattern and was considered a true preneoplastic condition (9). However, it has been suggested that LCD

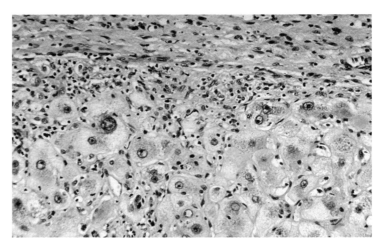

FIGURE 24.9 Liver cell dysplasia, large cell type (hematoxylin-eosin, original magnification ×200).

is not truly preneoplastic, instead reflecting a response to cholestasis in the failing liver (115). In our experience, LCD is only rarely associated with cholestasis. In an experimental model, LCD was a clear precursor to the development of HCC (62).

Small cell dysplasia (SCD) is less common than LCD. The liver cell nuclei are enlarged, but the hepatocytes remain relatively small, imparting the histologic appearance of an increased number of cells in a defined histologic field (e-Figs. 24.43. 24.44). There is general agreement that SCD is a reliable indicator of malignancy and, in biopsy, may not be distinguishable from well-differentiated HCC.

MRNs are also discussed in the chapters on benign liver lesions/tumors (Chapter 23) and cirrhosis (Chapter 20) (3,4,49,53,54,58,144, 152,172).

Hepatoblastoma

Hepatoblastoma (HB) is a primary liver cell tumor mostly affecting males younger than 3 years of age, only rarely seen in adults (33,80,104). There is failure to thrive, a growing abdominal mass, and high serum AFP values (33). The tumor may be associated with several congenital anomalies, including Down syndrome, Beckwith-Wiedemann syndrome, nephroblastoma, absence of right adrenal gland, fetal hydrops, Meckel diverticulum, and umbilical hernia. Familial cases have been described (33,81,102,161).

PATHOLOGY. Irregular tumor nodules composed of epithelial and mesenchymal components are usually separated by delicate fibrous strands and may initially resemble cirrhotic liver. Epithelial hepatoblastoma can show fetal and embryonal cells. Fetal cells resemble hepatocytes of the fetus at 6 to 8 weeks of gestation, arranged in two- to three-cell-thick liver cell cords. The

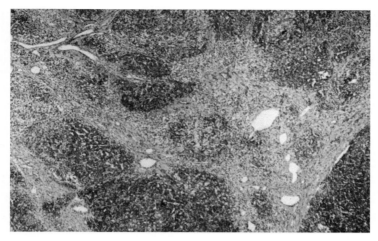

FIGURE 24.10 Hepatoblastoma, epithelial type with embryonal and fetal cells (hematoxylin-eosin, original magnification ×100).

fetal cells contain variable amounts of glycogen and neutral fat, giving a characteristic alternating light and dark histologic pattern of the tumor. Extramedullary hematopoiesis is often present (33,38,66). Embryonal cells are usually elongated or spindle cells, arranged in cords or rosette-like formations. Some epithelial HBs exhibit striking similarity to HCC, with so-called macrotrabecular growth pattern. These have a poorer prognosis (Fig. 24.10, e-Figs. 24.44–24.51) (38,66).

Mixed epithelial-mesenchymal HB has, in addition to its usual epithelial component, mesenchymal tissue composed of fibroblasts, colla-

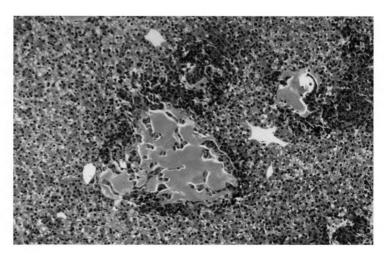

FIGURE 24.11 Hepatoblastoma, mixed type with osteoid-like formation (hematoxylin-eosin, original magnification ×100).

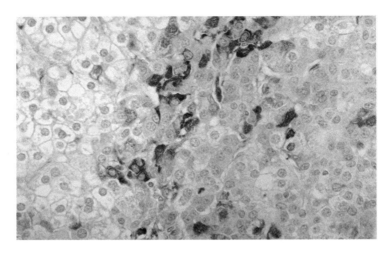

FIGURE 24.12   Hepatoblastoma, focal positivity for α-fetoprotein (AFP) (immunoperoxidase, antibody for AFP, original magnification ×200).

gen, and osteoid (Fig. 24.11). Sometimes these tumors are described as teratoid hepatoblastomas (125). Anaplastic hepatoblastoma is composed of small, undifferentiated cells with hyperchromatic nuclei and scant cytoplasm. The prognosis of this type is worse than that of other types (65,66). Combined hepatoblastoma and yolk sac tumor have also been described (35).

Immunohistochemical findings include positivity for low and high molecular weight keratins, CAM 5.2 and AE 1/3, and for AFP, S-100, and vimentin, particularly in embryonal spindle cells (Fig. 24.12). Endocrine differentiation within the tumor has been reported, and chromogranin and neuron-specific enolase may be positive (166). Some HBs secrete human chorionic gonadotropin demonstrable with immunostain (134). Melanin-containing HB has also been reported (167).

Untreated, the prognosis is dismal. Fetal pattern HB may respond to therapy. HB grows rapidly, invading adjacent tissues and organs with distant metastases often in lungs, brain, or bone marrow at diagnosis. Survival generally is better for HB after liver transplantation than for HCC (104).

Cholangiocarcinoma

This adenocarcinoma of bile duct origin can be intrahepatic (peripheral), hilar (Klatskin tumor), or extrahepatic (33). CCa is usually solitary and, unlike HCC, usually arises in a noncirrhotic liver. Factors associated with CCa include primary sclerosing cholangitis, infestation with various oriental flukes (77,169), and congenital biliary cysts, including Caroli disease and choledochal cyst (13,19,23,26,33,36,75), as well as after exposure to thorium dioxide (Thorotrast) (87,165,192). CCa usually develops between 50 and 70 years of age with both sexes equally affected (141). Peripheral

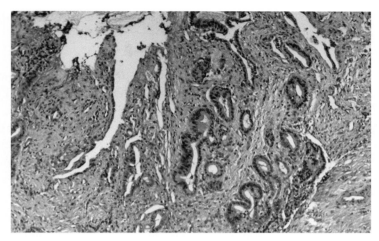

FIGURE 24.13   Cholangiocarcinoma in a patient with known primary sclerosing cholangitis (hematoxylin-eosin, original magnification ×200).

CCa is more common, involving the smaller intrahepatic bile ducts. By the time symptoms manifest, CCa is generally significantly large and unresectable. In contrast, hilar CCa presents relatively early with jaundice and other signs and symptoms of bile duct obstruction. Extrahepatic CCa arises anywhere between the hepatic duct and ampulla of Vater. Both hilar and extrahepatic variants of CCa affect mostly men in the sixth and seventh decades (141).

PATHOLOGY. CCa is a glandular tumor with abundant desmoplastic stromal reaction (Fig. 24.13, e-Figs. 24.52–24.55). There can be papillary or solid growth patterns. Tumor cells are columnar or cuboidal with mildly basophilic cytoplasm, round or ovoid nuclei, and indistinct nucleoli. Intracytoplasmic mucin is often seen.

There are several grades of differentiation. A signet ring component can be present in poorly differentiated, usually papillary CCa variants. Focal squamous differentiation can also occur, with the tumor resembling mucoepidermoid or adenosquamous carcinoma (105,141,157). The tumor locally infiltrates portal tracts and insidiously invades periportal sinusoids. Metastases are usually in regional lymph nodes at the time of diagnosis, and distant metastases to lungs and peritoneal surface may be seen. It may be impossible to distinguish this tumor from adenocarcinoma originating from pancreas or the extrahepatic portion of the biliary tree.

Differentiating between HCC with predominantly acinar architectural configuration and CCa is often difficult. Reactivity with antibodies for epithelial membrane antigen, high molecular weight keratins, carcinoembryonic antigen, blood group antigens, tissue polypeptide antigens, and carbohydrate antigen CA 19-9 can help establish the diagnosis of CCa (Table 24.3) (20,41,78,91,110,120).

Mixed Cholangiohepatocellular Carcinoma

Mixed cholangiohepatocellular carcinoma is an uncommon tumor with features of HCC and CCa. Patients present with elevated serum AFP values (67) (e-Figs. 24.56, 24.61).

HEPATOID TUMOR. Rare HCC-like malignancies, so-called hepatoid tumors, are histologically indistinguishable from usual HCC. They produce albumin, bile, fibrinogen, AFP, and other hepatocytes products. They have been described in the ovary, stomach, gallbladder, pancreas, lung, kidney, and endometrium (e-Fig. 24.62) (61,73, 84–86, 128,147).

Hepatobiliary Cystadenocarcinoma

Hepatobiliary mucinous cystadenocarcinoma with mesenchymal stroma is a rare malignant tumor, occurring almost exclusive in women, and is indistinguishable from that of the ovary (33,43,68). It can develop in congenital hepatic fibrosis, choledochal cyst, or in the setting of a pre-existing hepatobiliary cystadenoma (5,33) and also arises from ectopic gallbladder rests and bile duct epithelium. This concept is supported by ultrastructural similarities between stroma and epithelium.

PATHOLOGY. Hepatobiliary cystadenocarcinoma is a multilocular cystic neoplasm lined with either simple cuboidal or columnar epithelium, with or without mucin production. A distinctive stroma composed of densely packed spindle cells, resembling either ovarian stroma or fetal mesenchyme, is subjacent to the epithelium (Fig. 24.14, e-figs. 24.63–24.65).

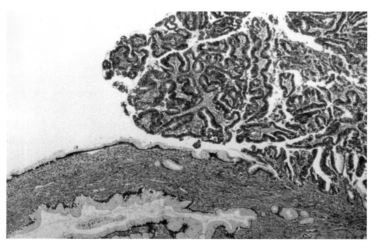

FIGURE 24.14   Hepatobiliary cystadenocarcinoma with mesenchymal stroma arising in cystadenoma (hematoxylin-eosin, original magnification ×100).

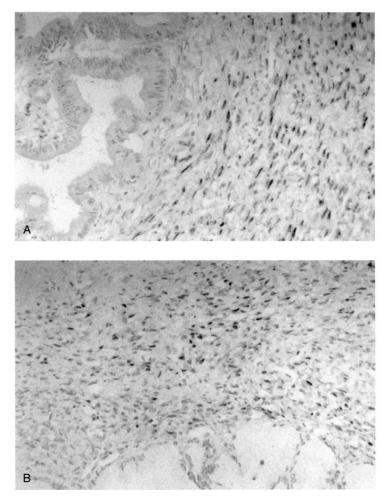

FIGURE 24.15 Hepatobiliary cystadenocarcinoma with mesenchymal stroma that expresses estrogen/progesterone receptors (immunoperoxidase, specific antibodies for estrogen **(A)** and progesterone **(B)** receptors, original magnification ×200).

In both hepatobiliary and pancreatic mucinous cystadenocarcinoma, stromal cells express estrogen and progesterone receptors (190) (Fig. 24.15).

Differential diagnosis includes CCa and CCa with hepatic cysts, both of which have invariably dismal prognosis. Hepatobiliary cystadenocarcinoma, in contrast, is a less aggressive neoplasm, and timely hepatic resection may be curative.

TABLE 24.4	Nonepithelial Primary Malignant Tumors of the Liver
1. Angiosarcoma	
2. Epithelioid hemangioendothelioma (EHE)	
3. Kaposi sarcoma (KS)	
4. Lymphomas	
5. Histiocytosis X	
6. Others	

NONEPITHELIAL PRIMARY MALIGNANT TUMORS OF THE LIVER (TABLE 24.4)

Angiosarcoma

Angiosarcoma is the commonest of the primary malignant mesenchymal neoplasms of the liver. Males are most often affected, and increasing age is a significant risk factor. Environmental risk factors include long-term exposure to monomeric vinyl chloride (56,159), thorium dioxide (Thorotrast) (82,87,126,159), arsenic (33), and steroids (49,74,133). Alcoholic cirrhosis and hemochromatosis may also be associated (33).

The biopsy diagnosis may be difficult, and differentiation from epithelioid hemangioendothelioma may be virtually impossible. Differentiation is important, however, since prognosis and treatment differ significantly. Epithelioid hemangioendothelioma can be cured by transplantation, whereas the prognosis of angiosarcoma is invariably dismal (82). There are four distinct gross patterns: diffuse micronodular, diffuse multinodular, massive, and mixed (82,159).

PATHOLOGY. Several patterns occur, often in combination. The sinusoidal or cavernous pattern has dilated sinusoid-like or vascular spaces lined by malignant spindle endothelial cells. The endothelial cells are enlarged, plump, with hyperchromatic, irregular nuclei, and often with bizarre nuclear features (Fig. 24.16, e-Figs. 24.66–24.70). Tumor cells are positive for various endothelial markers, including factor VIII, CD31, and CD34 (Fig. 24.17, e-Fig. 24.71) (82,159). Diagnostic problems arise when only solid areas, composed of spindle cells, are present without obvious vascular spaces. The less differentiated the tumor is, the less for positivity with specific endothelial markers. Other sarcomas have to be considered in the differential diagnosis, especially in biopsy samples.

Epithelioid Hemangioendothelioma

Epithelioid hemangioendothelioma (EHE) is a relatively rare, generally low- or intermediate-grade malignant vascular tumor. Usually slow growing,

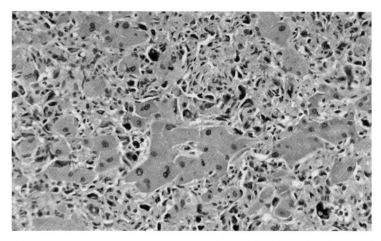

FIGURE 24.16   Angiosarcoma. Large, hyperchromatic endothelial cells line the vascular spaces (hematoxylin-eosin, original magnification ×200).

presentation is variable and often vague with abdominal pain, malaise, weight loss, jaundice, and sometimes Budd-Chiari syndrome (33,82). Females are affected twice as often as males, and the tumor may occur any time between the second and seventh decades of life.

The tumor is usually multinodular, but tumor nodules may be confluent giving the impression of one massive nodule. Two histologic patterns are recognized and described: dendritic and epithelioid (Fig. 24.18, e-Figs. 24.72–24.77).

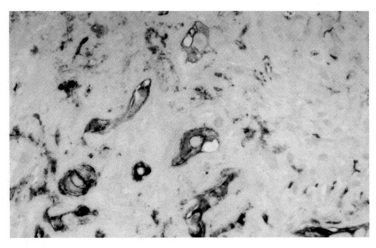

FIGURE 2.17   Angiosarcoma. Malignant endothelial cells are strongly positive for factor VIII (immunoperoxidase, specific antibody for factor VIII, original magnification ×400).

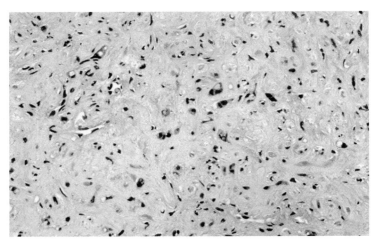

FIGURE 24.18 Epithelioid hemangioendothelioma showing many epithelioid cells (hematoxylin-eosin, original magnification ×200).

Spindle and stellate cells, embedded in a dense and myxoid fibrous stroma, characterize the dendritic pattern. Tumor cells show vacuolation and sometimes appear as if they are forming glands. Vacuoles, when present, are actually primitive vascular lumina (blister cells) (Fig. 24.19) (33,82,159). Cells react to factor VIII, CD31, and CD34 (e-Fig. 24.78). Ultrastructural analysis of the endothelial cells reveals endothelial differentiation, including tight junctions, pinocytotic vesicles, and Weibel-Palade bodies in about 30% of cases (179).

The epithelioid pattern shows enlarged, atypical cells with abundant cytoplasm and with more solid areas of growth. EHE has a propensity for

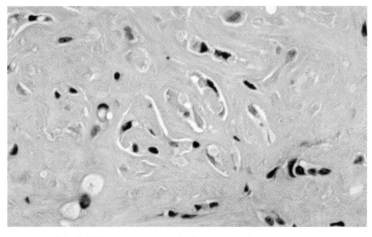

FIGURE 24.19 Epithelioid hemangioendothelioma. Small vascular lumina are formed by the endothelial cells (hematoxylin-eosin, original magnification ×400).

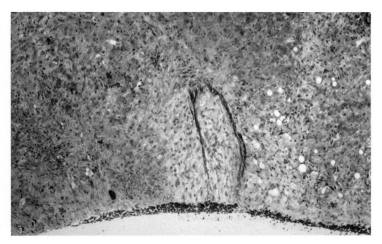

FIGURE 24.20   Epithelioid hemangioendothelioma growing into vascular spaces and mimicking venoocclusive disease (Masson trichrome, original magnification ×200).

vascular dissemination, often mimicking venoocclusive disease (Fig. 24.20). Tumor cells are surrounded by mild to moderate inflammatory infiltrate that is predominantly lymphocytic, but some polymorphonuclear and eosinophilic leukocytes may also be present.

Differentiation includes other vascular tumors such as angiosarcoma, Kaposi sarcoma, bacillary angiomatosis, and nontumorous conditions such as venoocclusive disease.

Kaposi Sarcoma

Kaposi sarcoma (KS) is a neoplastic proliferation of endothelial cells, most likely of lymphatic origin. Kaposi sarcoma appears as hemorrhagic ill-defined nodules in the liver. Tumor cells are spindle shaped, often containing intracytoplasmic inclusions, most likely representing phagocytosed erythrocytes (Fig. 24.21). The nuclei are relatively bland and do not show either significant cytologic atypia or many mitoses (176). In addition, slit-like spaces, not lined by endothelial cells, contain extravasated red blood cells. Hemosiderin-laden macrophages and lymphocytic cells are present. Immunostains for endothelial markers, including factor VIII, CD31, and CD34, are rarely positive, but human herpesvirus 8 is often demonstrable.

Differentiating between angiosarcoma and Kaposi sarcoma is important. Patients with hepatic KS are almost always seropositive for human immunodeficiency virus (HIV) and are usually in the advanced stage of acquired immune deficiency syndrome (AIDS). They often already have multiple lesions elsewhere in the body.

Bacillary angiomatosis, like KS, occurs in AIDS patients with HIV and is caused by *Bartonella quintana/henselae* organisms, which are demonstrated with Warthin-Starry stain and also by polymerase chain reaction or electron microscopy (112,174,176).

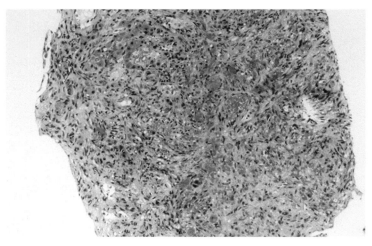

FIGURE 24.21 Kaposi sarcoma in the liver in a patient with acquired immune deficiency syndrome (hematoxylin-eosin, original magnification ×200).

Lymphoproliferative Disorders

The liver is often secondarily involved in leukemias and Hodgkin (HL) and non-Hodgkin (NHL) lymphomas. NHL is more prevalent and can be associated with AIDS, autoimmune hepatitis, and HBV and HCV infection. EBV-associated posttransplantation lymphoproliferative disorder (PTLD) occurs after liver transplantation (Fig. 24.22) (91,139,172,200).

Hepatic HL is usually seen when there is involvement of other sites, particularly the spleen. Primary HL of the liver is virtually nonexistent. Liver

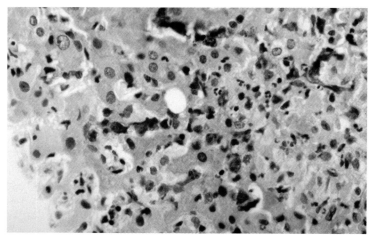

FIGURE 24.22 B-cell lymphoma, large cell type in an immunocompromised patient (hematoxylin-eosin, original magnification ×200).

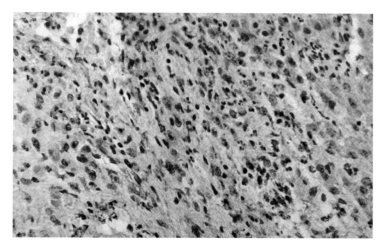

FIGURE 24.23   Histiocytosis X. Note numerous eosinophils (hematoxylin-eosin, original magnification ×200).

biopsy findings include various nonspecific and nondiagnostic lymphoid infiltrates and changes indicative of the vicinity of a mass lesion (21,91, 117,124,177,185). Unexplained liver granulomas in patients with persistent febrile illness should raise a suspicion for HL (170,171). Cholestasis in the absence of obstruction may be prominent. Lymphoproliferative processes can cause acute liver failure and may clinically mimic fulminant hepatic failure resulting from acute hepatitis, which can be an important consideration in the evaluation of liver transplantation patients (198).

Histiocytosis X

Histiocytosis X is an encompassing term for the spectrum of three diseases: Hand-Schüller-Christian, Letterer-Siwe, and eosinophilic granuloma of bone. Rarely, patients with histiocytosis X may present with a clinical picture mimicking sclerosing cholangitis, with jaundice and portal hypertension (187).

Abundant strongly S-100–positive Langerhans-type cells are seen, usually with many eosinophilic leukocytes (51) (Figs. 24.23, 24.24). Ultrastructurally, Langerhans cells contain Birbeck granules. Langerhans cells are present in the portal tracts but also extend into and replace variable portions of liver parenchyma. In addition, interlobular bile ducts show bile duct epithelial changes similar to those of primary sclerosing cholangitis, with focal ductular reaction (88,111,155,187). Liver transplantation has been performed (30).

Other Rare Tumors

Rare primary malignant neuroendocrine tumors, including hepatic gastrinoma and apudoma, have been described in the liver and in the biliary tree

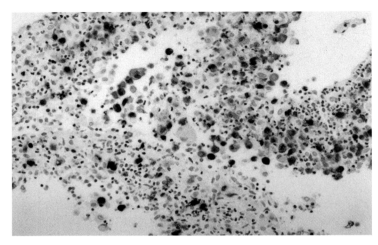

FIGURE 24.24   Histiocytosis X. Langerhans-type cells are strongly positive for S-100 (immunoperoxidase, specific antibody for S-100, original magnification ×200).

(10,138,168). Liver cell carcinoma may be ectopic in the abdominal cavity (8,37,108). Primary hepatic malignant melanoma has also been reported (45). Some rare primary malignant tumors of the liver include undifferentiated (embryonal, mesenchymal) sarcoma (Fig. 24.25) (60,107), choriocarcinoma (7), endodermal (yolk sac) tumor (60,72,142), adrenal or pancreatic rest tumor (32), rhabdomyosarcoma (129), leiomyosarcoma (Fig. 24.26) (55,123), fibrosarcoma (8), osteosarcoma (191),

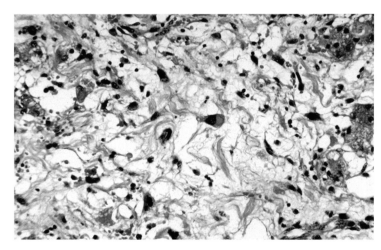

FIGURE 24.25   Mesenchymal undifferentiated sarcoma (hematoxylin-eosin, original magnification ×200).

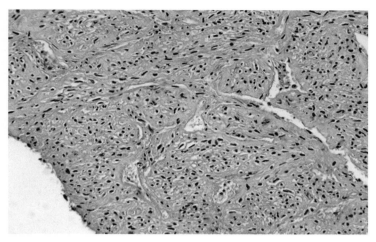

FIGURE 24.26   Primary leiomyosarcoma of the liver (hematoxylin-eosin, original magnification ×200).

liposarcoma (Fig. 24.27) (101), malignant schwannoma (114), hemangiopericytoma (195), malignant histiocytoma (6,94), and squamous cell carcinoma (70).

METASTATIC TUMORS

The liver is a particularly common site for metastases from almost any primary site. Liver biopsies are often performed to determine if a liver mass is

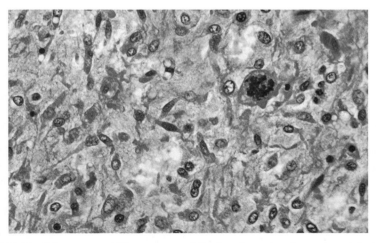

FIGURE 24.27   Primary myxoid liposarcoma of the liver (hematoxylin-eosin, original magnification ×200).

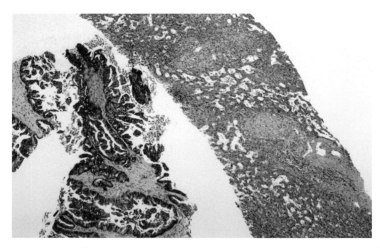

FIGURE 24.28   Liver adjacent to metastatic lesion, showing sinusoidal dilatation, cholestasis, and polymorphonuclear leukocytes (hematoxylin- eosin, original magnification ×200).

primary or secondary. Fine-needle aspiration of the liver is generally not very useful in the diagnosis of acute or chronic liver diseases but is valuable in tumor diagnosis (93), particularly with appropriate immunohistochemical studies (110).

Changes Associated with Mass Lesions

Liver parenchyma adjacent to a mass, neoplastic or nonneoplastic, shows typical changes, including bile ductular reaction with associated periductular acute inflammatory cell response, zone 1 sinusoidal dilatation, and cholestasis (Fig. 24.28) (63).

REFERENCES

1. Abbondanzo SL, Manz HJ, Klappenbach RS, et al. Hepatocellular carcinoma in an 11-year-old girl with Fanconi's anemia. Report of a case and review of the literature. Am J Pediatr Hematol Oncol 1986;8:334–337.
2. Adams PC. Hepatocellular carcinoma in hereditary hemochromatosis. Can J Gastroenterol 1993;7:37–41.
3. Aihara T, Noguchi S, Sasaki Y, et al. Clonal analysis of regenerative nodules in hepatitis C virus–induced liver cirrhosis. Gastroenterology 1994;107:1805–1811.
4. Aihara T, Noguchi S, Sasaki Y, et al. Clonal analysis of precancerous lesion of hepatocellular carcinoma. Gastroenterology 1996;111:455–461.
5. Akwari OE, Tucker A, Seigler HF, et al. Hepatobiliary cystadenoma with mesenchymal stroma. Ann Surg 1990;211:18–27.
6. Albert-Flor JJ, O'Hara MF, Weaver F, et al. Malignant fibrous histiocytoma of the liver. Gastroenterology 1985;39:890–893.
7. Alonso JF, Saez C, Perez P, et al. Primary pure choriocarcinoma of the liver. Pathol Res Pract 1992;188:375–377.

8. Alrenga DP. Primary fibrosarcoma of the liver. Case report and review of the literature. Cancer 1975;36:446–449.

9. An C, Petrovic LM, Reyter I, et al. The application of neural network technology to the study of large cell dysplasia and hepatocellular carcinoma. Hepatology 1997;26: 1224–1231.

10. Angeles A, Quintanilla-Martinez L, Larriva-Sahd J. Primary carcinoid of the common bile duct. Am J Clin Pathol 1991;96:341–344.

11. Anthony PP, Vogel CL, Barker LF. Liver cell dysplasia: a premalignant condition. J Clin Pathol 1973;26:217–233.

12. Anthony PP. Liver cell dysplasia: what is its significance? Hepatology 1987;7:394–396.

13. Azizah N, Paradinas FJ. Cholangiocarcinoma coexisting with developmental liver cysts: a distinct entity different from liver cystadenocarcinoma. Histopathology 1980;4: 391–400.

14. Barsky SH, Linnoila I, Triche TJ, et al. Hepatocellular carcinoma with carcinoid features. Hum Pathol 1984;15:892–894.

15. Bassendine MF. Alcohol: a major risk factor for hepatocellular carcinoma? J Hepatol 1986;2:513–519.

16. Beasly RP. Hepatitis B virus. The major etiology of hepatocellular carcinoma. Cancer 1988;61:1942–1956.

17. Berman MA, Burnham JA, Sheahan DG. Fibrolamellar carcinoma of the liver: an immunohistochemical study of nineteen cases and a review of the literature. Hum Pathol 1988;19:784–794.

18. Berman MM, Libbey NP, Foster JH. Hepatocellular carcinoma. Polygonal cell type with fibrous stroma—an atypical variant with favorable prognosis. Cancer 1980;46: 1448–1455.

19. Bloustein PA. Association of carcinoma of congenital cystic conditions of the liver and bile ducts. Am J Gastroenterol 1977;67:40–46.

20. Bonetti F, Chilosi M, Pisa R, et al. Epithelial membrane antigen expression in cholangiocarcinoma. An useful immunohistochemical tool for differential diagnosis with hepatocarcinoma. Virchows Archiv A 1983;401:307–313.

21. Bruguera M, Caballero T, Carreas E, et al. Hepatic sinusoidal dilatation in Hodgkin's disease. Liver 1987;7:76–80.

22. Buchanan TF Jr, Huvos AG. Clear-cell carcinoma of the liver. A clinicopathologic study of 13 patients. Am J Clin Pathol 1974;61:529–539.

23. Burns CD, Kuhns JG, Wieman J. Cholangiocarcinoma in association with multiple biliary microhamartomas. Arch Pathol Lab Med 1990;114:1287–1289.

24. Caballero T, Aneiros J, Lopez-Caballero J, et al. Fibrolamellar hepatocellular carcinoma. An immunohistochemical and ultrastructural study. Histopathology 1985;9: 445–456.

25. Chen C-J, Liang K-Y, Vajng A-S, et al. Effects of hepatitis B virus, alcohol drinking, cigarette smoking and familial tendency on hepatocellular carcinoma. Hepatology 1991;13:398–406.

26. Chen KTK. Adenocarcinoma of the liver. Association with congenital hepatic fibrosis and Caroli's disease. Arch Pathol Lab Med 1981;105:294–295.

27. Cheng WS, Govindarajan S, Redeker AG. Hepatocellular carcinoma in a case of Wilson's disease. Liver 1992;12:42–45.

28. Chisari FV, Klopchin K, Moriyama T, et al. Molecular pathogenesis of hepatocellular carcinoma in hepatitis B virus transgenic mice. Cell 1989;59:1145–1156.

29. Christensen WN, Boitnott JK, Kuhajda FP. Immunoperoxidase staining as a diagnostic aid for hepatocellular carcinoma. Mod Pathol 1989;2:8–12.

30. Concepcion W, Esquivel CO, Terry A, et al. Liver transplantation in Langerhans' cell histiocytosis (histiocytosis X). Semin Oncol 1991;18:24–28.

31. Conti JA, Kemeny N. Type Ia glycogenosis associated with hepatocellular carcinoma. Cancer 1992;69:1320–1322.

32. Contreras P. Altieri E, Liberman C, et al. Adrenal rest tumor of the liver causing Cushing's syndrome. J Clin Endocrinol Metab 1985;60:21–28.

33. Craig JR, Peters RL, Edmondson HA. Tumors of the liver and intrahepatic bile ducts. In: Atlas of Tumor Pathology, 2nd series, fascicle 26. Washington DC: Armed Forces Institute of Pathology, 1989.

34. Crawford JM. Pathologic assessment of liver cell dysplasia and benign liver tumors: differentiation from malignant tumors. Semin Diagn Pathol 1990;7:115–128.

35. Cross SS, Variend S. Combined hepatoblastoma and yolk sac tumor of the liver. Cancer 1992;69:1323–1326.

36. Darioca PJ, Tuthill R, Reed RJ. Cholangiocarcinoma arising in congenital hepatic fibrosis. Arch Pathol 1975;99:592–595.

37. Davison FD, Fagan EA, Portmann B, et al. HBV-DNA sequences in tumor and nontumor tissue in a patient with the fibrolamellar variant of hepatocellular carcinoma. Hepatology 1990;12:676–679.

38. Dehner LP., Manivel JC. Hepatoblastoma: an analysis of the relationship between morphologic subtypes and prognosis. Am J Pediatr Hematol Oncol 1988;10:301–307.

39. Dehner LP, Snover DC, Sharp HL, et al. Hereditary tyrosinemia type 1 (chronic form). Hum Pathol 1989;20:149–158.

40. Deprez C, Vangansbeke D, Fastrez R, et al. Nuclear DNA content, proliferative index, and nuclear size determination in normal and cirrhotic liver, and in benign and malignant primary and metastatic hepatic tumors. Am J Clin Pathol 1993;99: 558–565.

41. Desmet V, De Vos R. Ultrastructural characteristics of novel epithelial cell types identified in human pathologic liver specimens with chronic ductular reaction. Am J Pathol 1992;16:1327–1333.

42. De Souza A, Yamada T, Mills JJ, et al. Imprinted genes in liver carcinogenesis. FASEB J 1997;11:60–67.

43. Devaney K, Goodman ZD, Ishak KG. Hepatobiliary cystadenoma and cystadenocarcinoma. A light microscopic and immunohistochemical study of 70 patients. Am J Surg Pathol 1994;18:1078–1091.

44. Deugnier Y, Guyader D, Crantock L, et al. Primary liver cancer in genetic hemochromatosis: a clinical, pathological and pathogenetic study of 54 cases. Gastroenterology 1993;104:228–234.

45. Deugnier Y, Turlin B, Lehry D, et al. Malignant melanoma of the hepatic and common bile ducts. Arch Pathol Lab Med 1991;115:915–917.

46. Eckstein RP, Bambach CP, Stiel D, et al. Fibrolamellar carcinoma as a cause of bile duct obstruction. Pathology 1988;20:326–331.

47. Edmondson HA, Steiner PE. Primary carcinoma of the liver. A study of 100 cases among 48,900 necropsies. Cancer 1954;7:462–403.

48. Eriksson S, Carlson J, Velez R. Risk of cirrhosis and primary liver cancer in alpha 1-antitrypsin deficiency. N Engl J Med 1986;314:736–739.

49. Falk H, Thomas LB, Popper H, et al. Hepatic angiosarcoma associated with androgenic-anabolic steroids. Lancet 1979;2:1120–1123.

50. Farinati F, Faginoli S, De Maria N, et al. Anti-HCV positive hepatocellular carcinoma in cirrhosis. J Hepatol 1992;14:183–187.

51. Favara BE, Jaffe R. Pathology of Langerhans cell histiocytosis. Hematol Oncol Clin North Am 1987;1:75–97.

52. Fellows IW, Stewart M, Jefcoate WJ, et al. Hepatocellular carcinoma in primary hemochromatosis in the absence of cirrhosis. Gut 1988;29:1603–1606.

53. Ferrell LD, Crawford JM, Dhillon AP, et al. Proposal for standardized criteria for the diagnosis of benign, borderline and malignant hepatocellular lesions arising in chronic advanced liver disease. Am J Surg Pathol 1993;17:1113–1123.

54. Ferrell L, Wright T, Lake J, et al. Incidence and diagnostic features of macroregenerative nodules vs. small hepatocellular carcinoma in cirrhotic liver. Hepatology 1992;16:1372–1381.

55. Fong JA, Ruebner BH. Primary leiomyosarcoma of the liver. Hum Pahol 1974;5:115–119

56. Fortwengler HP Jr, Jones D, Espinosa E, et al. Evidence for endothelial cell origin of vinyl chloride-induced hepatic angiosarcoma. Gastroenterology 1981;80:1415–1419.

57. Fujimoto J, Okamoto E, Yamanak N, et al. Flow cytometric DNA analysis of hepatocellular carcinoma. Cancer 1991;67:939–944.

58. Furuya K, Nakamura M, Yamamoto Y, et al. Macroregenerative nodule of the liver: a clinicopathologic study of 345 autopsy cases of chronic liver disease. Cancer 1988;61:99–105.

59. Gaffey MJ, Joyce JP, Carlson GS, et al. Spontaneous regression of hepatocellular carcinoma. Cancer 1990;65:2779–2783.

60. Gallivan MVE, Lack EE, Chun B, et al. Undifferentiated (embryonal) sarcoma of the liver. Pediatr Pathol 1983;1:291–300.

61. Gardiner GW, Lajoie G, Keith R. Hepatoid adenocarcinoma of the papilla of Vater. Histopathology 1992;20:541–544.

62. Geller SA, Nichols WS, Kim SS, et al. Hepatocarcinogenesis is the sequel to hepatitis in the Z#2 alpha 1-antitrypsin transgenic mouse. Hepatology 1994;19:389–397.

63. Geller SA, Dhall D, Alsabeh R. Application of immunochemistry to liver and gastrointestinal neoplasms. Arch Pathol Lab Med 2008;132:490–499.

64. Gerber MA, Thung SN, Bodenheimer HC, et al. Characteristic histologic triad in liver adjacent to metastatic neoplasm. Liver 1986;6:85–88.

65. Goldblum JR, Bartos RE, Carr KA, et al. Hepatitis B and alterations of the p53 tumor suppressor gene in hepatocellular carcinoma. Am J Surg Pathol 1993;17:1244–1251.

66. Goldstein RM, Stone M, Tillery GW, et al. Is liver transplantation indicated for cholangiocarcinoma? Am J Surg 1993;166:768–772.

67. Gonzales-Crussi F, Upton MP, Maurer HS. Hepatoblastoma. Attempt at characterization of histologic subtypes. Am J Surg Pathol 1982;6:599–612.

68. Goodman ZD, Ishak KG, Langloss JM, et al. Combined hepatocellular-cholangiocarcinoma. A histologic and immunohistochemical study. Cancer 1985;55:124–135.

69. Gourley WK, Kumar D, Bouton MS, et al. Cystadenoma and cystadenocarcinoma with mesenchymal stroma of the liver. Immunohistochemical analysis. Arch Pathol Lab Med 1992;116:1047–1050.

70. Grasl-Kraupp B, Ruttkay-Nedecky B, Mullauer L, et al. Inherent increase in apoptosis in liver tumors: implications for carcinogenesis and tumor regression. Hepatology 1997;25:906–913.

71. Gresham GA, Rue LW. Squamous cell carcinoma of the liver. Hum Pathol 1985;16:413–416.

72. Haagsma EB, Smit GPA, Niezen-Koning KE, et al. Type IIIb glycogen storage disease associated with end-stage cirrhosis and hepatocellular carcinoma. Hepatology 1997;25:537–541.

73. Hart WR. Primary endodermal sinus (yolk sac) tumor of the liver. First reported case. Cancer 1975;35:1453–1458.

74. Hasebe C, Sekiya C, Satoh H, et al. A case of alpha-fetoprotein-producing gallbladder carcinoma. Acta Hepatol Jpn 1984;25:1180–1186.

75. Hoch-Ligeti C. Angiosarcoma of the liver associated with diethylstilbestrol. JAMA 1978;240:1510–1511.

76. Honda N, Cobb C, Lechago J. Bile duct carcinoma associated with multiple von Meyenburg complexes in the liver. Hum Pathol 1986;17:1287–1290.

77. Hood DL, Bauer TW, Leibel SA, et al. Hepatic giant cell carcinoma. An ultrastructural and immunohistochemical study. Am J Clin Pathol 1990;93:111–116.

78. Hou P-C. The relationship between primary carcinoma of the liver and infestation with *Clonorchis sinensis*. J Pathol Bacteriol 1956;72:239–246.

79. Hurlmann J, Gardiol D. Immunohistochemistry in the differential diagnosis of liver carcinomas. Am J Surg Pathol 1991;15:280–288.

80. International Working Party. Terminology of nodular hepatocellular lesions. Hepatology 1995;22:983–993.

81. Ishak KG, Anthony PP, Sobin LH. Histological typing of tumors of the liver. In: World Health Organization International Histological Classification of Tumors, 2nd Ed. Berlin: Springer-Verlag, 1994.

82. Ishak KG, Glunz PR. Hepatoblastoma and hepatocarcinoma in infancy and childhood. Report of 4 cases. Cancer 1967;20:396–422.

83. Ishak KG, Sesterhenn IA, Goodman ZD, et al. Epithelioid hemangioendothelioma of the liver: a clinicopathologic and follow-up study of 32 cases. Hum Pathol 1984;15: 839–852.

84. Ishak KG. Malignant mesenchymal tumors of the liver. In: Okuda K, Ishak KG, eds. Neoplasms of the Liver. Tokyo: Springer-Verlag, 1987:159–176.

85. Ishikura H, Ishiguro T, Enatsu C, et al. Hepatoid adenocarcinoma of the renal pelvis producing alpha-fetoprotein of hepatic type and bile pigment. Cancer 1991;67: 3051–3056.

86. Ishikura H, Kanda M, Nosaka K, et al. Hepatoid adenocarcinoma: a distinctive histological subtype of alpha-fetoprotein-producing lung carcinoma. Virchows Archiv A 1990;417:73–80.

87. Ishikura H, Scully RE. Hepatoid carcinoma of the ovary. Cancer 1987;60:2775–2784.

88. Ito Y, Kojiro M, Nakashima T, Mori T. Pathomorphologic characteristics of 102 cases of Thorotrast-related hepatocellular carcinoma, cholangiocarcinoma, and hepatic angiosarcoma. Cancer 1988;62:1153–1162.

89. Iwai M, Kashiwadani M, Okuno T, et al. Cholestatic liver disease in a 20-year old woman with histiocytosis X. Am J Gastroenterol 1988;83:164–168.

90. Jaffe ES. Malignant lymphomas: pathology of hepatic involvement. Semin Liver Dis 1987;7:257–268.

91. Jameson CF. Primary hepatocellular carcinoma in hereditary hemorrhagic telangiectasia. Histopathology 1989;15:550–552.

92. Jovanovic R, Jagirdar J, Thung SN, et al. Blood-group-related antigen Lewis(x) and Lewis(y) in the differential diagnosis of cholangiocarcinoma and hepatocellular carcinoma. Arch Pathol Lab Med 1989;113:139–142.

93. Kakizoe S, Kojiro M, Nakashima T. Hepatocellular carcinoma with sarcomatous change. Cancer 1987;59:310–316.

94. Kaklamani E, Trichopoulos D, Tzonou A, et al. Hepatitis B and C and their interaction in the origin of hepatocellular carcinoma. JAMA 1991;265:1974–1976.

95. Katsuda S, Kawahara E, Matsui Y, et al. Malignant fibrous histiocytoma of the liver: a case report and review of the literature. Am J Gastroenterol 1988;83:1278–1282.

96. Kaufman SS, Wood P, Shaw B, et al. Hepatocarcinoma in a child with the Alagille syndrome. Am J Dis Child 1987;141:698–700.

97. Kawahara E, Kitamura T, Ueda H, et al. Hepatocellular carcinoma arising in the abdominal cavity. Acta Pathol Jpn 1988;38:1575–1581.

98. Kawakita N, Seki S, Sakaguchi H, et al. Analysis of proliferating hepatocytes using a monoclonal antibody against proliferating nuclear antigen/cyclin in embedded tissue from various liver diseases fixed in formalin. Am J Pathol 1992;140:513–520.
99. Kawano Y. Localization of hepatitis B surface antigen in hepatocellular carcinoma. Acta Pathol Jpn 1983;33:1087–1093.
100. Kew MC, McKnight A, Hodkinson H, et al. The role of membranous obstruction of the inferior vena cava and hepatocellular carcinoma in Southern African blacks. Hepatology 1989;9:121–125.
101. Kim CM, Koike K, Saito I, et al. HBx gene of hepatitis B virus induces liver cancer in transgenic mice. Nature 1991;351:317–320.
102. Kim YI, Yu ES, Lee KW, et al. Dedifferentiated liposarcoma of the liver. Cancer 1985; 60:2785–2790.
103. Kingston JE, Herbert A, Draper GJ, et al. Association between hepatoblastoma and polyposis coli. Arch Dis Child 1983;58:959–962.
104. Kolars JC. Aflatoxin and hepatocellular carcinoma: a useful paradigm for environmentally induced carcinogenesis. Hepatology 1992;16:848–851.
105. Koneru B, Flye MW, Busuttil RW, et al. Liver transplantation for hepatoblastoma: the American experience. Ann Surg 1991;213:118–121.
106. Koo J, Ho J, Wong J, et al. Mucoepidermoid carcinoma of the bile duct. Ann Surg 1982;196:140–148.
107. Kung ITM, Chan S-W, Gung K-H. Fine-needle aspiration in hepatocellular carcinoma. Combined cytologic and histologic approach. Cancer 1991;67:673–680.
108. Lack EE, Scloo BL, Azumi N, et al. Undifferentiated (embryonal) sarcoma of the liver. Clinical and pathologic study of 16 cases with emphasis on immunohistochemical features. Am J Surg Pathol 1991;15:1–16.
109. Laferla G, Kaye SB, Crean GP. Hepatocellular and gastric carcinoma associated with familial polyposis coli. J Surg Oncol 1988;38:19–21.
110. Lai Y-S, Thung SN, Gerber MA, et al. Expression of cytokeratins in normal and diseased liver and in primary liver carcinomas. Arch Pathol Lab Med 1989;113:134–138.
111. Lau S, Prakash S, Geller SA, et al. Comparative immunohistochemical profile of hepatocellular carcinoma, cholangiocarcinoma, and metastatic adenocarcinoma. Hum Pathol 2002;33:1175–1181.
112. Leblanc A, Hadchouel M, Jehan P, et al. Obstructive jaundice in children in histiocytosis X. Gastroenterology 1981;80:134–139.
113. Leboit PE, Berger TG, Egbert BM, et al. Bacillary angiomatosis: the histopathology and differential diagnosis of a pseudoneoplastic infection in patients with human immunodeficiency virus disease. Am J Surg Pathol 1989;13:909–920.
114. LeBrun DP, Silver MM, Freedman MH, et al. Fibrolamellar carcinoma of the liver in a patient with Fanconi anemia. Hum Pathol 1991;22:396–398.
115. Lederman SM, Martin EC, Laffey KT, et al. Hepatic neurofibromatosis, malignant schwannoma and angiosarcoma in von Recklinghausen's disease. Gastroenterology 1987;92:234–239.
116. Lee GR, Tsamndas AC, Demetris AJ. Large cell change (liver cell dysplasia) and hepatocellular carcinoma in cirrhosis: matched case-control study, pathological analysis and pathogenic hypothesis. Hepatology 1997;26:1415–1423.
117. Lefkowitch JH, Apfelbaum TF. Liver cell dysplasia and hepatocellular carcinoma in non-A, non-B hepatitis. Arch Pathol Lab Med 1987;111:170–173.
118. Leslie KO, Colby TV. Hepatic parenchymal lymphoid aggregates in Hodgkin's disease. Hum Pathol 1984;15:808–809.
119. Lithner F, Wetterberg L. Hepatocellular carcinoma in patients with acute intermittent porphyria. Acta Med Scand 1984;215:271–274.

120. Ljubimova JY, Petrovic LM, Wilson SE, et al. Gene expression of HGF, its receptor (c-met), c-myc, and albumin in cirrhotic and neoplastic human liver tissue. J Histochem Cytochem 1997;45:79–87.

121. Lok ASF, Lai C-L. Factors determining the development of hepatocellular carcinoma in hepatitis B surface antigen carriers. Cancer 1988;61:1287–1291.

122. Lones MA, Shintaku IP, Weiss LM, et al. Post-transplant lymphoproliferative disorder in liver allograft biopsies: a comparison of three methods for the demonstration of Epstein-Barr virus. Hum Pathol 1997;28:533–539.

123. Ma CK, Zarbo RJ, Frierson HF, et al. Comparative immunohistochemical study of primary and metastatic carcinomas of the liver. Am J Clin Pathol 1993;99:551–557.

124. Maki HS, Hubert BC, Sajjad SM, et al. Primary hepatic leiomyosarcoma. Arch Surg 1987;122:1193–1196.

125. Man KM, Drejet A, Keefe EB, et al. Primary sclerosing cholangitis and Hodgkin's disease. Hepatology 1993;18:1127–1131.

126. Manivel C, Wick MR, Abenoza P, et al. Teratoid hepatoblastoma. Cancer 1986;57: 2168–2174.

127. Manning JT Jr, Ordonez NG, Barton JH. Endothelial cell origin of thorium oxide–induced angiosarcoma of liver. Arch Pathol Lab Med 1983;107:456–458.

128. Manowski Z, Silver MM, Roberts EA, et al. Liver cell dysplasia and early liver transplantation in hereditary tyrosinemia. Mod Pathol 1990;3:694–701.

129. Matsukuma K, Tsukamoto N. Alpha-fetoprotein-producing endometrial adenocarcinoma. Gynecol Oncol 1988;29:370–377.

130. McArdle JP, Hawley I, Shevland J, et al. Primary rhabdomyosarcoma of the adult liver. Am J Surg Pathol 1989;13:961–965.

131. Melia WH, Johnson PJ, Neuberger J, et al. Hepatocellular carcinoma in primary biliary cirrhosis. Gastroenterology 1984;87:660–663.

132. Michalopoulos G. Liver regeneration and growth factors: old puzzle and new perspectives. Lab Invest 1992;67:413–415.

133. Miura K, Shirasawa H. Primary carcinoid tumor of the liver. Am J Clin Pathol 1988;89:561–564.

134. Monroe PS, Riddell RH, Siegler M, et al. Hepatic angiosarcoma. Possible relationship to long-term oral contraceptive ingestion. JAMA 1981;246:64–65.

135. Morinaga S, Yamagouchi M, Watanabe I, et al. An immunohistochemical study of hepatoblastoma producing human chorionic gonadotropin. Cancer 1983;51: 1647–1652.

136. Mzeako UC, Goodman ZD, Ishak KG. Comparison of tumor pathology with duration of survival of North American patients with hepatocellular carcinoma. Cancer 1995;76:579–588.

137. Naccarato R, Farinati F. Hepatocellular carcinoma, alcohol and cirrhosis: facts and hypothesis. Dig Dis Sci 1991;36:1137–1142.

138. Nagasue N, Kohno H, Chang Y, et al. Androgen and estrogen receptors in hepatocellular carcinoma and the surrounding liver in women. Cancer 1989;63:112–116.

139. Nagasue N, Yamanoi A, Takemoto Y, et al. Comparison between diploid and aneuploid hepatocellular carcinomas: a flow cytometric study. Br J Surg 1992;79:667–670.

140. Nagasue N, Kohno H, Hayashi T, et al. Lack of intratumoral heterogeneity in DNA ploidy pattern of hepatocellular carcinoma. Gastroenterology 1993;105:1449–1454.

141. Nagorney DM, Adson MA, Weiland LH, et al. Fibrolamellar hepatoma. Am Surg 1985;149:113–119.

142. Nakajima T, Knodo Y, Miyazaki M, et al. A histopathologic study of 102 cases of intra-hepatic cholangiocarcinoma: histologic classification and modes of spreading. Hum Pathol 1988;19:1228–1234.

143. Nakanuma Y, Ohta G. Expression of Mallory bodies in hepatocellular carcinoma in man and its significance. Cancer 1986;62:558–563.
144. Nakanuma Y, Terada T, Doishita K, et al. Hepatocellular carcinoma in primary biliary cirrhosis: an autopsy study. Hepatology 1990;11:1010–1016.
145. Nakanuma Y, Terada T, Ueda K, et al. Adenomatous hyperplasia of the liver as a pre-cancerous lesion. Liver 1993;13:1–9.
146. Nalpas B, Driss F, Pol S, et al. Association between HCV and HBV infection in hepatocellular carcinoma and alcoholic liver disease. J Hepatol 1991;12:70–74.
147. Narita T, Moriyama Y, Ito Y. Endodermal sinus (yolk sac) tumor of the liver. A case report and review of the literature. J Pathol 1988;155:41–47.
148. Nojima T, Kojima T, Kato H, et al. Alpha-fetoprotein-producing acinar cell carcinoma of the pancreas. Hum Pathol 1992;23:828–830.
149. Ojanguren I, Ariza A, Llatos M, et al. Proliferating cell nuclear antigen in normal, regenerative and neoplastic liver. Hum Pathol 1993;24:905–908.
150. Okuda K. Hepatocellular carcinoma: recent progress. Hepatology 1992;15:948–963.
151. Omata M, Petres RL, Tatter D. Sclerosing hepatic carcinoma: relationship to hypercalcemia. Liver 1981;1:33–49.
152. Ordonez NG, Manning JT Jr. Comparison of alpha-1-antitrypsin and alpha-1-antichymotrypsin in hepatocellular carcinoma: an immunoperoxidase study. Am J Gastroenterol 1984;79:959–963.
153. Orsatti G, Thiese ND, Thung SN, et al. DNA image cytometric analysis of macroregenerative nodules (adenomatous hyperplasia) of the liver: evidence in support of their preneoplastic nature. Hepatology 1993;17:621–627.
154. Otsuru A, Nagataki S, Koji T, et al. Analysis of alpha-fetoprotein gene expression in hepatocellular carcinoma and liver cirrhosis by in situ hybridization. Cancer 1988;62:1105–1112.
155. Parker-Ponder K. Analysis of liver development, regeneration, and carcinogenesis by genetic marking studies. FASEB J 1996;10:673–684.
156. Pirovino M, Jeaneret C, Lang RH, et al. Liver cirrhosis in histiocytosis X. Liver 1988;8:293–298.
157. Pistoi S, Morello D. Prometheus myth revisited: transgenic mice as a powerful tool to study liver regeneration. FASEB J 1996;10:819–828.
158. Pliskin A, Cauling H, Stenger RJ. Primary squamous cell carcinoma originating in congenital cysts of the liver. Arch Pathol Lab Med 1985;116:105–107.
159. Polio J, Enriquez RE, Chow A, et al. Hepatocellular carcinoma in Wilson's disease. J Clin Gastroenterol 1989;11:220–224.
160. Popper H, Thomas LB, Telles NC, et al. Development of hepatic angiosarcoma in man induced by vinyl chloride, thorotrast, and arsenic. Comparison with cases of unknown etiology. Am J Pathol 1978;92:349–369.
161. Rabinowitz M, Imperial JC, Schade RR, et al. Hepatocellular carcinoma in Alagille's syndrome: a family study. J Pediatr Gastroenterol Nutr 1989;8:26–30.
162. Riikonen P, Tuominen L, Seppa A, et al. Simultaneous hepatoblastoma in identical male twins. Cancer 1990;66:2429–2431.
163. Ringe B, Wittekind C, Weimann A, et al. Results of hepatic resection and transplantation for fibrolamellar carcinoma. Surg Gynecol Obstet 1992;175:299–305.
164. Rojter SE, Villamil FG, Petrovic LM, et al. Malignant vascular tumors of the liver presenting as liver failure and portal hypertension. Liver Transplant Surg 1995;1:156–161.
165. Roth JA, Berman E, Befler D, et al. A black hepatocellular carcinoma with Dubin-Johnson–like pigment and Mallory bodies: a histochemical and ultrastructural study. Am J Surg Pathol 1982;6:375–382.

166. Rubel LR, Ishak KG. Thorotrast-associated cholangiocarcinoma. An epidemiologic and clinicopathologic study. Cancer 1982;50:1408–1415.
167. Ruck P, Harms D, Kaiserling E. Neuroendocrine differentiation in hepatoblastoma: an immunohistochemical investigation. Am J Surg Pathol 1990;14:847–855.
168. Ruck P, Keiserling E. Melanin-containing hepatoblastoma with endocrine differentiation. Cancer 1993;72:361–368.
169. Rugge M, Sonego F, Militello C, et al. Primary carcinoid tumor of the cystic and common bile ducts. Am J Surg Pathol 1992;16:802–807.
170. Ruiz J, Sangro B, Cuende JI, et al. Hepatitis B and C viral infections in patients with hepatocellular carcinoma. Hepatology 1992;16:637–641.
171. Sacks E, Donaldson SS, Gordon J, et al. Epithelioid granulomas associated with Hodgkin's disease. Cancer 1979;41:562–567.
172. Saito K, Nakanuma Y, Ogawa S, et al. Extensive hepatic granulomas associated with peripheral T-cell lymphoma. Am J Gastroenterol 1991;86:1243–1246.
173. Sakamoto M, Hisrohashi S, Shimosato Y. Early stages of multistep hepatocarcinogenesis: adenomatous hyperplasia and early hepatocellular carcinoma. Hum Pathol 1991;22:172–178.
174. Sato Y, Fujiwara K, Kakagawa S, et al. A case of spontaneous regression of hepatocellular carcinoma with bone metastases. Cancer 1985;56:667–671.
175. Schneiderman DJ, Arenson DM, Cello JP, et al. Hepatic disease in patients with acquired immune deficiency syndrome. Hepatology 1987;7:925–930.
176. Schrimacher P, Rogler CE, Dienes HP. Current pathogenetic and molecular concepts in viral liver carcinogenesis. Virchows Archiv B 1993;63:71–89.
177. Scoazec J-Y, Degott C, Reynes M, et al. Epithelioid hemangioendothelioma of the liver: an ultrastructural study. Hum Pathol 1989;20:673–681.
178. Scoazec J-Y, Degott C, Brousse N, et al. Non-Hodgkin's lymphoma presenting a primary tumor of the liver: presentation, diagnosis and outcome in eight patients. Hepatology 1991;13:870–875.
179. Scully PA, Steinman HK, Kennedy C, et al. AIDS-related Kaposi's sarcoma displays differential expression of endothelial surface antigens. Am J Pathol 1988;130:244–251.
180. Sell S. Is there a liver stem cell? Cancer Res 1990;50:3811–3815.
181. Sheu J-C, Huang G-T, Chou H-C, et al. Multiple hepatocellular carcinomas at the early stage have different clonality. Gastroenterology 1993;105:1471–1476.
182. Simonetti RG, Camma C, Fiorello F, et al. Hepatitis C virus infection as a risk factor for hepatocellular carcinoma in patients with cirrhosis. Ann Intern Med 1992;116:97–102.
183. Slersema PD, Ten Kate FJW, Mulder PGH, et al. Hepatocellular carcinoma in porphyria cutanea tarda: frequency and factors related to its occurrence. Liver 1992;12:56–61.
184. Strom SC, Faust JB. Oncogene activation and hepatocarcinogenesis. Pathobiology 1990;58:153–167.
185. Theise ND, Schwartz M, Miller C, et al. Macroregenerative nodules and hepatocellular carcinoma in forty four sequential adult liver explants with cirrhosis. Hepatology 1992;16:949–955.
186. Thomas FB, Clausen KP, Greenberger NJ. Liver disease in multiple myeloma. Arch Intern Med 1973;132:195–202.
187. Thomas RM, Berman JJ, Yetter RA, et al. Liver cell dysplasia: a DNA aneuploid lesion with distinct morphologic features. Hum Pathol 1992;23:496–503.
188. Thompson HH, Pitt HA, Lewin KJ, et al. Sclerosing cholangitis and histiocytosis X. Gut 1984;25:526–530.
189. Trao K, Ohkawa S, Shimizu A, et al. The male preponderance in incidence of hepatocellular carcinoma in cirrhotic patients may depend on the higher DNA synthetic activity of cirrhotic tissue in men. Cancer 1993;72:369–374.

190. Ueki T, Fujimoto J, Suzuki T, et al. Expression of hepatocyte growth factor and its receptor, the c-met proto-oncogene in hepatocellular carcinoma. Hepatology 1997;25:619–631.
191. Van Eyken P, Sciot R, Patereson A, et al. Cytokeratin expression in hepatocellular carcinoma: an immunohistochemical study. Hum Pathol 1988;19:562–568.
192. Von Hochstetter AR, Hattenschwiler J, Vogt M. Primary osteosarcoma of the liver. Cancer 1987;60:2312–2317.
193. Wakely PE Jr, Krummel TM, Johnson DE. Yolk sac tumor of the liver. Mod Pathol 1991;4:121–125.
194. Wakely PE Jr, Silverman JF, Geisinger KR, et al. Fine needle aspiration biopsy cytology of hepatoblastoma. Mod Pathol 1990;3:688–693.
195. Weihing RR, Shintaku IP, Geller SA, et al. Hepatobiliary and pancreatic mucinous cystadenocarcinomas with mesenchymal stroma: analysis of estrogen and progesterone receptors and expression of tumor associated antigens. Mod Pathol 1997;10:372–379.
196. Weitzner S. Primary hemangiopericytoma of the liver associated with hypoglycemia. Am J Dig Dis 1970;15:673–678.
197. Wenming C, Mengchao W. The biopathologic characteristics of DNA content of hepatocellular carcinomas. Cancer 1990;66:498–501.
198. Wennerberg AE, Nalesnik MA, Coleman WB. Hepatocyte paraffin 1: a monoclonal antibody that reacts with hepatocytes and can be used for differential diagnosis of hepatic tumors. Am J Pathol 1993;143:1050–1054.
199. Woolf GM, Petrovic LM, Rojter SE, et al. Acute liver failure due to lymphoma: a diagnostic concern when considering liver transplantation. Dig Dis Sci 1994;39:1351–1358.
200. Yu M-W, You S-L, Chang AS, et al. Association between hepatitis C virus antibodies and hepatocellular carcinoma in Taiwan. Cancer Res 1991;51:5621–5625.
201. Zafrani ES, Gaulard P. Primary lymphoma of the liver. Liver 1993;13:57–61.

25

TRANSPLANTATION PATHOLOGY

Liver transplantation (LT) is the treatment of choice for fulminant and sub-fulminant liver failure, cirrhosis, congenital biliary diseases, several meta-bolic diseases, and some primary neoplasms of the liver (30,37,45,57). Changes in liver biopsy must be evaluated in the context of the posttrans-plant setting, including effects of immunosuppressive therapy, as well as other therapies. Three distinct posttransplantation periods are recognized (Table 25.1).

WEEK ONE FOLLOWING LIVER TRANSPLANTATION

Primary Graft Failure

Primary graft nonfunction/failure (PGF) occurs in as many as 9% of trans-plants. Significant donor liver macrovesicular steatosis (30% to 50%) is an important contributing factor (5,8,33,53). PGF is unlikely when donor liv-ers with more than 30% steatosis are excluded (14,49,54,63). If PGF does not occur after transplantation with more than 30% macrovesicular steato-sis, 5-year survival is not affected (4). Other factors contributing to primary graft failure include a relatively small allograft, use of older donor livers, and prolonged cold ischemic preservation time greater than 12 hours. Biopsy shows extensive ischemic coagulative.

Histopathologic Changes Associated with Postperfusion State

Biopsies taken at the end of the transplantation operation (postperfusion) can show transient, nonimmunologically mediated cellular injury, thought to have no significant prognostic value, including so-called surgical hepati-tis (see Chapter 7), with focal liver cell necrosis or liver cell dropout and focal, usually mild, macrovesicular steatosis.

Preservation (Harvesting) Injury

Various factors contribute, including donor hypotension immediately prior to death. Ischemia also occurs during donor liver harvesting or trans-port. Posttransplantation hypotension or hepatic artery or portal vein

TABLE 25.1	Posttransplantation Histopathologic Complications

Day 1–Day 7
Primary graft failure
Harvesting injury
Reperfusion injury
Vascular/biliary anastomotic problems (e.g., dehiscence, stenosis)

Day 7–3 months
Harvesting injury
Acute allograft rejection
Opportunistic infections
Drug effect
Biliary anastomatotic problems (e.g., bile leak, stricture)
Recurrent disease
Acute vanishing bile duct syndrome

3 months+
Recurrent disease
Chronic ductopenic rejection
Drug effect

thrombosis can also lead to the changes of harvesting injury. These changes can persist for as long as 3 months.

PATHOLOGY. The earliest changes are in perivenular zone 3 (centrilobular), with hepatocyte balloon degeneration and variable architectural disarray with canalicular and hepatocellular cholestasis (Fig. 25.1). Acidophilic bodies are common, and mitoses may be frequent (32). True zone 3 necrosis can be seen. In severe cases, there may be hemorrhagic and confluent necrosis. When portal tracts are affected, bile ductular reaction (proliferation) is accompanied by a variable number of polymorphonuclear leukocytes around both the bile ducts and proliferated bile ductules (ischemic cholangitis) (e-Figs. 25.1–25.3).

Features suggesting bile duct stenosis or obstruction may be the first sign of arterial thrombosis. Biopsy is not specifically diagnostic, and arterial visualization with Doppler ultrasound and angiography may be needed. Children are especially at high risk (31,69).

Centrilobular necrosis is seen in as many as 30% of liver allografts. Etiologic and pathogenic factors are not completely understood. Acute allograft rejection (AAR) can manifest as isolated perivenular and

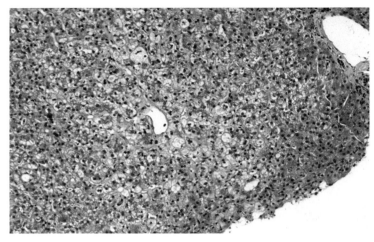

FIGURE 25.1   Preservation (harvesting) injury several days following orthotopic liver transplantation. Note ballooning of the hepatocytes in zone 3 and the associated cholestasis (hematoxylin-eosin, original magnification ×200).

subendothelial terminal hepatic venule (central vein) inflammation without portal tract inflammation or bile duct damage, not affected by calcineurin inhibitors (32).

Hyperacute Rejection (Antibody-Mediated Rejection)

Hepatic hyperacute rejection is exceedingly rare and usually occurs with ABO blood group incompatibility (17). Preformed antibodies preferentially affect arterial endothelial cells. Hyperacute rejection occurs in the first few days after transplantation with the development of liver failure (1,17,35). Irregular areas of coagulative necrosis, resembling those of eclampsia and preeclampsia, are seen (see Chapter 21).

PATHOLOGY. Zone 1 coagulative necrosis with fibrinoid necrosis of hepatic arterioles is typical (13), with scattered areas of hemorrhage and infarction and focal or widespread deposition fibrin thrombi (Fig. 25.2). Immunofluorescent studies demonstrate immunoglobulins IgG, IgM, C3, and C1q in sinusoids. Early changes of acute cellular rejection can also be seen.

ONE WEEK TO THREE MONTHS FOLLOWING TRNSPLANTATION

Acute Allograft Rejection (AAR)

The classic triad of AAR is (a) a mixed portal tract inflammatory infiltrate, (b) variable degrees of bile duct injury, and (c) endothelialitis (venulitis). AAR is less common with current immunosuppressive therapy than in past

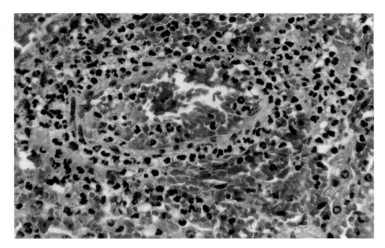

FIGURE 25.2   Hyperacute rejection affecting a porcine allograft transplanted into a young woman with fulminant hepatic failure, showing extensive hemorrhage and infarction (hematoxylin-eosin, original magnification ×200).

years and is usually mild. Multiple episodes of AAR, associated with patient noncompliance or intercurrent viral infections, are also less frequently seen (1,35,36).

PATHOLOGY. The portal tract inflammatory infiltrate includes mostly mature lymphocytes, proliferating lymphoblasts, histiocytes, and a variable number of eosinophils (Fig. 25.3, e-Figs. 25.4–25.11). Eosinophils are virtually

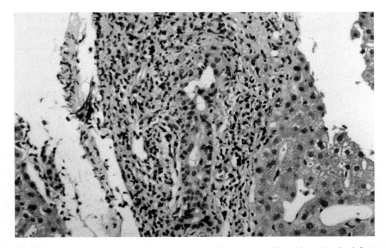

FIGURE 25.3   Acute allograft rejection 2 weeks after transplantation. Typical features are present, including mixed immunoinflammatory infiltrate rich in eosinophils with a moderate degree of bile duct injury (hematoxylin-eosin, original magnification ×200).

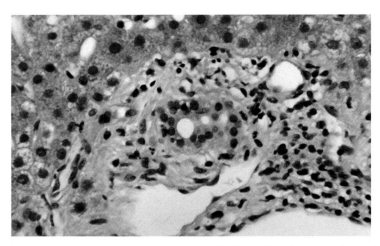

FIGURE 25.4   Acute allograft rejection, showing bile duct injury (hematoxylin-eosin, origi-nal magnification ×400).

always present, and their absence should make the diagnosis suspect. Polymorphonuclear leukocytes (PMNs) are also occasionally seen, espe-cially in children. With significant numbers of portal PMNs, early posttrans-plantation ischemic injury (ischemic cholangitis) should be considered (47).

The exuberant inflammatory infiltrate of severe AAR spills into adja-cent liver parenchyma, sometimes with true portal–portal bridging and extensive lobular necrosis. Despite this, graft failure rarely occurs. Increased number of CD8$^+$ T cells are seen, particularly in the portal tracts, as well as an increase of CD45RO$^+$ (memory) T cells.

Interlobular bile ducts show variable degrees of injury (e-Figs. 25.7, 25.9–25.11), ranging from mild to severe, including vacuolation of the epithelial cytoplasm, overlapping nuclei, nuclear pyknosis, infiltration of the epithelium with lymphocytes and occasional eosinophils, and true epithelial necrosis with subsequent disruption of the basement membrane (Fig. 25.4).

Endothelialitis involves mostly portal veins, but terminal hepatic venules (central veins) can also show changes (e-Figs. 25.4–25.7). Endothelialitis can be subtle, with only endothelial cell swelling and focal subendothelial lymphocytic infiltration (Fig. 25.5). When fully developed, there is lifting and detachment of endothelial cells under-mined by lymphocytic infiltrate followed by sloughing into the lumen.

In addition to the typical AAR features, zone 3 hepatocyte ballooning (preservation injury) can be seen. The most important and clinically rele-vant indicator of AAR severity is the response to supplemental immuno-suppression. Endothelialitis resolves first; then the immunoinflammatory infiltrate diminishes and the bile duct injury becomes less severe. Rebiopsy after treatment is useful to ensure adequate immunosuppression and to avoid excessive immunosuppression.

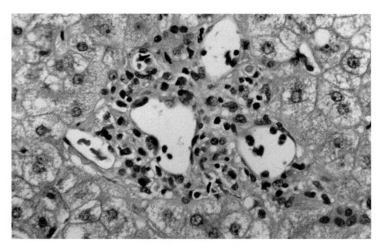

FIGURE 25.5   Acute allograft rejection, showing endothelialitis (hematoxylin-eosin, original magnification ×200).

Earlier criteria for histologic grading of AAR were based on the degree of bile duct injury, severity and extent of portal infiltrate, and endothelialitis. One of the earliest grading systems (75) has four categories of rejection: (a) relatively mild mixed portal inflammatory infiltrate and bile duct injury involving less than 50% of all interlobular bile ducts and without endothelialitis; (b) grade 1 rejection, similar to the first category, but also showing endothelialitis; (c) grade 2 rejection, with more than 50% of interlobular bile ducts showing injury; and (d) grade 3 rejection, including all features from the previous category, but also demonstrating arteritis and paucity of bile ducts with associated ballooning of hepatocytes in zone 3 of the acinus.

A multicenter study attempted to standardize the grading and nomenclature of AAR, with moderate to excellent intraobserver and interobserver agreement (14,18). Recently, an international panel of pathologists reached consensus regarding a standardized nomenclature and grading system of allograft rejection in the liver (Table 25.2) (37,38).

MORE THAN THREE MONTHS FOLLOWING LIVER TRANSPLANTATION

Chronic Allograft Rejection

Chronic (ductopenic) rejection, affecting both bile ducts and arteries, may become obvious as early as a few months following transplantation (48,52,60).

PATHOLOGY. Vascular rejection implies changes in the intima of medium-sized arteries, which lead to obliterative endarteritis or "foamy"

TABLE 25.2	Banff Schema for Grading Liver Allograft Rejection
Global Assessment[a]	Criteria
Indeterminate	Portal inflammatory infiltrate that fails to meet the criteria for the diagnosis of acute rejection[b]
Mild	Rejection infiltrate in a minority of the triads, which is generally mild and confined within the portal spaces
Moderate	Rejection infiltrate, expanding most or all of the triads
Severe	As above for mild, with spillover into periportal areas and moderate to severe perivenular inflammation that extends into the hepatic parenchyma and its associated perivenular hepatocyte necrosis

[a]Global assessment of rejection grade made on a review of the biopsy and after the diagnosis of rejection has been established.
[b]See Harrison RF, Davies MH, Goldin RD, et al. Recurrent hepatitis B in liver allografts: a distinctive form of rapidly developing cirrhosis. Histopathology 1993;23:21–28.

arteriopathy (48) (Fig. 25.6, e-Figs. 25.12–25.14). These changes, usually not seen in biopsy material, include intimal accumulation of histiocytes and subsequent fibrosis and lumen obliteration. Zone 3 (centrolobular) ballooning and, eventually, perivenular fibrosis are seen. These changes are similar to those of schemia of other causes, which must be excluded. Chronic vascular rejection may be reversible after therapy (33,75).

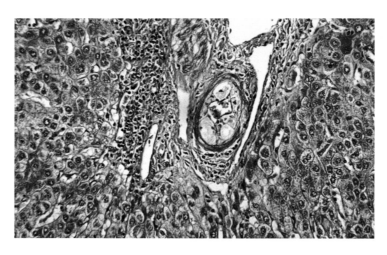

FIGURE 25.6 Chronic ductopenic rejection, showing transplant (foamy) subintimal arteriopathy (hematoxylin-eosin, original magnification ×200).

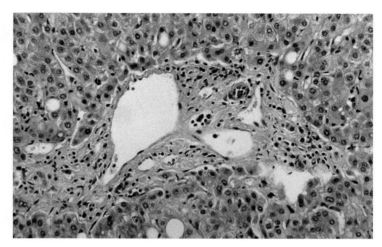

FIGURE 25.7   Chronic ductopenic rejection (vanishing bile duct syndrome). Note complete absence of the original interlobular bile ducts as well as the absence of bile ductular proliferation (hematoxylin-eosin, original magnification ×200).

Potential etiologic roles for cytomegalovirus (CMV) and human leukocyte antigen incompatibility have been suggested but are controversial (5,50).

Chronic ductopenic rejection (vanishing bile duct syndrome, VBDS) manifests as progressive bile duct injury and subsequent reduction in the number of bile ducts (paucity) with eventual loss of virtually all interlobular bile ducts (Fig. 25.7, e-Fig. 25.15) (48,52). This develops with or without features of chronic vascular rejection. The biopsy shows virtually complete absence of interlobular bile ducts, without significant bile ductular proliferation, but with extensive zone 3 canalicular cholestasis (e-Fig. 25.16). Inflammatory infiltrate is usually not prominent.

Early paucity may not be easily appreciated unless markers for biliary epithelium, including CK19 and keratin AE 1,3, are used (Fig. 25.8). An acute form of chronic ductopenic rejection can develop within a month of liver transplantation (Fig. 25.9). Criteria for grading and reporting of chronic rejection have been proposed (Table 25.3) (39).

RECURRENT DISEASES

Hepatitis B

The recurrence rate of hepatitis B virus (HBV) infection was once high, with severe progressive disease, ultimately resulting in graft failure (40,51). In the last 20 years, however, hepatitis B immunoglobulin (HBIG) post-transplantation clears hepatitis B surface antigen (HBsAg) from serum, with HBV DNA still detectable in serum or circulating mononuclear cells, potentially sustaining a low level of viral replication (58).

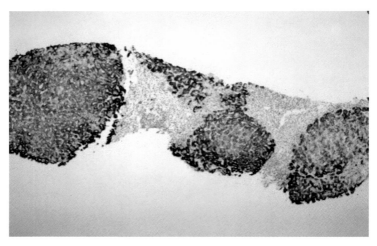

FIGURE 25.8 Ductopenic rejection, showing complete absence of interlobular bile ducts (immunoperoxidase, using antibody against keratin AE1/3, original magnification ×200).

In recurrence, various histologic changes are seen. As many as 80% show chronic hepatitis changes including cirrhosis, which can develop within a few years. In approximately 10% there are only nonspecific changes. Fibrosing cholestatic hepatitis (FCH) is a unique and usually rapidly progressive and fatal form of recurrent HBV infection.

PATHOLOGY. Recurrent HBV in the allograft may be indistinguishable from HBV in the nontransplant patient. Typical chronic hepatitis, with

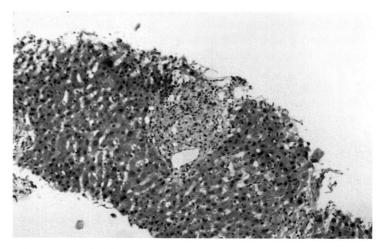

FIGURE 25.9 Ductopenic rejection developing within a month after transplantation, showing loss of interlobular bile ducts as well as portal tract edema (hematoxylin-eosin, original magnification ×200).

TABLE 25.3	Rejection Activity Index[a]	
Category	Criteria	Score[b]
Portal	Mostly lymphocytic inflammation involving, but not noticeably expanding, a minority of the triads.	1
	Expansion of most or all of the triads, by a mixed infiltrate containing lymphocytes with occasional blasts, neutrophils, and eosinophils.	2
	Marked expansion of most or all of the triads by a mixed infiltrate containing numerous blasts and eosinophils with inflammatory spillover into the periportal parenchyma.	3
Bile duct	A minority of the ducts are cuffed and infiltrated by inflammatory cells and show only mild reactive changes such as increased nuclear cytoplasmic ratio of the epithelial cells.	1
	Most or all of the ducts infiltrated by inflammatory cells. More than an occasional duct shows degenerative changes such as nuclear pleomorphism, disordered polarity, and cytoplasmic vacuolization of the epithelium.	2
	As above, with most or all of the ducts showing degenerative changes or focal luminal disruption.	3
Venous	Subendothelial lymphocytic infiltration involving some, but not most, of the portal and/or hepatic venules.	1
	Subendothelial infiltration involving most or all of the portal and/or hepatic venules.	2
	As above, with moderate or severe perivenular inflammation that extends into the perivenular parenchyma and is associated with perivenular hepatocytes necrosis.	3

[a]Criteria that can be used to score liver allograft biopsies with acute rejection, as defined by the World Gastroenterology Consensus Document (37,38).
[b]Total score equals sum of components.

many "ground glass" hepatocytes filled with HBsAg can be seen (see Chapter 8) (Fig. 25.10). FCH variant has portal, periportal, and perisinusoidal/pericellular fibrosis, canalicular and intracellular cholestasis, severe ballooning of hepatocytes, relatively mild portal inflammatory infiltrate, and usually, significant expression of HBsAg and HbcAg in hepatocytes (Fig. 25.11). Excessive intracellular accumulation of HBsAg may be directly cytopathic (16).

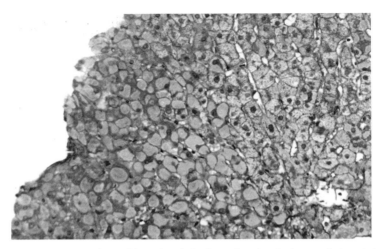

FIGURE 25.10   Recurrent hepatitis B virus infection, showing features of chronic hepatitis with numerous "ground glass" (hepatitis B surface antigen–containing) cells (hematoxylin-eosin, original magnification ×200).

Patients who undergo transplantation for fulminant HBV or with simultaneous HBV and hepatitis delta virus (HDV) infection have a recurrence rate of 50% to 70%. Paradoxically, the clinical course is usually relatively mild. In contrast with the nontransplantation population, patients develop recurrent HDV without associated HBV markers of infection, suggesting that HDV replicates in the absence of HBV and is

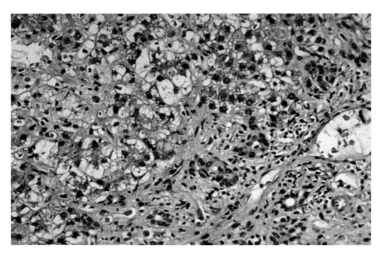

FIGURE 25.11   Recurrent hepatitis B virus infection with histopathologic features of fibrosing cholestatic cholangitis (hematoxylin-eosin, original magnification ×100).

not necessarily cytopathic, instead requiring HBV to cause liver cell injury (46). Coagulative necrosis of zone 1 is seen, with associated fibrinoid necrosis of hepatic arterioles (13,15).

Hepatitis C

Hepatitis C virus (HCV) recurrence following liver transplantation is virtually universal and is confirmed by serologic tests or polymerase chain reaction (PCR). Reinfection is usually with the same HCV strain as the original disease. Although the natural history of the posttransplant recurrent HCV hepatitis is variable, recurrent HCV hepatitis is generally more rapidly progressive when compared to the patients who underwent LT years ago (68). Newer therapies, such as pegylated interferon, may be altering this. Risk factors associated with more aggressive HCV recurrence include treated prior acute allograft rejection, cytomegalovirus (CMV) infection, and use of OKT3.

Five risk factors possibly contributing to severe recurrent disease within 2 years are the following: donor age older than 50 years, HCV genotype 1b, use of OKT3, mycophenolate mofetil (MMF) immunosuppression induction, and short-term prednisone and azathioprine (AZT) use (68).

Some patients develop HCV as an acquired infection following transplantation, either from blood products or from the organ donor (23,62). Recurrent HCV is often relatively mild (22). In spite of this, 5% to 10% of patients develop cirrhosis and, ultimately, graft failure. In some patients, HCV recurs within weeks of transplantation, and in others recurrence takes months to years. Levels of circulating HCV are much higher in individuals experiencing early recurrence (10,20,21). Furthermore, immunosuppression may contribute to high viral levels. HCV can be directly cytopathic for bile duct epithelium, but there is no correlation between levels of circulating HCV and degree of liver cell or bile duct injury. A donor–recipient match at one or two human leukocyte antigen DQ loci has been associated with more severe recurrent HCV. Other factors include cytokine gene polymorphism and chemokine effects (68). Patients infected with HCV type 1 genotype seem to have higher recurrence risk. As many as 30% of treated patients have features of ductopenic rejection.

PATHOLOGY. Typical chronic HCV changes are seen in as many as 80% of patients with recurrent HCV. Various findings not typically associated with HCV in the nontransplantation setting can also be seen, including severe bile duct injury and bile ductular proliferation, mimicking large duct obstruction (23). Cholestasis and ischemic changes may be prominent. When HCV recurs early in the posttransplantation period, before 6 weeks, the features are quite subtle (Fig. 25.12) and differentiation from AAR can be difficult (Table 25.4) (61,67,68). Multiple serial posttransplantation biopsies can be helpful as portal tract inflammation, lymphoid

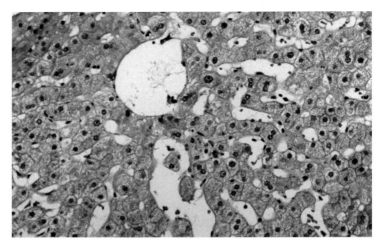

FIGURE 25.12   Recurrent hepatitis C virus infection developing within 3 months of trans-plantation. Note sinusoidal dilatation and only focal lobular inflammation (hematoxylin-eosin, original magnification ×200).

TABLE 25.4	Histopathologic Features Useful to Differentiate Acute Cellular Rejection from Early Recurrent Hepatitis C (2–3 Months following LT)
Features	***p* Value**
Features favoring acute cellular rejection	
1. Portal eosinophils	0.0038
2. Bile duct epithelial cell overlap	0.0107
3. Bile duct lymphocytic infiltration	0.0262
4. Endothelialitis	0.0248
5. Bile duct necrosis	0.0329
6. Portal inflammation	0.0366
7. Portal histiocytes	0.0415
8. Zone 3 cholestasis	0.0415
9. Hepatocyte mitoses	0.0490
10. Canalicular cholestasis	0.0490
Feature favoring early recurrent hepatitis C (<3 months)	
1. Sinusoidal dilatation (in the absence of other features of AAR)	0.0366

LT, liver transplantation; AAR, acute allograft rejection.
Reprinted with permission from Petrovic LM, Villamil FG, Vierling JM, et al. Comparison of histopathology in acute allograft rejection and recurrent hepatitis C after liver transplanta-tion. Liver Transpl Surg 1997;3:398–406.

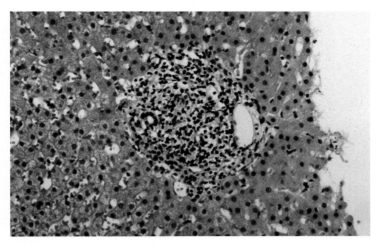

FIGURE 25.13 Recurrent hepatitis C virus infection occurring more than a year following transplantation and histologically indistinguishable from chronic hepatitis C in the nontransplantation setting (hematoxylin-eosin, original magnification ×200).

aggregate formation, and lobular activity become more evident (25,27). Early HCV recurrence can be predominantly lobular hepatitis with little or no portal inflammation.

One of the most important features of HCV is bile duct injury (Fig. 25.13) (Table 25.5). The precise mechanism for this is unclear.

Nodular regenerative hyperplasia (NRH) has been described in the setting of recurrent HCV infection (Fig. 25.14).

TABLE 25.5	**Differentiating Early Recurrent HCV (<3 Months following LT) from AAR Liver Biopsy Findings**	
	AAR	*Early HCV*
Portal tract/inflammation	Mixed (variable number of eosinophils)	Mononuclear
Bile duct injury	Present, prominent	No/Minimal
Endothelialitis	Present	Absent
Sinusoidal dilatation	Absent	Present
Parenchymal changes	Mild	Present
Inflammation/liver cell necrosis	Minimal/mild	Present
Steatosis	Absent	Present
Cholestasis	Present	May be present

HCV, hepatitis C virus; LT, liver transplantation; AAR, acute allograft rejection.

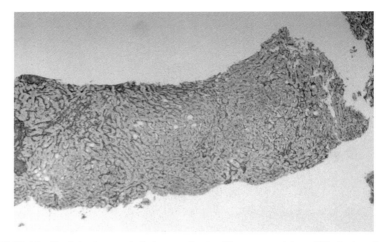

FIGURE 25.14   Nodular hyperplasia in a patient with recurrent hepatitis C virus infection (reticulin silver preparation, original magnification ×100).

Primary Biliary Cirrhosis

Primary biliary cirrhosis (PBC) can recur (6,34,59,64), generally after many years. It can be exceedingly difficult to distinguish early recurrent PBC from AAR because of the similarity of bile duct injury. Typical early granulomatous bile duct injury and features of florid bile duct injury are usually not seen. Mild bile duct injury, with predominantly mononuclear inflammatory infiltrate, is more usual. Recurrent PBC progresses slowly, and advanced stages are uncommon.

Primary Sclerosing Cholangitis

Primary sclerosing cholangitis (PSC) also recurs (31). Infectious and non-infectious causes, including ischemia, CMV, and technical complications, may cause secondary sclerosing cholangitis, which can be difficult to distinguish from PSC. If these and other potential etiologic factors can be excluded, the finding of imaging and pathology features of PSC (Fig. 25.15) can be considered diagnostic. Features compatible with PSC that become apparent at least a year after LT are considered more significant, since the other potential factors (including ischemia) are less likely at that time (28,40,74). Recurrent PSC is generally histologically indistinguishable from usual PSC.

Other Conditions

Recurrence of alcoholic liver disease, Budd-Chiari syndrome, and autoimmune hepatitis are well recognized (30,37). Some patients with recurrent autoimmune hepatitis can have concurrent HCV. Nonalcoholic steatohepatitis (NASH)/nonalcoholic fatty liver disease (NAFLD) also recurs,

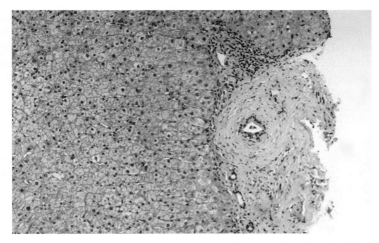

FIGURE 25.15 Recurrent primary sclerosing cholangitis. Note the characteristic periductal concentric fibrosis (Masson trichrome, original magnification ×200).

especially in patients who have undergone prior jejunoileal bypass (Fig. 25.16). The course may be more rapidly progressive.

Extrahepatic biliary atresia has not been shown to recur, but metabolic diseases, including glycogenosis IV, may.

Hepatocellular Malignancies

Malignant tumors, including hepatocellular carcinoma and hepatoblastoma, can recur (39,57). Cholangiocarcinomas can recur relatively quickly

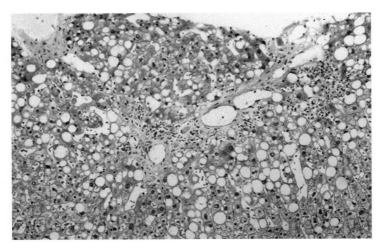

FIGURE 25.16 Recurrent nonalcoholic steatohepatitis in a patient who had previously undergone jejunoileal bypass (hematoxylin-eosin, original magnification ×200).

with a 2-year posttransplant survival less than 50%. Epithelioid heman-gioendothelioma, even when extensive, is not a contraindication for LT. Long-term survival occurs when the tumor is limited to the liver, even with lymph node metastasis. Metastatic neoplasms, even if solitary, can also recur relatively quickly, and transplantation is generally considered inappropriate (26).

Hepatitis G and Hepatitis E in Liver Transplantation Patients

Hepatitis G virus (HGV) can be present in as many as 20% of HCV patients, but apparently has little or no clinical impact (3,12,24). It has recently been suggested that hepatitis E is associated with clinically chronic disease in the posttransplant setting, but HEV is quite rare (41).

OPPORTUNISTIC INFECTIONS

Infection with opportunistic organisms is a common problem because all liver transplantation patients undergo immunosuppressive therapy. The most common viral infections are CMV, herpes simplex virus and varicella zoster virus, adenovirus (especially in children), and Epstein-Barr virus (EBV).

Viruses

CMV is the most commonly encountered posttransplantation infectious agent (34,38). Scattered collections of PMNs (microabscesses) can be seen (Fig. 25.17), but they are not necessarily CMV and confirmation with immunostains is needed. Their presence, however, should be taken as

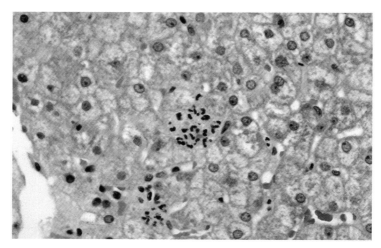

FIGURE 25.17 Microabscesses in the posttransplantation allograft. A specific etiologic factor was not identified (hematoxylin-eosin, original magnification ×200).

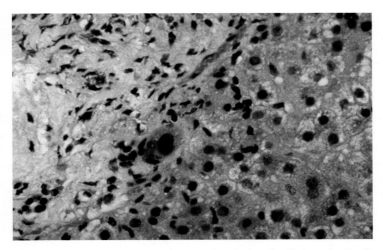

FIGURE 25.18   Cytomegalovirus hepatitis occurring during the first week after liver transplantation, showing characteristic cell enlargement and typical intranuclear inclusion (hematoxylin-eosin, original magnification ×200).

presumptive evidence of CMV pending confirmation. Characteristic intranuclear viral inclusions can also be seen (Fig. 25.18, e-Figs. 25.17–25.19).

Other viral infections, such as herpes simplex (e-Figs. 25.20, 25.21), can be seen. Herpes has varying degrees of liver cell necrosis, and viral inclusions may not always be appreciated until immunostains are used. In adenovirus, necrosis may be extensive (9) (e-Fig. 25.22).

Fungal Infection and Bacterial Infections

Fungal infection is only rarely seen in the posttransplantation liver biopsy.

Bacterial infection, with associated septicemia and sepsis, develops in patients after LT. Similar to the nontransplantation setting, a mild mononuclear and polymorphonuclear portal infiltrate is seen, with focal bile ductular proliferation.

Other Infectious Agents

Toxoplasma gondii, *Pneumocystis carinii*, and *Bartonella quintana* can occur in the posttransplantation setting.

Posttransplantation Lymphoproliferative Disorders

Most posttransplantation lymphoproliferative disorders (PTLDs) occurring after liver transplantation are associated with EBV infection and can occur as early as 4 to 6 weeks following transplantation. The incidence in the pediatric population is approximately 8% and in the adult population is 1% to 2%. EBV may develop de novo or may represent viral reactivation. The presence of the viral genome can be confirmed by in situ hybridization or polymerase chain reaction of serum or tissue. In situ hybridization for EBER-1 gene in tissue is sufficiently sensitive and specific for the detection of the viral genetic material. Immunostain for latent membrane protein seems to be somewhat less sensitive (44).

PATHOLOGY. The findings are similar to those in the nontransplantation setting. Sinusoidal and portal tract infiltration with B lymphocytes, including immunoblastic forms, is characteristic. Initially, B-cell proliferation is polyclonal and, at this stage, will resolve with reduction of immunosuppression and antiviral therapy. Monoclonal proliferation is likely to be malignant and unresponsive to treatment. Most cases of PTLD are usually of recipient origin. Rarely, proliferating lymphoid cells of donor origin have been demonstrated. T-cell PTLD can also occur.

Histopathologic features of EBV-associated PTLD may be difficult to recognize and differentiate from AAR, especially in the early, polyclonal phase (2,42). Portal tracts are mildly to moderately expanded with a predominantly mononuclear lymphoid infiltrate composed of small, mature lymphocytes and transformed cells, including lymphoblasts and immunoblasts (Fig. 25.19, e-Figs. 25.23–25.26). Plasma cells may be prominent. The absence of eosinophils is striking and may be helpful in excluding AAR. Bile duct injury, if present, is minimal, with only mild irregularity of epithelial cells, without evidence of lymphocytic infiltration or bile duct disruption, despite being surrounded by a dense lymphoid infiltrate. The lymphoid infiltrate often has angiocentric (perivenular) distribution, mimicking endothelialitis, but no true endothelialitis. The histopathologic features may be exceedingly subtle, may mimic bile duct obstruction with focal bile ductular proliferation, or may be quite patchy

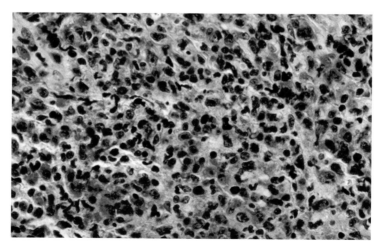

FIGURE 25.19   Posttransplantation Epstein-Barr virus–related lymphoproliferative disorder (hematoxylin-eosin, original magnification ×200).

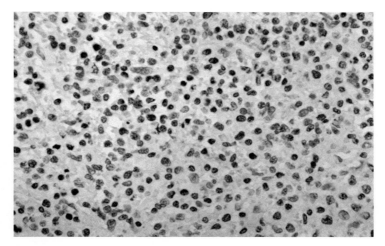

FIGURE 25.20   Posttransplantation Epstein-Barr virus–related lymphoproliferative disorder with numerous cells demonstrating positive reaction for EBER-1 gene (in situ hybridization with a probe for EBER-1 gene, original magnification ×200).

and not seen in any given biopsy (2,65,66). Immunohistochemical and molecular methods for demonstrating EBV should be performed (Fig. 25.20, e-Fig. 25.26) (44).

FUTURE DEVELOPMENTS

Although LT is only about 30 years old, newer modalities are being applied, with their own sets of problems. There is growing use of split donor livers, use of living-related donor livers, heterotopic grafts, and xenografts using porcine and baboon livers as bridge grafts until a donor is obtained (8,19). Various bioartificial liver devices are being evaluated, also serving as therapeutic bridges in critically ill patients with fulminant or subfulminant liver failure.

LIVER BIOPSY FOLLOWING BONE MARROW TRANSPLANTATION

Acute Graft Versus Host Disease

Graft versus host disease (GVHD) is commonly associated with bone marrow transplantation but can develop following orthotopic liver transplantation (11). Changes primarily involve skin and colon, and the liver is affected in only the most severe cases. Rarely, liver is the single affected organ (55,70,71). GVHD is an immunologically mediated condition and develops from the effects of the immunocompetent donor cells on liver cells.

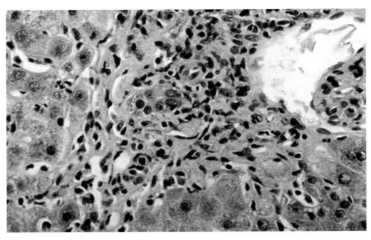

FIGURE 25.21   Graft versus host disease in a patient who had undergone liver transplantation, showing bile duct epithelial necrosis (hematoxylin-eosin, original magnification ×200).

PATHOLOGY. Acute GVHD manifests as interlobular bile duct injury and cholestasis (55,71) (Fig. 25.21, e-Figs. 25.27–25.29). Bile duct epithelium appears irregular and shows cytoplasmic vacuolation, overlapping nuclei, and nuclear pleomorphism sometimes with increased nuclear/cytoplasmic ratio. Numerous apoptotic nuclei with scattered nuclear debris may be seen. Endothelialitis of both portal and hepatic veins is seen in as many as approximately 10% of patients, as well as true venous occlusion. Endothelialitis is not invariable, as it is in AAR, and hence does not seem to have the same diagnostic and prognostic importance. Focal liver cell necrosis with acidophilic body formation occurs. Kupffer cells and sinusoidal endothelial cells may contain abundant hemosiderin.

There may be associated nodular hyperplasia (NH) (see Chapter 23) with portal hypertension (72). Furthermore, patients with GVHD may have concomitant hepatitis, either viral or drug induced, and establishing the correct diagnosis may be quite difficult.

Chronic Graft Versus Host Disease

Chronic GVHD usually develops after more than 100 days following bone marrow transplantation, and manifestations may be seen in multiple organs.

PATHOLOGY. Chronic GVHD is characterized by progressive bile duct injury and ultimate bile duct loss with marked cholestasis (Fig. 25.22). Eventually, there is portal and septal fibrosis. A few patients become cirrhotic (38,43). Arteriopathic changes, frequently seen in ductopenic allograft rejection, are not common.

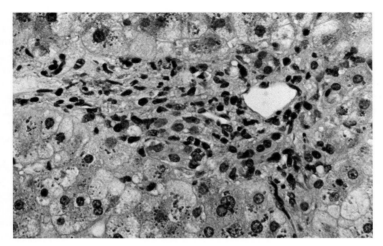

FIGURE 25.22   Chronic graft versus host disease involving the liver in a patient following bone marrow transplantation (hematoxylin-eosin, original magnification ×200).

Differential diagnosis includes various types of hepatitis. However, in most hepatitis severed bile duct and injury and bile duct loss are not seen, even with marked hepatocellular injury and necrosis. GVHD can, of course, have concurrent hepatitis.

OTHER FINDINGS. Venoocclusive disease (VOD) and NH occur in patients who have undergone cytoreductive therapy. VOD is most common during the first 30 days after bone marrow transplantation. VOD and HN can have similar manifestations, and differentiation generally requires liver biopsy. Furthermore, although NH does not necessarily have a significant immediate effect, patients develop portal hypertension (72).

LIVER BIOPSY FOLLOWING RENAL TRANSPLANTATION

After renal transplantation, various conditions affecting the liver have been described, including steatosis, NH, peliosis hepatis, infection with hepatitis B and C viruses, and hepatocellular carcinoma (53). Secondary hemosiderosis is common in patients who underwent hemodialysis or received multiple transfusions. After long-standing hemodialysis, silicone from the dialysis tubing may elicit a foreign-body reaction, with subsequent hepatic fibrosis. Silicone may be seen as a birefringent crystalloid foreign material in the tissue.

Drug-induced changes, including cholestasis, sinusoidal dilatation, and VOD associated with azathioprine, are also well recognized after renal transplantation (53). Superimposed bacterial infection with associated septicemia and sepsis and various opportunistic infections may also occur.

REFERENCES

1. Adams DH, Neuberger JM. Patterns of graft rejection following liver transplantation. J Hepatol 1990;10:113–119.
2. Alshak NS, Jimenez AM, Gedebou M, et al. Epstein-Barr virus infection in liver transplantation patients: correlation of histopathology and semi-quantitative Epstein-Barr virus-DNA recovery using polymerase chain reaction. Hum Pathol 1993;24:1306–1312.
3. Alter HJ. The cloning and clinical implications of HGV and HGBV-C. N Engl J Med 1996;334:1536–1537.
4. Angele MK, Rentsch M, Wittmann B, et al. Effect of steatosis on liver function and organ survival after liver transplantation. Am J Surg 2008;195(2):214–220.
5. Arnold JC, Portman BC, O'Grady JG, et al. Cytomegalovirus infection persists in the liver graft in the vanishing bile duct syndrome. Hepatology 1992;16:285–292.
6. Balan V, Batts KP, Porayko MK, et al. Histologic evidence of recurrence of primary biliary cirrhosis after liver transplantation. Hepatology 1993;18:1392–1398.
7. Bizzolon T, Palazzo U, Ducerf C, et al. Pilot study of the combination of interferon alpha and ribavirin as therapy of recurrent hepatitis C after liver transplantation. Hepatology 1997;26:500–505.
8. Broelsch CE, Whitington PF, Emond JC, et al. Liver transplantation in children from living related donors: surgical techniques and results. Ann Surg 1994;214:428–439.
9. Cames B, Rahier J, Burtomboy G, et al. Acute adenovirus hepatitis in liver transplant patients. J Pediatr 1992;120:33–37.
10. Chazouilleres O, Kim M, Combs C, et al. Quantitation of hepatitis C virus RNA in liver transplant recipients. Gastroenterology 1994;106:994–999.
11. Collins RH Jr, Cooper B, Nikaein A, et al. Graft-versus-host disease in a liver transplant recipient. Ann Intern Med 1992;116:391–392.
12. Cotler SJ, Gretch DR, Bronner MP, et al. Hepatitis G virus co-infection does not alter the course of recurrent hepatitis C virus infection in liver transplantation recipients. Hepatology 1997;26:432–437.
13. Craig FE, Gulley ML, Banks PM. Posttransplant lymphoproliferative disorders. Am J Clin Pathol 1993;99:265–276.
14. D'Alessandro AM, Kalayoglu M, Sollinger HW, et al. The predictive value of donor liver biopsies for the development of primary nonfunction after orthotopic liver transplantation. Transplantation 1991;51:157–163.
15. David E, Rahier J, Pucci A, et al. Recurrence of hepatitis D (delta) in liver transplants: histopathologic aspects. Gastroenterology 1991;104:1122–1128.
16. Davies SE, Portmann BC, O'Grady JG, et al. Hepatic histologic findings after transplantation for chronic hepatitis B virus infection, including a unique pattern of fibrosing cholestatic hepatitis. Hepatology 1992;13:150–157.
17. Demetris AJ, Jaffe R, Tzakis A, et al. Antibody-mediated rejection of human orthotopic liver allografts: a study of liver transplantation across ABO blood group barriers. Am J Pathol 1988;132:489–502.
18. Demetris AJ, Belle SH, Hart J, et al. Intraobserver and interobserver variation in the histopathologic assessment of liver allograft rejection. Hepatology 1991;14:949–951.
19. Demetriou AA, Whiting J, Levenson SM, et al. New method of hepatocyte transplantation and extracorporeal liver support. Ann Surg 1986;204:259–271.
20. Faust TW. Recurrent primary biliary cirrhosis, primary sclerosing cholangitis, and autoimmune hepatitis after transplantation. Liver Transplant 2001;7:99–108.
21. Ferey C, Samuel D, Thiers V, et al. Reinfection of liver graft by hepatitis C virus after liver transplantation. J Clin Invest 1992;89:1361–1365.
22. Ferey C, Gigou M, Samuel D, et al. The course of hepatitis C virus infection after liver transplantation. Hepatology 1994;20:1137–1143.

23. Ferey C, Gigou M, Samuel D, et al. Influence of the genotypes of hepatitis C virus on the severity of recurrent liver disease after liver transplantation. Gastroenterology 1995;108: 1088–1096.

24. Freese DK, Snover DC, Sharp HL, et al. Chronic rejection after liver transplantation: a study of clinical, histopathological and immunological features. Hepatology 1991;13: 882–891.

25. Fried MW, Khudyakov YE, Smallwood GA, et al. Hepatitis G co-infection in liver transplantation recipients with chronic hepatitis C and nonviral chronic liver disease. Hepatology 1997;25:1271–1276.

26. Gane EJ, Portmann BC, Naoumov NV, et al. Long-term outcome of hepatitis C infection after liver transplantation. N Engl Med 1996;334:815–820.

27. Geubel AP, Cnudde A, Ferrant A, et al. Diffuse biliary tract involvement mimicking primary sclerosing cholangitis after bone marrow transplantation. J Hepatol 1990;10:23–28.

28. Graziadei IW, Wiesner RH, Batts KP, et al. Recurrence of primary sclerosing cholangitis following liver transplantation. Hepatology 1999;29:1050–1056.

29. Greenson JK, Svoboda-Newman SM, Merion RM, et al. Histologic progression of recurrent hepatitis C in liver transplant allografts. Am J Surg Pathol 1996;20:731–738.

30. Gretch DR, Bacchi CE, Corey L, et al. Persistent hepatitis C virus infection after liver transplantation: clinical and virological features. Hepatology 1995;22:1–10.

31. Halff G, Todo S, Tzakis AG, et al. Liver transplantation for the Budd-Chiari syndrome. Ann Surg 1990;202:43–49.

32. Harrison RF, Davies MH, Goldin RD, et al. Recurrent hepatitis B in liver allografts: a distinctive form of rapidly developing cirrhosis. Histopathology 1993;23:21–28.

33. Hartman GG, Gordon R, Lerut J, et al. Intrahepatic bile duct strictures in a liver allograft recipient mimicking recurrent primary sclerosing cholangitis. Transplant Int 1991;4: 191–192.

34. Hertzler G, Milikan WJ. The surgical pathologist's role in liver transplantation. Arch Pathol Lab Med 1991;115:273–382.

35. Hubscher SG, Buckels JAC, Elias E, et al. Reversible vanishing bile duct syndrome after liver transplantation. Report of 6 cases. Transplant Proc 1991;23:1415–1416.

36. Hubscher SG, Elias E, Buckels JAC, et al. Primary biliary cirrhosis: histologic evidence of disease recurrence after liver transplantation. J Hepatol 1993;18:173–184.

37. International Working Party. Terminology of hepatic allograft rejection. Hepatology 1995; 22:648–655.

38. International Panel. Banff schema for grading liver allograft rejection; an international consensus document. Hepatology 1997;25:658–664.

39. International Panel. Update of the international Banff schema for liver allograft rejection: working recommendations for the histopathologic staging and reporting of chronic rejection. Hepatology 2000;31:792–799.

40. Jeyarajah DR, Netto GJ, Lee SP, et al. Recurrent primary sclerosing cholangitis after orthotopic liver transplantation: is chronic rejection part of the process? Transplantation 1998;66:1300–1306.

41. Kamar N, Selves J, Mansuy JM, et al. Hepatitis E virus and chronic hepatitis in organ-transplant recipients. N Engl J Med 2008;358(8):811–817.

42. Keeffe EB. Milestones in liver transplantation for alcoholic liver disease. Liver Transplant Surg 1997;3:197–199.

43. Knapp AB, Crawford JM, Rappaport JM, et al. Cirrhosis as a consequence of graft-versus-host disease. Gastroenterology 1997;92:513–519.

44. Koneru B, Flye MM, Busittil RW, et al. Liver transplantation for hepatoblastoma: the American experience. Ann Surg 1991;213:118–121.

45. Lake JR, Wright T, Ferrell L, et al. Hepatitis C and B in liver transplantation. Transplant Proc 1993;25:2006–2009.

46. Langnas AN, Castaldo P, Markin RS, et al. The spectrum of Epstein-Barr infection with hepatitis following liver transplantation. Transplant Proc 1991;23:1513–1514.

47. Lee RG. Recurrence of alcoholic liver disease after liver transplantation. Liver Transplant Surg 1997;3:292–296.

48. Lones MA, Shintaku IP, Weiss LM, et al. Posttransplant lymphoproliferative disorder in liver allograft biopsies: a comparison of three methods for the demonstration of Epstein-Barr virus. Hum Pathol 1997;28:533–539.

49. Lucey MR, Merion RM, Henley KS, et al. Selection for and outcome of liver transplantation in alcoholic liver disease. Gastroenterology 1992;102:1736–1741.

50. Lucey MR, Graham DM, Martin P, et al. Recurrence of hepatitis B and delta hepatitis after orthotopic liver transplantation. Gut 1992;33:1390–1396.

51. Ludwig J, Batts KP, MacCarty RL. Ischemic cholangitis in hepatic allografts. Mayo Clin Proc 1992;67:519–526.

52. Ludwig J, Wiesner RH, Batts KP, et al. The acute vanishing bile duct syndrome (acute irreversible rejection) after orthotopic liver transplantation. Hepatology 1987;7:476–483.

53. Manez R, White LT, Linden P, et al. The influence of HLA matching on cytomegalovirus hepatitis and chronic rejection after liver transplantation. Transplantation 1993;55:1067–1071.

54. Markin RS, Wisecarver JL, Radio SJ, et al. Frozen section evaluation of donor livers before transplantation. Transplantation 1990;56:1403–1409.

55. Marubbio AT, Danielson B. Hepatic veno-occlusive disease in renal transplant patient receiving azathioprine. Gastroenterology 1975;69:739–743.

56. Mason AL, Wick M, White HM, et al. Increased hepatocyte expression of hepatitis B virus transcription in patients with features of cholestatic fibrosing hepatitis. Gastroenterology 1993;105:237–244.

57. Matsumoto Y, McCaughan GW, Painter DM, et al. Evidence that portal tract microvascular destruction precedes bile duct loss in human liver allograft rejection. Transplantation 1993;56:69–75.

58. McDonald GB, Sharma P, Matthews DE, et al. Venoocclusive disease of the liver after bone marrow transplantation: diagnosis, incidence and predisposing factors. Hepatology 1984;4:116–122.

59. McPeake JR, O'Grady JG, Zaman S, et al. Liver transplantation for primary hepatocellular carcinoma: tumor size and number determine outcome. J Hepatol 1993;18:226–234.

60. Milkiewicz P, Hubscher SG, Skiba G, et al. Recurrence of autoimmune hepatitis after liver transplantation. Transplantation 1999;68:253–256.

61. Nalesnik MA. Lymphoproliferative disease in organ transplant recipients. Springer Semin Immunopathol 1991;13:199–216.

62. Neuberger J. Recurrent primary biliary cirrhosis. Liver Transplant 2001;7:596–599.

63. Noack KB, Wiesner RH, Batts K, et al. Severe ductopenic rejection with features of vanishing bile duct syndrome: clinical, biochemical and histologic evidence for spontaneous resolution. Transplant Proc 1991;23:1448–1451.

64. Palazzo J, Lundquist K, Mitchell D, et al. Rapid development of lymphoma following liver transplantation in a recipient with hepatitis B and primary hemochromatosis. Am J Gastroenterol 1993;88:102–104.

65. Paya C, Wiesner R, Hermans P, et al. Lack of association between cytomegalovirus infection, HLA matching and the vanishing bile duct syndrome after liver transplantation. Hepatology 1992;16:66–70.

66. Pereira BJG, Milford EL, Kirkman RL, et al. Prevalence of hepatitis C virus RNA in organ donors positive for hepatitis C antibody and in the recipients of their organs. N Engl J Med 1992;327:910–915.

67. Petrovic LM, Villamil FG, Vierling JM, et al. Comparison of histopathology in acute allograft rejection and recurrent hepatitis C infection after liver transplantation. Liver Transpl Surg 1997;3:398–406.

68. Petrovic LM. Early recurrent hepatitis C virus infection after liver transplantation Liver Transplantation. 2006;12(11 Suppl 2):S32–37.

69, Ploeg RJ, D'Alessandro AM, Knechtle SJ, et al. Risk factors for primary dysfunction after liver transplantation: a multivariate analysis. Transplantation 1993;55:807–813.

70. Randhawa PS, Jaffe R, Demetris AJ, et al. The systemic distribution of Epstein-Barr virus genomes in fatal posttransplantation lymphoproliferative disorders. An in situ hybridization study. Am J Pathol 1991;138:1027–1033.

71. Randhawa PS, Jaffe R, Demetris AJ, et al. Expression of Epstein-Barr virus–encoded small RNA (by the EBER-1 gene) in liver specimens from transplant recipients with posttransplantation lymphoproliferative disease. N Engl J Med 1992;327:1710–1714.

72. Roberts JP, Ascher NL, Lake J, et al. Graft vs. host disease after liver transplantation: a report of four cases. Hepatology 1991;14:274–281.

73. Sanchez-Urdazpal L, Gores GJ, Ward EM, et al. Diagnostic features and clinical outcome of ischemic-type biliary complications after liver transplantation. Hepatology 1993;17:605–609.

74. Sheng R, Campbell WI, Zajki AB, et al. Cholangiographic features of biliary stricture liver transplantation for primary sclerosing cholangitis: evidence of recurrent disease. AJR Am J Roentgenol 1996;166:1109–1113.

75. Snover DC, Freese DK, Sharp HL, et al. Liver allograft rejection. An analysis of the use of the biopsy in determining outcome of rejection. Am J Surg Pathol 1987;11:1–10.

26

EVALUATION OF CHOLESTASIS

Cholestasis is the result of either a functional defect in bile formation at the level of the hepatocyte or a defect in bile secretion and flow at the bile duct level (37). Factors contributing to hepatocyte defects include the viral hepatitides, drugs (19), alcohol, and sepsis. Bile duct obstruction can be intrahepatic (e.g., primary biliary cirrhosis, vanishing bile duct syndrome (28), paucity of interlobular bile ducts) and extrahepatic (e.g., primary sclerosing cholangitis, large duct stones, tumors).

Bile secretion depends on the activities of hepatocytes and bile duct epithelial cells, including many membrane transport systems, and on the morphologic and functional integrity of the bile secretory apparatus (11,17,25,33).

Jaundice is the biochemical and physiologic result of the accumulation in the circulation of bilirubin and other bile constituents. Jaundice is usually, but not always, associated with morphologic changes in the liver. Sometimes the changes reflect primary liver injury, as in cholestatic hepatitis, and sometimes they are secondary to some other condition, such as extrahepatic large duct obstruction (LDO). In some patients jaundice may be clinically and biochemically apparent, but the liver biopsy is essentially unchanged (e.g., increased serum unconjugated bilirubin value in hemolysis).

Jaundice can be a reflection of increase of either unconjugated or conjugated bilirubin, or both, and there are various potential contributing causes (Table 26.1), many of which are discussed in other chapters of this book. This chapter concentrates on the liver biopsy features in conditions not discussed elsewhere in the text and in which there is a disturbance in bilirubin metabolism or in bile flow.

CHOLESTASIS

In the normal liver, bile is almost never visible in the usual histologic preparations. *Cholestasis* is the term used to describe bile when it is visible in the histologic section, and its presence should be regarded as abnormal. Bile can vary in color from orange or yellow, to green and even brown. Sometimes bile is pale and can be overlooked. With Perls iron stain, it is light green; with Fouchet bile stain or Sirius red, it is more olive-green.

TABLE 26.1	**Causes of Jaundice with or without Cholestasis**

I. Jaundice, with predominantly unconjugated bilirubin in the serum

    A. Decreased hepatic glucuronosyltransferase activity (decreased conjugation)

       1. Hereditary transferase deficiency

          Gilbert syndrome

          Crigler-Najjar disease

          Transient transferase deficiency (neonatal jaundice)

          Acquired transferase deficiency

       2. Drug effect

       3. Breast milk jaundice

       4. Hepatocellular disease

       5. Sepsis

    B. Decreased hepatic uptake

       1. Prolonged fasting

       2. Sepsis

    C. Overproduction of unconjugated bilirubin

       1. Hemolysis

       2. Impaired erythropoiesis

II. Jaundice, with predominantly conjugated bilirubin

    A. Impaired excretion

       1. Hereditary

          Dubin-Johnson syndrome

          Rotor syndrome

          Recurrent intrahepatic cholestasis

          Cholestatic jaundice of pregnancy

          Congenital

             Paucity of intrahepatic bile ducts, syndromatic (Alagille)

             Paucity of intrahepatic bile ducts, nonsyndromatic

             Ductal plate malformation

             Bile duct hamartoma (von Meyenburg complex)

       2. Acquired

          Hepatocellular diseases

          Drug effect:

             Alcohol

             Parenteral nutrition

             Other

(continued)

TABLE 26.1	Causes of Jaundice with or without Cholestasis (Continued)

Sepsis

Postoperative state

Cholangiopathies

    Primary biliary cirrhosis

    Autoimmune cholangitis

Paraneoplastic

    Hodgkin lymphoma

B. Large duct (extrahepatic biliary) obstruction

    Congenital

        Biliary atresia

        Choledochal cyst

        Infectious

        Parasitic

        Hemobilia

        Primary sclerosing cholangitis

        Malignancy

            Cholangiocarcinoma

            Ampullary carcinoma

        Large duct compression

        Inflammatory

        Malignancy

        Pancreatic adenocarcinoma

        Portal lymph node metastasis

        Hodgkin lymphoma

        Non-Hodgkin lymphoma

These stains are usually not needed except in the setting of purely intra-hepatocytic cholestasis or to find bile production in hepatocellular carcinoma. Cholestasis can be canalicular (Figs. 26.1 to 26.3) and/or intrahepatocytic (Figs. 26.4 and 26.5, e-Figs. 26.1–26.4).

Canalicular cholestasis is seen most often and is easiest to recognize. It is usually most prominent in zone 3 (centrilobular) in acute cholestasis and first seen as accentuation of the usual canalicular structure (Fig. 26.1). Later, globular droplets form (bile plugs, bile thrombi) in dilated canaliculi, which, with surrounding hepatocytes, form an acinus-like structure (Fig. 26.3). With prolonged acute cholestasis, cholestatic rosettes form (e-Fig. 26.1), often appearing empty because larger bile plugs are lost during processing. Canalicular cholestasis is often, but not

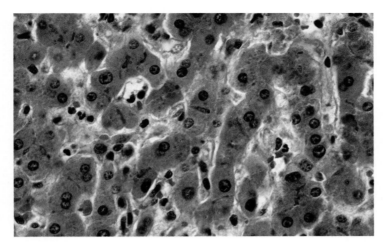

FIGURE 26.1   Canalicular cholestasis (hematoxylin-eosin, original magnification ×400).

always, accompanied by the accumulation of bile in hepatocytes and, eventually, Kupffer cells. The principal causes of canalicular cholestasis are summarized in Table 26.2.

Intrahepatocytic cholestasis is seen as cytoplasmic brown granularity that is initially quite fine and delicate, initially difficult to see, resembling lipofuscin or ceroid (Fig. 26.4). When cholestasis is severe or prolonged, it resembles coarser hemosiderin. In chronic liver diseases, especially those

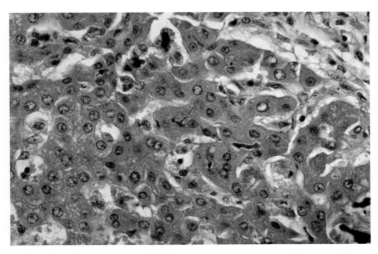

FIGURE 26.2   Canalicular cholestasis, showing canalicular rupture (hematoxylin-eosin, original magnification ×400).

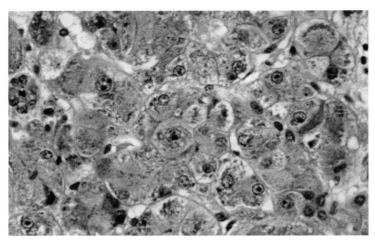

FIGURE 26.3   Canalicular cholestasis, showing acinus formation with a bile plug (hematoxylin-eosin, original magnification ×400).

involving the bile duct system, various hepatocyte changes can be seen. Swollen and pale hepatocytes ("feathery degeneration") become prominent, particularly in zone 1 (periportal) (e-Fig. 26.2). Bile is seen as delicate brown cytoplasmic granularity (Fig. 26.4). This stage is referred to as "cholate stasis" because abnormal bile salts have been implicated in its pathogenesis (25). Copper and copper-associated protein, histochemically demonstrated, and Mallory hyalin can be seen. The connective tissue

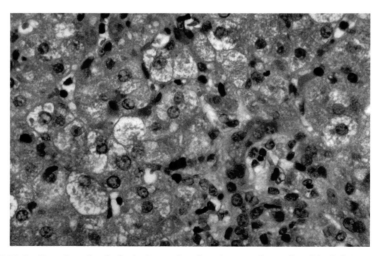

FIGURE 26.4   Hepatocytic cholestasis, acute, showing swollen cells with delicate cytoplasmic granularity (hematoxylin-eosin, original magnification ×400).

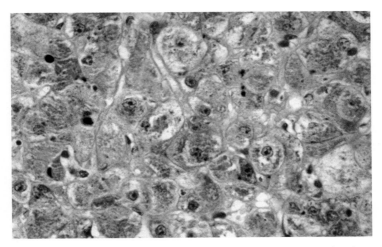

FIGURE 26.5 Prolonged Hepatocytic cholestasis, showing coarse granules (hematoxylin-eosin, original magnification ×400).

adjacent to cholate stasis is also often edematous, imparting a halo-like appearance to the cirrhotic nodules of chronic cholestatic disorders (Fig. 26.6). Ductular reaction may be prominent at the interface between portal tracts or cirrhotic septa and the limiting plate of hepatocytes (ductular piecemeal necrosis) (Fig. 26.7) (26).

Isolated or Predominantly Canalicular Cholestasis

Canalicular cholestasis, without hepatocytic cholestasis, is seen in various conditions. Isolated canalicular cholestasis may be caused by idiosyncratic reaction to various drugs (Table 26.3). Biopsy in those cases may show many eosinophils in the inflammatory portal tract infiltrate.

TABLE 26.2	Causes of Isolated or Predominantly Canalicular Cholestasis
Large duct obstruction	
Drugs	
Cholestasis of pregnancy	
Sepsis	
Acute hepatitis	
Recurrent intrahepatic cholestasis (benign recurrent cholestasis)	

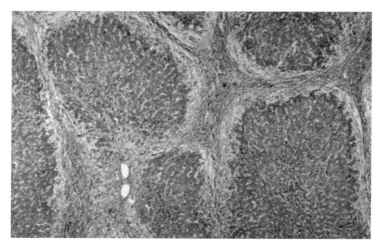

FIGURE 26.6 Prolonged cholate stasis seen as pale hepatocytes at the periphery of a cirrhotic nodule in secondary biliary cirrhosis (Masson trichrome, original magnification ×100).

LARGE DUCT OBSTRUCTION (LDO). With contemporary clinical laboratory testing and imaging methods, the diagnosis of LDO rarely requires biopsy confirmation. Biopsy is needed when imaging studies fail to demonstrate obstruction or when laboratory tests are equivocal or suggest parenchymal disease. There is almost always portal inflammation, but it can be relatively mild (see Chapter 18). Portal edema may not be prominent in the posttransplantation biopsy. Cholestasis first affects zone 3 canaliculi but

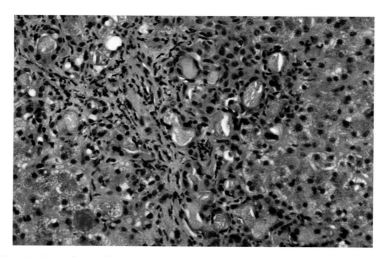

FIGURE 26.7 Ductular proliferation at the interface between portal tract and lobule (ductular piecemeal necrosis) in large duct obstruction (hematoxylin-eosin, original magnification ×100).

TABLE 26.3	**Some Drugs That Cause Cholestasis**
Fluconazole	
Mestranol	
Methyltestosterone	
Norethindrone	
Norethynodrel	
Norgestrel	
Prochlorperazine	
Stanozolol	
Testosterone	
Trimethoprim/sulfamethoxazole	
Warfarin	

if unrelieved is seen progressively in the other zones. Eventually canaliculi are destroyed and bile lakes, with variable numbers of acute inflammatory cells, develop (e-Figs. 26.3, 26.4). Ductular reaction is typical. Intrahepatocytic cholestasis is also seen with longstanding LDO.

DRUG-ASSOCIATED CHOLESTASIS. Drugs should always be considered as a cause of canalicular cholestasis, particularly in nonpregnant patients without other contributing conditions. Drugs and toxins are discussed in greater detail in Chapter 11. Cholestasis is almost always seen first in zone 3 (centrilobular) and then can involve the entire lobule. In general, the liver is otherwise unremarkable. Several medications can cause cholestasis (Table 26.3).

CHOLESTASIS OF PREGNANCY. Pregnancy-associated cholestasis generally becomes manifest in the third trimester as painless pruritus and, with rare exceptions, resolves after delivery (23,37). There may be a familial tendency (14). The cholestasis is primarily in zone 3 hepatocytes, predominantly canalicular or also intrahepatocytic (30). There may be mild inflammatory changes, most likely a result of the cholestasis itself. After delivery, the condition regresses and the liver is entirely normal. These patients may develop cholestasis if they take oral contraceptives, however (2).

SEPSIS. Cholestasis is common in sepsis (see Chapter 22). The cholestasis is most often ductular, involving ductules and canals of Hering, but can also manifest as centrilobular (zone 3) and midzonal (zone 2) predominantly canalicular cholestasis (12).

ACUTE HEPATITIS. Acute hepatitis may initially be seen as isolated canalicular cholestasis, before there is significant liver cell necrosis or inflammatory cell reaction.

TABLE 26.4	Causes of Isolated or Predominantly Hepatocytic Cholestasis
Drugs	
Cholestasis of pregnancy	
Recurrent intrahepatic cholestasis (benign recurrent cholestasis)	
Lymphomas	

Predominantly Hepatocytic Cholestasis

Hepatocytic cholestasis is generally accompanied by at least focal canalicular cholestasis. However, in a limited sample, the canalicular component may not always be seen (Table 26.4).

BENIGN RECURRENT INTRAHEPATIC CHOLESTASIS (BRIC). This exceedingly rare condition occurs principally in adults and is almost never biopsied (5). The changes resemble LDO, with both portal and lobular changes, although portal tract edema is normally not prominent. Sometimes there is only isolated, predominantly hepatocytic cholestasis. This condition can be associated with cholestasis of pregnancy and with the use of oral contraceptives (10). A gene locus, similar to that of Byler disease (see below), has been identified (5).

LYMPHOMAS. Cholestasis may be seen as a paraneoplastic phenomenon in patients with malignant lymphomas, particularly Hodgkin lymphoma (20,24), as well as in patients with non-Hodgkin lymphoma (35). Isolated cholestasis in Hodgkin lymphoma may reflect adult-onset bile duct paucity (16). Cholestasis in Hodgkin lymphoma can also be from extrahepatic bile duct compression by enlarged, often fibrotic lymph nodes.

Familial Syndromes and Other Conditions Associated with Intrahepatic Cholestasis

Familial disorders of cholestasis are usually related to mutations in genes controlling hepatocellular transport systems involved in bile formation. (29,33).

PROGRESSIVE FAMILIAL INTRAHEPATIC CHOLESTASIS (PFIC). The group of disorders termed progressive familial intrahepatic cholestasis is characterized by (a) chronic, unremitting cholestasis; (b) a characteristic constellation of clinical, biochemical, and histologic features; (c) absence of a specific anatomic abnormality; (d) absence of an identifiable metabolic disorder; and (e) an autosomal recessive inheritance pattern of occurrence. PFIC generally presents in neonates or early childhood with cholestasis, pruritus, growth failure, hepatomegaly, pancreatic deficiency, and fat-soluble vitamin deficiency (36). Typically other clinical manifestations are seen. One or more defects in the genes expressing proteins contribute (11,21).

BYLER DISEASE AND BYLER SYNDROME. The gene for Byler disease has been mapped to the 19-cM region of chromosome 18q21-q22 (7), the same site for the genes of BRIC (15). Early, the liver biopsy is similar in the two conditions, with intracanalicular cholestasis the predominant feature, with little or no inflammatory or other tissue reaction. Later Byler disease, in contrast with BRIC, has progressive portal tract fibrosis and portal-to-portal bridging. Death from cirrhosis and liver failure occurs in childhood and early adolescence. Liver transplantation is curative. A similar, but ultrastructurally different, disorder occurs in non-Amish kindred and is known as Byler syndrome (6), with various abnormal gene loci (33,37).

PEROXISOMAL DISORDERS

Zellweger (Cerebrohepatorenal) Syndrome

In classic Zellweger syndrome the liver biopsy may be unremarkable initially, but there may be portal inflammation, focal necrosis, progressive fibrosis, and ultimately, cirrhosis (9,22,27). The only constant finding is the absence of peroxisomes when the liver is studied with the electron microscope (13).

Recurrent Cholestasis with Lymphedema (Norwegian Cholestasis; Aagenaes Syndrome)

This form of neonatal jaundice may clear in childhood but can recur throughout life. Profound lower extremity lymphedema begins in childhood or during adolescence (1,31), and there may be familial lymphangiomas and hemangiomas (29). Biopsies vary, with changes including paucity of intrahepatic bile ducts, canalicular cholestasis, giant cell transformation of hepatocytes, and, in adults, cirrhosis (29).

CONGENITAL HYPERBILIRUBINEMIA SYNDROMES

Physiologic Jaundice of the Newborn

During the first few days of life, the capacity of the liver to clear hepatic bilirubin is not yet fully developed. There may also be increased bilirubin production because of accelerated red blood cell destruction in this period. Biopsy is virtually never required.

Unconjugated Hyperbilirubinemia Syndromes

CRIGLER-NAJJAR SYNDROMES I AND II. In type I Crigler-Najjar syndrome, there is lifelong, severe nonhemolytic unconjugated hyperbilirubinemia caused by congenital deficiency of bilirubin–uridine diphosphate–

glucuronyl transferase. The less severe type II is responsive to therapy with phenobarbital (32). In both forms, the liver biopsy is unremarkable except for occasional bile plugs (8).

GILBERT SYNDROME. Gilbert syndrome is a relatively common condition that affects more than 5% of the adult population. Liver biopsy is not helpful because there are no recognizable microscopic changes other than increased lipofuscin pigment (4).

Conjugated Hyperbilirubinemia Syndromes

DUBIN-JOHNSON SYNDROME. Dubin-Johnson syndrome has a point mutation of the gene responsible for the canalicular multispecific organic-anion transporter (33). Patients have chronic or intermittent hyperbilirubinemia rather than cholestasis (36). Biopsy is almost always obtained incidental to a surgical procedure in which the surgeon sees the mahogany-colored liver. The liver biopsy is characteristic, with large, coarse, dark brown, iron-negative, Fontana-Masson–positive nonmelanin granules in hepatocytes, primarily in zone 3 (Fig. 26.8, e-Figs. 26.5, 26.6) (3,34). The biopsy is otherwise unremarkable.

ROTOR SYNDROME. This benign familial disorder is clinically similar to Dubin-Johnson syndrome, but there are no macroscopic or microscopic liver changes.

METABOLIC DISORDERS

The principal metabolic disorders contributing to cholestasis are discussed in Chapter 14.

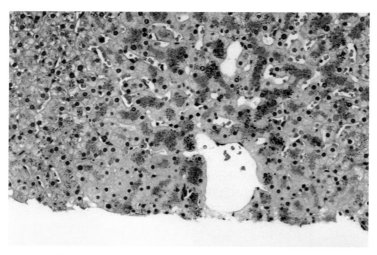

FIGURE 26.8 Dubin-Johnson syndrome, showing the typical coarse intrahepatocytic granules, predominantly in zone 3 (hematoxylin-eosin, original magnification ×100).

ACQUIRED CONDITIONS

Various acquired conditions can contribute to the development of cholestasis, including viral hepatitis, sepsis, total parenteral nutrition, infiltrative disorders, and infectious and granulomatous disorders.

Benign Postoperative Cholestasis

Cholestasis, with and without jaundice, in the postoperative period is a result of various factors, including sepsis, LDO, shock, hemolysis, drug-induced hepatitis, and other conditions. Characterized by predominantly conjugated hyperbilirubinemia, it generally occurs in the first 2 days after major surgery and may last as long as 2 weeks. It is thought to be caused by bilirubin overload of the liver, with or without reduced secretory capacity of the liver; biopsy shows predominantly zone 3 canalicular cholestasis without inflammation (e-Figs. 26.7, 26.8). With hemolysis, Kupffer cells contain hemosiderin (18).

REFERENCES

1. Aagenae Ø, Van der Hagen CB, Refsum S. Hereditary recurrent intrahepatic cholestasis from birth. Arch Dis Child 1968;43:646–657.
2. Adlercreutz H, Tenenbaum R. Some aspects of the interaction between natural and synthetic female sex hormones and the liver. Am J Med 1970;49:630–649.
3. Barone P, Inferrera C, Carrozza G. Pigments in the Dubin-Johnson syndrome. In: Wolman M, ed. Pigments in Pathology. New York: Academic Press, 1969:307–325.
4. Barth RF, Grimley PM, Berk PD, et al. Excess lipofuscin accumulation in constitutional hepatic dysfunction (Gilbert's syndrome). Arch Pathol 1971;91:41–47.
5. Bijleveld CAM, Vomnk RJ, Kuipers F, et al. Benign recurrent intrahepatic cholestasis: a long-term follow-up study of two patients. Hepatology 1989;9:532–537.
6. Bull LN, Carlton VE, Stricker NL, et al. Genetic and morphologic findings in progressive familial intrahepatic cholestasis (Byler disease [PFIC 1] and Byler syndrome); evidence for heterogeneity. Hepatology 1997;26:155–164.
7. Carlton VE, Knisely As, Freimer NB. Mapping of a locus for progressive familial intrahepatic cholestasis (Byler disease) to 18q21–q22, the benign recurrent intrahepatic cholestasis region. Hum Mol Genet 1995;4:1049–1053.
8. Crigler JF, Najjar VA. Congenital familial nonhemolytic jaundice associated with kernicterus. Pediatrics 1952;10:169–179.
9. Danks DM, Tippett P, Adams C, et al. Cerebro-hepato-renal syndrome of Zellweger: a report of eight cases with comments upon the incidence, the liver lesion, and a fault of pipecolic acid metabolism. J Pediatr 1975;86:382–387.
10. DePagter AGF, van Berge Henegouwen FP, ten Bokkel Huinink JA, et al. Familial benign recurrent intrahepatic cholestasis: interrelation with intrahepatic cholestasis of pregnancy and from oral contraceptives? Gastroenterology 1976;71:202–207.
11. Fitz JG. Regulation of cholangiocyte secretion. Semin Liver Dis 2002;22:241–258.
12. Fuchs M, Sanyal AJ. Sepsis and cholestasis. Clin Liver Dis 2008;12:151–172.
13. Goldfischer S, Moore CL, Johnson AB, et al. Peroxisomal and mitochondrial defects in the cerebro-hepato-renal syndrome. Science 1973;182:62–64.

14. Holzbach RT, Sivak, DA, Braun WE. Familial recurrent intrahepatic cholestasis of pregnancy: a genetic study providing evidence for a sex-linked, dominant trait. Gastroenterology 1983;85:175–179.

15. Houwen RHJ, Baharloo S, Blankenship K, et al. Genome screening by searching for shared segments: mapping a gene for benign recurrent intrahepatic cholestasis. Nat Genet 1994;8:380–386.

16. Hubscher SG, Lumley MA, Elias E. Vanishing bile duct syndrome: a possible mechanism for intrahepatic cholestasis in Hodgkin's lymphoma. Hepatology 1993;17:70–77.

17. Jansen PLM. The pathophysiology of cholestasis with special reference to primary biliary cirrhosis. Ballières Clin Gastroenterol 2000;14:571–583.

18. Kantrowitz PA, Jones WA, Greenberger NJ, et al. Severe postoperative hyperbilirubinemia simulating obstructive jaundice. N Engl J Med 1967;276:591–598.

19. Kass GEN, Price SC. Role of mitochondria in drug-induced cholestatic injury. Clin Liv Dis 2008;12:27–51.

20. Lieberman DA. Intrahepatic cholestasis due to Hodgkin's disease: an elusive diagnosis. J Clin Gastroenterol 1986;8:304–307.

21. Muller M, Jansen PLM. Molecular aspects of hepatobiliary transport. Am J Physiol 1997;272:G1285–G1303.

22. Nakamura K, Takenouchi T, Aizawa M, et al. Cerebro-hepato-renal syndrome of Zellweger. Clinical and autopsy findings and a review of previous cases in Japan. Acta Pathol Jpn 1986;36:1727–1735.

23. Ollson R, Tysk C, Aldenborg F, et al. Prolonged postpartum course of intrahepatic cholestasis of pregnancy. Gastroenterology 1993;105:267–271.

24. Perera DR, Greene ML, Fenster LF. Cholestasis associated with extrabiliary Hodgkin's disease. Report of three cases and review of four others. Gastroenterology 1974;67:680–685.

25. Popper H. Cholestasis: the future or a past and present riddle. Hepatology 1981;1:187–191.

26. Portmann B, Popper H, Neuberger J, et al. Sequential and diagnostic features in primary biliary cirrhosis based on serial histologic study in 209 patients. Gastroenterology 1985;88:1777–1790.

27. Powers JM, Moser HW, Moser AB, et al. Fetal cerebrohepatorenal (Zellweger) syndrome. Dysmorphic, radiologic, biochemical, and pathologic findings in four affected fetuses. Hum Pathol 1985;16:610–620.

28. Reau NS, Jensen DM. Vanishing bile duct syndrome. Clin Liver Dis 2008;12:203–217.

29. Riely CA. Familial intrahepatic cholestatic syndromes. Semin Liver Dis 1987;7:119–133.

30. Rolfes DB, Ishak KG. Liver disease in pregnancy. Histopathology 1986;10:555–570.

31. Sharp HL, Krivit W. Hereditary lymphedema and obstructive jaundice. J Pediatr 1971;78:491–496.

32. Sorrentino D, Jones EA, Berk PD. Familial hyperbilirubinemia syndromes: kinetic approaches. Ballières Clin Gastroenterol 1989;3:313–336.

33. Trauner M, Meier PJ, Boyer JL. Molecular pathogenesis of cholestasis. N Engl J Med 1998;339:1217–1227.

34. Varma RR, Sarna T. Hepatic pigments in Dubin-Johnson syndrome and mutant Corriedale sheep are not melanin. Gastroenterology 1986;84:1401.

35. Watterson J, Priest JR. Jaundice as a paraneoplastic phenomenon in a T-cell lymphoma. Gastroenterology 1989;97:1319–1322.

36. Wolkoff AW. Inheritable disorders manifested by conjugated hyperbilirubinemia. Semin Liver Dis 1993;3:65–72.

37. Zollner G, Trauner M. Mechanisms of cholestasis. Clin Liv Dis 2008;12:1–26.

27

DIFFERENTIAL DIAGNOSIS: COMMON LIVER BIOPSY PROBLEMS

A definitive diagnosis is not always established after liver biopsy review, even with the most complete clinical information and comprehensive laboratory testing. Biopsy findings are not always diagnostic. Often the sample size is inadequate (see Chapters 5 and 7). This chapter is a condensed review of some commonly encountered problems, emphasizing features useful in differentiating morphologically similar disorders.

ACUTE VIRAL HEPATITIS VERSUS ACUTE DRUG-INDUCED HEPATITIS (TABLE 27.1)

Portal tract inflammation can be variable. In general, however, inflammation is more prominent in acute viral hepatitis (AVH). In viral hepatitis, a predominantly mononuclear inflammatory infiltrate composed of lymphocytes, histiocytes, and occasional plasma cells predominates. In acute hepatitis A (HAV), for reasons not fully understood, plasma cells may outnumber other inflammatory cells, resembling autoimmune hepatitis, although clinical data usually resolve this question. Eosinophils can be present in viral hepatitis but, in contrast to many drug-induced hepatitis cases, are generally few. Not every drug-induced hepatitis will have increased numbers of eosinophils.

Interface hepatitis (piecemeal necrosis) is usually not prominent in acute viral or acute drug-induced hepatitis, except for acute hepatitis A where it can be significant. Lobular inflammation and necrosis can be variable in both acute and drug-induced hepatitis. Both show lobular inflammation, focal liver cell necrosis with acidophilic body formation, at least some degree of ballooning degeneration, and Kupffer cell prominence, and it is often impossible to distinguish between the two. Some drugs cause massive or submassive necrosis; acetaminophen toxicity is the best example. Bile duct injury is usually mild in drug-induced

TABLE 27.1	Acute Viral Hepatitis versus Acute Drug-Induced Hepatitis				
Type	Portal Inflammation	Lobular Inflammation	Granulomas	Cholestasis	Bile Duct Injury
Acute viral	+ − + +	+ − + + +	+/−	+	+/−
Acute drug-induced	+ − + +	+ +	+ +	+ +	+ +

hepatitis. Rarely, drug-induced bile duct injury leads to true ductopenia, as with chlorpromazine-induced bile duct injury. Mild ductal epithelial changes, including pleomorphism of nuclei and vacuolization of cytoplasm, is often seen with AVH, particularly in HAV and HCV virus infection, but also, rarely, in hepatitis B (HBV). Cholestasis, canalicular or intracellular or both, is more often seen with drug-induced hepatitis. HAV can be morphologically indistinguishable from drug hepatitis when present in the cholestatic form. Granulomas are uncommon in viral hepatitis but are seen with some drugs such as phenylbutazone and allopurinol. Granulomas rarely form in chronic viral hepatitis. Some drugs (e.g., diclofenac) can give the picture of autoimmune hepatitis, with prominent interface and lobular hepatitis.

Fibrosis is not associated with either acute viral or acute drug-induced hepatitis. When acute hepatitis, either viral or drug induced, is superimposed on already existing chronic liver disease, interpretation of histopathology can be exceedingly difficult.

Detailed clinical information is required, including time of onset of symptoms and duration, serologic studies, and history of exposure to new and traditional medications and herbal products, including teas. The clinical picture of an acute hepatitis can be seen in alcoholics at any time in their disease course, including when they are already cirrhotic, and acute inflammatory changes can be seen in the background of chronic injury.

ACUTE VIRAL HEPATITIS VERSUS ACUTE ALCOHOLIC HEPATITIS (TABLE 27.2)

Portal inflammation in acute alcoholic hepatitis is usually relatively mild. The inflammatory infiltrate is predominantly mononuclear, but polymorphonuclear leukocytes (PMNs) are also seen. True interface hepatitis is usually not present, although some spillover of inflammatory cells into the liver parenchyma may be present.

Lobular inflammatory activity in alcoholic hepatitis is characterized by ballooned and distended hepatocytes, often containing Mallory hyalin and surrounded by PMNs. These hallmarks of alcoholic hepatitis can be

TABLE 27.2	Acute Viral Hepatitis versus Acute Alcoholic Hepatitis					
Type	Portal Inflammation	Lobular Inflammation	Acidophilic Bodies	Steatosis	Fibrosis	Mallory Hyaline
Acute viral	+ − ++	+ − +++	++ − +++	−	−	−
Alco-holic	+	+ − ++	+	+ − ++	+	+

seen in nonalcoholic steatohepatitis (NASH), associated with obesity, diabetes mellitus, and jejunoileal bypass. In contrast to AVH, acidophilic bodies are unusual. Mallory hyalin is not seen in AVH. Steatosis, predominantly macrovesicular, typically zone 3, is a hallmark of alcoholic hepatitis, although it can be variable. Steatosis is uncommon in AVH. Pure microvascular steatosis rarely occurs. Cholestasis occurs in both acute HAV and alcoholic hepatitis.

Fibrosis, perivenular (central hyaline sclerosis) and pericellular ("chicken-wire"), is typical of alcoholic hepatitis. AVH, by definition, does not show changes of chronicity. Clinical data including symptoms, biochemistry, and serologic markers are invaluable. A careful social history, inquiring about exposure to alcohol and other drugs and toxins is mandatory.

ACUTE VIRAL HEPATITIS VERSUS CHRONIC HEPATITIS (TABLE 27.3)

Portal inflammation is generally mild in the early stages of AVH. In chronic hepatitis (CH), portal inflammation predominates. The inflammatory infiltrate in CH is predominantly mononuclear, including lymphocytes, histiocytes, and occasional plasma cells. In autoimmune CH, plasma cells may be particularly prominent. Lymphoid aggregates, often with true germinal center formation, are typical of chronic HCV but are not specific and can also be seen in autoimmune hepatitis (AIH) as well as in CH resulting from HBV. Interface hepatitis is the hallmark of CH and is usually

TABLE 27.3	Acute Viral Hepatitis versus Chronic Hepatitis			
Type	Portal Inflammation	Lobular Inflammation	Lobular Disarray	Fibrosis
Acute	+ − ++	+ − +++	++ − +++	−
Chronic	+ − +++	+ − ++	+/−	+ − +++

variable. Focal interface hepatitis and spillover of inflammatory cells is sometimes seen in AVH.

Lobular activity is typical of acute hepatitis, including lobular inflammation and acidophilic body formation. The constellation of hepatocyte pleomorphism, with ballooned cells, pyknotic cells, acidophilic bodies, and patchy inflammation imparts a disordered look to the lobules, so-called lobular disarray, sometimes also described as dirty appearing. Reticulin stain helps demonstrate focal liver cell loss (dropout).

Immunohistochemistry and histochemistry can be helpful. In chronic HBV infection, viral antigens, hepatitis B surface antigen (HBsAg), and hepatitis B core antigen (HBcAg) can be demonstrated. HBsAg can also be seen with Victoria blue or orcein stains.

Wilson disease can present as a CH. Some hepatocytes exhibit deeply eosinophilic cytoplasm, whereas others may be distended with Mallory or Mallory-like material. Macrovesicular steatosis and glycogenated nuclei are often seen without any particular zonal distribution. Special stains, rhodanine and rubeanic acid, can confirm the presence of copper but are not always positive, and quantitative copper assay is often needed.

Fibrosis is a feature of CH regardless of cause. Fibrosis varies from mild portal/periportal fibrosis to extensive fibrosis, bridging fibrosis, and then cirrhosis. Minimal fibrosis is best seen with reticulin silver stain.

LARGE BILE DUCT OBSTRUCTION VERSUS CHOLESTATIC HEPATITIS (TABLE 27.4)

Portal edema is characteristic of large duct obstruction (LDO), developing a few days after obstruction. The inflammatory infiltrate is usually mild and predominantly mononuclear cells, with a variable number of PMNs surrounding, but not usually infiltrating, bile ducts (pericholangitis). PMNs increase with persistence of obstruction when ductules proliferate secondarily (marginal bile ductular proliferation). Interlobular bile ducts and bile ductules may be dilated. True ascending cholangitis can develop with PMNs seen in the bile duct lumen. If obstruction persists, portal fibrosis and then portal–portal bridging fibrosis develops. These changes are not

TABLE 27.4	Large Bile Duct Obstruction versus Cholestatic Hepatitis				
Type	Portal Edema	Portal PMNs	Lobular Inflammation	Cholestasis	Ductular Reaction
Large duct obstruction	++ − +++	+ − ++	+ − ++	++ − +++	++ − +++
Cholestatic hepatitis	−	−	+ − +++	+	−

PMNs, polymorphonuclear leukocytes.

seen in AVH or CH, although ductular reaction (proliferation) is common in severe hepatitis.

Portal edema is less prominent in posttransplant LDO, in which the principal manifestations are acute pericholangitis and ductular reaction (proliferation).

Lobular activity is not prominent in LDO except in zone 3 when cholestasis is prominent. Cholestatic changes include hepatocyte ballooning with a foamy cytoplasm (feathery degeneration).

Zone 3 canalicular cholestasis is the first sign of LDO, progressing rapidly during the first week to include other zones when obstruction is not relieved. Numerous bile plugs (bile thrombi) are seen in zone 3. Intracellular cholestasis and hypertrophied Kupffer cells are also seen. In long-standing LDO, bile lakes and bile infarcts form when dilated bile ducts rupture with extravasation of bile into the liver parenchyma. Consequently, hepatocytes undergo degeneration and necrosis and become surrounded by reactive, foamy macrophages.

In contrast, cholestatic hepatitis has only mild intracanalicular and intracellular cholestasis. Bile lakes or bile infarcts are not seen.

Helpful clinical information includes onset (acute versus gradual onset), duration of symptoms, jaundice, epigastric pain, biochemistry (e.g., disproportionately elevated alkaline phosphatase and bilirubin would be more indicative of LDO), serologic markers, and endoscopic and radiologic findings.

CHRONIC HEPATITIS VERSUS PRIMARY BILIARY CIRRHOSIS (TABLE 27.5)

Portal inflammation in primary biliary cirrhosis (PBC) is variable in intensity. The inflammatory cell infiltrate is predominantly mononuclear and consists of lymphocytes, histiocytes, some plasma cells, and some eosinophils. Interface hepatitis is often present, although the inflammatory infiltrate is often intermingled with ductular reaction (proliferation), referred to as *ductular interface hepatitis*. Granulomas and granulomatous occur with

TABLE 27.5	Chronic Hepatitis versus Primary Biliary Cirrhosis			
Type	Portal Inflammation	Lobular Inflammation	Bile Duct Injury/Loss	Cholestasis
Chronic hepatitis	+ − +++	+ − +++	− − +	−
Primary biliary cirrhosis	+ − +++	+ − ++	+++	+ − ++

bile duct injury in early (stage 1) PBC. So-called florid bile duct injury is typical of early PBC. Variable degrees of destructive bile duct injury are seen, ultimately leading to bile duct loss. Cholate stasis with ballooning of the periportal and periseptal hepatocytes, often with Mallory material and copper-associated protein, is almost invariable in late PBC (stages 2 to 4).

Mild lobular inflammation and focal liver cell necrosis are not common in PBC in contrast with CH. Granulomas are often in the PBC portal tract but may be scattered throughout the parenchyma.

Differentiating between CH and early PBC can be problematic. In late stage PBC, bile duct loss and biliary-type fibrosis are seen, features not seen in CH. In contrast, AIH and early PBC can be histologically quite similar. Indeed, a true overlap syndrome with clinical and morphologic features of both AIH and PBC exists.

Helpful clinical information includes patient's gender (PBC is rare in men) and age, onset of symptoms, pruritus, biochemistry, serologic and autoimmune markers, and antimitochondrial antibody (AMA) titer.

CHRONIC HEPATITIS VERSUS PRIMARY SCLEROSING CHOLANGITIS (TABLE 27.6)

The liver biopsy may be normal in primary sclerosing cholangitis (PSC) (see Chapter 17), and differentiating from chronic hepatitis will not be an issue.

When liver changes are seen, portal inflammation is generally mild to moderate. The inflammatory cell infiltrate is predominantly mononuclear, with lymphocytes, histiocytes, and some plasma cells. Interface hepatitis is not prominent, in contrast to both CH and PBC.

Bile duct injury is always present, but the degree is variable and often very subtle in early PSC. Cholangiography is the standard for diagnosing PSC. Biopsy changes are variable and scattered, and even multiple biopsies may fail to show a typical lesion. Instead of necrosis, bile ducts more often show progressive atrophy, with periductal concentric fibrosis ("onion

TABLE 27.6	Chronic Hepatitis versus Primary Sclerosing Cholangitis			
Type	Portal Inflammation	Lobular Inflammation	Bile Duct Injury/Loss	Cholestasis
Chronic hepatitis	++ − +++	+ − +++	− − +	−
Primary sclerosing cholangitis	+ − ++	+	+++	+ − ++

skinning"). Complete bile duct loss, sometimes leaving a resultant fibrous scar that characteristically has a smudgy appearance with trichrome and is a hallmark of PSC. Bile ductular reaction is more prominent in late PSC than in PBC. In CH, ductular reaction (proliferation) is generally not seen until cirrhosis ensues.

Granuloma is exceedingly rare in PSC. Cholate stasis in periportal and periseptal hepatocytes, with ballooning, Mallory material, and copper-associated protein is similar in late PSC and PBC and is not seen in CH.

Clinical information of value includes include gender, time of onset and duration of symptoms, other associated conditions (e.g., inflammatory bowel disease, especially ulcerative colitis), biochemistry, serologic and autoimmune markers, and antineutrophil cytoplasmic antibody (ANCA) status.

LARGE BILE DUCT OBSTRUCTION VERSUS PRIMARY CHOLANGIOPATHIES (PRIMARY BILIARY CIRRHOSIS AND PRIMARY SCLEROSING CHOLANGITIS) (TABLE 27.7)

Portal edema is typical of LDO and not seen in PBC or PSC. The predominantly mononuclear portal tract inflammatory infiltrate is more prominent in the cholangiopathies. Interface hepatitis is not seen in LDO, in contrast with PBC.

TABLE 27.7 Large Bile Duct Obstruction versus Primary Cholangiopathies

Type	Portal Edema	Portal Inflammation	Lobular Inflammation	Bile Duct Injury/Loss	Fibrosis	Granulomas
Large duct obstruction	+ + − + + +	+ + (mixed, including PMNs)	+	+/−	+ − + + +	−
Primary tbiliary cirrhosis	−	+ + (mononuclear)	+/−	+ − + + +	+ − + + +	+ + − + + +
Primary sclerosing cholangitis	−	+ + (mononuclear)	+/−	+ − + + +	+ − + + +	Rare

PMNs, polymorphonuclear leukocytes.

TABLE 27.8	Conditions Characterized by Progressive Bile Duct Injury and Bile Duct Loss
Primary biliary cirrhosis	
Primary sclerosing cholangitis	
Autoimmune cholangitis	
Chronic, ductopenic rejection (vanishing bile duct syndrome)	
Graft versus-host disease	
Sarcoidosis	
Drug-induced ductopenia (e.g., chlorpromazine)	
Paucity of intrahepatic bile ducts (Alagille syndrome and nonsyndromatic paucity)	

Bile duct injury is the most important histologic feature of both PBC and PSC.

Bile duct loss, characteristic of late PBC and PSC, is not seen in LDO even when long-standing (Tables 28.8 and 28.9). In LDO, a true necroinflammatory and destructive bile duct injury is not seen. Marginal bile ductular reaction is typical of LDO.

Granulomas and granulomatous bile duct injury are characteristic of PBC and not seen in LDO

Cholestasis may be present in all three conditions. In LDO, cholestasis is centrolobular and intracanalicular. Bile lakes and bile infarcts are virtually pathognomonic. Cholate stasis is common in both PBC and PSC in periportal and paraseptal hepatocytes and is not seen in LDO.

The pattern of fibrosis is the same in LDO and the cholangiopathies. Portal–portal fibrous bridging, with irregular islands of liver parenchyma surrounded by relatively paucicellular fibrous septa, imparts a so-called jigsaw pattern. In the primary cholangiopathies, there is widespread bile duct loss, not seen in secondary biliary cirrhosis caused by LDO.

TABLE 27.9	Conditions with Relatively Mild and Nonprogressive Bile Duct Injury But No Bile Duct Loss
	Large bile duct obstruction
	Viral hepatitis C
	Viral hepatitis A
	AIDS-associated bile duct injury
	Drug-induced hepatitis
	Parasitic biliary disease

TABLE 27.10 Alcoholic Steatohepatitis versus Nonalcoholic Steatohepatitis			
Type	Steatosis	Mallory Hyaline	Fibrosis
Alcoholic steatohepatitis	+ − +++	+ − +++ (zone 3)	+ − +++ (pericellular pattern early)
Nonalcoholic steatohepatitis	+ − ++	+ − ++ (zone 1)	+ − +++ (pericellular pattern early)

ALCOHOLIC STEATOHEPATITIS VERSUS NONALCOHOLIC STEATOHEPATITIS (TABLE 27.10)

Steatosis in both alcoholic steatohepatitis (ASH) and nonalcoholic steatohepatitis (NASH) is similar. It can be macrovesicular, mixed microvesicular and macrovesicular, or, rarely, purely microvesicular with foamy cells. Zone 3 is typically affected, but steatosis can be diffuse in severe cases.

Mallory material tends to be more abundant and prominent in ASH. In NASH, Mallory material, fat, and glycogenated nuclei, when seen, are prominent mostly in zone 1. Glycogenated nuclei occur in both conditions. Fibrosis, including central hyaline and pericellular (chicken wire) fibrosis, may be identical in both with progression to cirrhosis. Detailed clinical history is crucial.

ALCOHOLIC STEATOHEPATITIS VERSUS DRUG-INDUCED PHOSPHOLIPIDOSIS (TABLE 27.11)

Drug-induced changes caused by amiodarone and perhexiline maleate mimic alcoholic hepatitis. Amiodarone, and sometimes high-dose estrogen therapy, causes drug-induced phospholipidosis, mimicking Niemann-Pick

TABLE 27.11 Alcoholic Steatohepatitis versus Drug-Induced Phospholipidosis					
Type	Lobular Inflammation	Steatosis	Mallory Hyaline	Fibrosis	Ultrastructural Myelin Figures
Alcoholic steatohepatitis	+ − ++	+ − +++	+ − ++	+ − +++	−
Drug-induced phospholipidosis	+	+ − ++	++ − +++	+ − +++	+− ++

disease. Clinical setting and history are crucial to understanding the biopsy.

Steatosis, predominantly macrovesicular, is generally more prominent in ASH. Mallory material is usually abundant in drug-induced phospholipidosis and can be diffuse in contrast to ASH in which it is usually in zone 1. Portal and pericellular fibrosis may be similar in both conditions. Central hyaline sclerosis is typically not seen in drug-induced steatosis. Electron microscopy in amiodarone-induced phospholipidosis shows characteristic myelin figures. They are not seen in ASH.

INDEX

Page numbers followed by an "f" indicate figures and images; page numbers followed by "t" indicate tables.

portal vein related
  hepatoportal sclerosis, 257
  hereditary hemorrhagic telangiectasia, 258
  intrahepatic portal vein obstruction, 257
  prehepatic obstruction, 257
  Zahn infarcts, 257–258
sinusoids related
  peliosis hepatis, 259
  sinusoidal dilatation, 258–259
  sinusoidal thrombosis, 259
terminal hepatic venules/ central veins
  hepatic venous outflow obstruction,
    260–262
  left heart failure and systemic hypotension,
    260
  right heart failure, 259
  viral hepatitides, 288–289
Vascular lesions, 7, 144
Venoocclusive disease (VOD), 144, 144t, 174f,
    253, 258, 260–262, 262f, 363, 399
Vicinity of mass lesion, 68, 68f
Victoria blue, 36, 39f, 65, 76, 106, 226, 227t, 235,
    249, 250, 271, 420
Visceral Larva Migrans, 314

von Gierke disease. *See* Type 1 glycogenosis
von Meyenburg Complex, 14, 47, 53, 54, 329, 330f

W
Weber-Christian disease, 175, 302
Weil disease. *See* Leptospirosis
Wilson disease (WD)
  definition, 220
  genetics, 222
  histochemistry of, 226
  key features of, 227t
  laboratory tests, 221t
  pathology, 222–225
  patterns of presentation in, 221t
  showing ductular reaction, 226f
  showing mallory hyalin in zone 1 hepatocytes,
    226f

Y
Yellow fever, 90–91, 90t, 91f

Z
Zellweger syndrome, 196, 413
Zellweger-like syndrome, 196